Studies in the METABOLISM

of VITAMIN B₁₂

BY

Alfred Doscherholmen, M.D., Ph.D.

The University of Minnesota Press

MINNEAPOLIS

Library of Congress Catalog Card Number: 65-12097

PUBLISHED IN GREAT BRITAIN, INDIA, AND PAKISTAN BY THE OXFORD UNIVERSITY
PRESS, LONDON, BOMBAY, AND KARACHI, AND IN CANADA BY THE
COPP CLARK PUBLISHING CO. LIMITED, TORONTO

ACKNOWLEDGMENTS

I AM grateful to my friend and adviser, the late Dr. Paul S. Hagen, who was a perpetual stimulus to me in my work. His help, guidance, and encouragement throughout this study were immense and it is therefore with great pleasure that this acknowledgment is made.

I should like to express my thanks also to my co-adviser, Dr. C. J. Watson, for his interest in my work and for his valuable help and advice in the preparation of papers resulting from my studies.

S. Sandhaus, R. Baskin, F. E. Christensen, and E. Zumwalde gave valuable advice and assistance in the use of the isotopic equipment for which acknowledgment is hereby given.

Especial thanks should go to the countless patients who took part in the various studies included in this work. Without their helpful cooperation the metabolic studies would have been impossible to carry out.

Ann Alar, Margaret Liu, Lois Olin, Donna Ripley, and Margaret Stronks have at various times given technical assistance, which is hereby acknowledged.

I am grateful to Merck and Company for supplying radio-labeled vitamin B_{12} without charge and to Eli Lilly and Company for financial support of part of this work. Both of these companies also donated intrinsic factor concentrates.

The experimental work was performed in the research laboratories of the Veterans Administration Hospital, Minneapolis, and part of the work was done during the author's tenure as a Veterans Administration clinical investigator. The Veterans Administration also contributed financial support toward the publication costs of this book, for which the author is very grateful.

I wish to express my thanks to Dr. Ananda S. Prasad for his help and advice in working out the method for the measurement of the serum vitamin B$_{12}$ binding capacity using the ultrafiltration technique.

I should like finally to thank Mary Miller for typing the manuscript; Mrs. Jean McMahon for valuable assistance rendered during its preparation; Lawrence B. Benson for his work on the illustrations; and Jane McCarthy, Marcia Strout, and the rest of the staff of the University of Minnesota Press.

TABLE OF CONTENTS

Miscellaneous Studies

Introduction and Methods Used in This Study

INTRODUCTION AND METHODS

In 1948 a group of investigators led by Rickes in the laboratories of Merck and Company announced that they had isolated from liver a crystalline compound which in microgram quantities had produced hematologic remissions in patients with Addison's pernicious anemia (535). About the same time and independently of the above group, E. Lester Smith of the Glaxo Laboratories reported on the purification of the antipernicious anemia principle in the liver (589, 591). The discovery of this new substance, vitamin B_{12} or cyanocobalamin, was regarded as a great accomplishment because biochemists had tried in vain for years to isolate the active compound in liver extracts.

Since pure crystalline vitamin B_{12} is able to induce as well as maintain hematologic and neurologic remissions in patients with pernicious anemia, one may now regard this disease as a form of avitaminosis (90, 92). The low serum concentrations (206, 261, 290, 292, 298, 344, 345, 347, 363, 441, 442A, 443, 443B, 464, 483, 496, 511, 599, 632) and liver stores (167, 208, 459, 550, 612, 663) of cyanocobalamin and hematopoietic activity of the liver (280, 533) in subjects with pernicious anemia in relapse lend justification to such a point of view. Because the diet is not deficient in vitamin B_{12} in Addison's pernicious anemia, Castle has used the term "conditioned deficiency disease" for this type of avitaminosis (90, 96).

The pathogenesis of pernicious anemia has for many years centered on a theory based on the brilliant observations of Castle and his colleagues (90, 91, 97, 98). Castle discovered that beef muscle and normal gastric juice given together induced hematologic remissions in patients with pernicious anemia in relapse whereas there was no response when normal gastric juice and beef muscle were fed separately or more than 6 hours apart. The essential substance in normal gastric juice was termed "intrinsic factor," and the food factor was

3

called "extrinsic factor." The antianemia principle of liver was thought to be formed through an interaction of these two factors. According to Castle's theory, the hematopoietic factor could not be formed in subjects with pernicious anemia because they lacked intrinsic factor in their gastric juice.

Vitamin B_{12} has been identified as the extrinsic (food) factor of Castle (28), and it is also the active factor in liver (190, 535, 589, 591). It is no longer necessary to assume the existence of a third factor, the antianemia principle formed by interaction of the extrinsic and the intrinsic factor, since extrinsic factor given alone parenterally is very effective in pernicious anemia in relapse (203). The intrinsic factor has not yet been isolated in pure form (301), but it is believed to be a mucoprotein or mucopolypeptide (213, 223, 358, 360, 651, 656). The purpose of the intrinsic factor is to bring about the absorption from the food, by some mechanism still unknown (90), of the small amount of cyanocobalamin needed.

The stomach thus appears to be the organ primarily responsible for the development of pernicious anemia. A connection between the stomach and the development of pernicious anemia had been suspected a long time before the discovery of the intrinsic factor (194, 195). In fact, it was the high incidence of achylia gastrica in pernicious anemia that constituted the main stimulus to Castle in his search for the cause of pernicious anemia (91, 96, 97). Though it is now generally agreed that gastric atrophy with its concomitant achylia gastrica is a basic defect in pernicious anemia (90), several cases have been described recently which definitively prove that genuine pernicious anemia can exist even in the absence of gastric atrophy (118, 275, 435, 552, 601). These latter patients show a functional loss of the ability to secrete the intrinsic factor despite a normal histologic picture of the gastric mucosa (118, 275, 435, 552) and a preserved ability to secrete hydrochloric acid (118, 275, 435, 552, 601). One outstanding feature of these cases has been that they all developed their pernicious anemia in childhood or early adulthood. It will be of great interest to follow these patients with gastroscopy and gastric biopsies as the years go by, to learn whether they will develop the picture of gastric atrophy as typically observed in the pernicious anemia that develops in middle life or in the older group.

Since genuine pernicious anemia appears to be a proved fact in the juvenile form of the disease in the absence of gastric atrophy, a question naturally arises about the role gastric atrophy plays in the pernicious anemia of later life. Is it really true, as is commonly believed, that gastric atrophy is the cause of the disease in the elderly? If that is so, a fundamental difference exists between juvenile and adult or old-age pernicious anemia. It is possible that both the inability to produce intrinsic factor and gastric atrophy are expressions of the same genetic defect, because both forms of the disease have been found in the same family (435, 552). In the juvenile form, then, the defective production of intrinsic factor would make itself apparent before the development of the grastric atrophy, whereas in the adult type the gastric atrophy might precede or develop simultaneously with the loss of the ability to produce intrinsic factor. Rubin states that his data from eight cases of juvenile pernicious anemia suggest that this disease is the homozygous state for adult Addison's pernicious anemia (552).

The various causes which might be implicated in the development of Addison's pernicious anemia have been reviewed recently by Victor Herbert (301). The possibility that prolonged vitamin B_{12} deficiency in itself might lead to gastric atrophy has been discussed (301), because patients with pernicious tapeworm anemia may show atrophic mucosal lesions (582, 583) which in some instances were reversible with therapy (582). The finding of an impaired vitamin B_{12} absorption in fish tapeworm carriers before and even during the first week after worm cure, but normal absorption one to six weeks after worm expulsion, may also indicate a reversible functional damage of the intrinsic-factor-secreting organ (471). Other evidences exist for impairment in the secretory function of the stomach in pernicious tapeworm anemia, as summarized recently (338). Since pernicious tapeworm anemia is regarded as a pure form of vitamin B_{12} deficiency (55, 56, 58, 466), injury to the gastric mucosa from prolonged B_{12} avitaminosis can therefore not be excluded. Whether such an injury, if it really exists, can proceed all the way to a total mucosal atrophy with achylia gastrica remains to be proved, for subjects with pernicious tapeworm anemia, while they have a higher incidence of achlorhydria than control subjects (55), can as a rule produce intrinsic factor (314, 315), although this production may be lower than normal (338). The previously mentioned findings in juvenile pernicious anemia have also led to the conclusion that the gastric lesion of Addison's pernicious anemia may be the result rather than the cause of vitamin B_{12} deficiency (435, 552, 601).

Knud Faber many years ago called attention to the association of achylia gastrica with simple hypochromic anemia (183, 186). After many years, patients with hypochromic anemia may develop pernicious anemia (130, 186). This observation was strengthened by the finding of impaired secretion of intrinsic factor in iron deficiency (277A). The relation among iron deficiency, changes in the stomach, and vitamin B_{12} metabolism has recently been re-explored (16, 130, 137). Undoubtedly iron deficiency can be associated with histological alterations in the stomach (130, 335) and functional impairment of this organ similar to the condition seen in Addison's pernicious anemia (16). Thus the clinical observations made by Faber so many years ago were confirmed by later findings. Since in the United States the usual patient with Addison's pernicious anemia does not suffer from iron deficiency (659), it is unlikely that these findings are of importance in the pathogenesis of pernicious anemia, at least in this country.

Recently it has been demonstrated that antibodies can be produced against intrinsic factor (217A, 618) and that antibodies, presumably autoantibodies, against this factor may be found in the blood of patients with pernicious anemia (217A, 615). Furthermore, antibodies against gastric mucosa have also been found in patients with pernicious anemia (386A, 618A). At present the role these antibodies play, if any, in the development of the gastric atrophy in pernicious anemia can only be speculated about (217A).

Although it is more difficult to assess the exact role of the gastric atrophy in the development of Addison's pernicious anemia today than it was a few years ago, the finding of gastric mucosal atrophy with achylia gastrica is so common, at least in the adult form of the disease, that the diagnosis should be questioned in its absence unless special studies have been performed, such as serum vitamin B$_{12}$ determination, vitamin B$_{12}$ absorption tests, gastric mucosal biopsy, and determination of the presence or absence of intrinsic factor in the gastric juice.

Defective secretion of intrinsic factor is the most commonly encountered etiologic factor in the development of vitamin B$_{12}$ deficiency outside Finland. Subjects suffering from this defect are unable to absorb in a normal manner test doses of labeled vitamin B$_{12}$. The absorption of cyanocobalamin is corrected in the presence of an exogenous source of intrinsic factor. All patients with Addison's pernicious anemia and total gastrectomy belong to this group. A few patients who have undergone gastric resection or gastroenterostomy may also develop pernicious anemia because they lose the ability to secrete the intrinsic factor (17, 171, 351, 377). They will therefore be included in this group, as will rare cases where the intrinsic-factor-secreting apparatus has been destroyed or damaged by corrosion (8), cancer (235), or gastritis (584, 586). An intrinsic-factor inhibitor in the gastric juice was thought to be the cause for the vitamin B$_{12}$ malabsorption in one case (366A), but the validity of this finding has been questioned (301).

Lack of cyanocobalamin in the diet over a prolonged period can also lead to a depletion of the body's stores of this vitamin, as is seen in food faddists and vegetarians (21, 63, 276, 301, 504, 660, 661), although not all subjects with a poor intake of animal proteins have low serum vitamin B_{12} levels (268, 660). The clinical picture in persons with dietary lack of vitamin B_{12} may be entirely indistinguishable from that in persons with Addison's pernicious anemia (504). Subacute combined degeneration of the spinal cord may also be found in such patients (12). Vitamin B_{12} absorption is, however, normal in patients who develop vitamin B_{12} deficiency because of defective diet, indicating a normal secretion of intrinsic factor (12, 276, 504).

A third group of patients may develop vitamin B_{12} deficiency secondary to intestinal malabsorption of vitamin B_{12}. This group includes patients with sprue (200, 214, 218, 436, 485, 519, 532), steatorrhea (436, 485, 494), resection of the small intestine (61, 116, 352, 354, 436, 485), regional ileitis (214, 354, 436), blind loop of the small intestine (157, 271, 392, 436, 485), strictures and anastomoses of the small intestine (271, 273), diverticula of the small intestine (14, 205, 271, 445, 568, 596), agammaglobulinemia (200), cystic fibrosis of the pancreas (200), and pernicious tapeworm anemia (66, 337, 467, 468, 471). Isolated intestinal defects in the absorption of cyanocobalamin have also been observed (243, 246, 247, 519, 568). A characteristic feature of patients in this group is their inability to absorb test doses of labeled vitamin B_{12} even in the presence of amounts of intrinsic factor adequate to correct the defect in Addison's pernicious anemia. Sterilization of the gut with tetracycline or its related compounds (14, 392, 436, 485, 568), but not with neomycin (157, 271), will usually correct the malabsorption of cyanocobalamin associated with intestinal stasis. Some improvement may be found in the absorption of vitamin B_{12} in patients with sprue when intrinsic factor is administered in doses far in excess of what is needed to correct the absorptive defect of patients with Addison's pernicious anemia (81). Improvement in the absorption of cyanocobalamin has also been achieved in some instances of steatorrhea with calcium given orally (248); this is of great interest, because it has been shown that vitamin B_{12} absorption is a calcium-dependent process (306). For this reason, subjects on long-term therapy with calcium-chelating agents may possibly develop vitamin B_{12} deficiency (301). Patients with pernicious anemia who have been treated with preparations containing hog intrinsic factor may develop resistance against this heterologous factor (31, 48, 176, 197, 339, 373, 492, 565–567, 587, 602, 608). They may wrongfully be thought to have intestinal malfunction until their vitamin B_{12} absorption is tested with homologous intrinsic factor, to which they respond normally (31, 197, 339, 566, 567, 602). Normal vitamin B_{12} absorption has been found in megaloblastic anemias associated with pregnancy and the puerperium (15, 182) and as a rule also in those associated with anticonvulsant therapy (12, 87, 100,

104, 238, 283, 316, 341, 364, 375, 376). Treatment with folic acid is usually very effective in these conditions (15, 114, 204, 634).

A deficiency of a specific B_{12}-binding protein in the serum may conceivably also lead to vitamin B_{12} deficiency. However, only one such possible case has been described (301, 317A).

The separation of the various etiological groups of vitamin B_{12} deficiency has become a routine procedure in well-equipped laboratories because methods have been devised for measuring the gastrointestinal absorption of vitamin B_{12} (60, 162–164, 221, 289, 557). With the help of the absorption tests, a vast body of information has been gathered within in a short span of time about the absorption of cyanocobalamin under various conditions in health and disease, as testified to by the large number of papers on this subject in recent years. The methods in question all rely upon the use of radio-labeled vitamin B_{12} for testing purposes. The development of radiocyanocobalamin (99) was therefore a scientific event of great importance. It not only opened the way for the study of the absorption of vitamin B_{12}, but it also made possible many other kinds of metabolic study which would otherwise have been difficult or impossible.

Vitamin B_{12} has a complex molecular structure with a nucleus of four pyrrol rings and a cobalt atom in the center (62, 317, 588). The molecular weight of the vitamin is 1355 (27A). Besides cobalt it contains carbon, hydrogen, oxygen, nitrogen, and phosphorus. Cyanocobalamin can be made radioactive by neutron bombardment in the atomic pile (588), but this is not the customary way of producing radioactive vitamin B_{12}. The commercially available cyanocobalamin is obtained through biosynthesis by B_{12}-producing bacteria (588), primarily *Streptomyces griseus* (534). In fact, it can be obtained as a by-product of the spent fermentation broths of streptomycin and chlortetracycline manufacture (588). P^{32} and C^{14} both have been incorporated into vitamin B_{12} by biosynthesis (590, 592, 649), although this type of radio-labeled vitamin B_{12} has had very limited use (588). It is the cobalt-labeled cyanocobalamin that has been employed almost exclusively in biology and medicine. By incorporating the cobalt isotope in the fermentation broth, radio-labeled vitamin B_{12} of high specific activity has been obtained (588). Co^{60} is made by neutron bombardment of cobalt in the atomic pile. It has a physical half-life of 5.3 years. This relatively long physical half-life limits the body burden of this isotope to 3 μc according to the Atomic Energy Commission (635) or to 1 μc according to the British Medical Research Council (64). Some liberalization in the body burden of the cobalt isotopes has recently been published (538). Besides its long physical half-life, $Co^{60}B_{12}$ has another disadvantage: a relatively low upper limit for its highest obtainable specific activity. Both these disadvantages were removed by the creation of several new cobalt isotopes by transmutation reactions. Co^{58} (half-life 72 days) was made by neutron bombardment of nickel (64). Co^{57} (half-life of 270 days) was made by proton bombardment of iron in a cyclotron under certain conditions, whereas under different conditions mainly Co^{56} (half-life of 72 days) was obtained (588). With these latter isotopes it was possible to make radio-cyanocobalamin with a much higher specific activity than was possible with Co^{60}. Furthermore, their lower physical half-life permitted a larger body burden of these isotopes as compared with Co^{60} (538).

In the studies of the metabolism of vitamin B_{12} to be reported in this book extensive use has been made of Co^{60}-, Co^{58}-, and Co^{57}-labeled cyanocobalamin. The book opens with a review of the literature. Chapters 2 through 4 have to do with the absorption of cyanocobalamin under varying conditions in health and disease. An assessment was made of the value of the most commonly used method for testing the absorption of cyanocobalamin, the urinary excretion test. Attempts were made to improve the urinary recovery of radioactivity and the basic mechanism of the test was investigated. An entirely new technique for the measurement of the absorption of cyanocobalamin was worked out — the plasma absorption method — and its clinical value was assessed. In conjunction with the other absorption tests this technique was used to get basic information about the absorption of vitamin B_{12}. An autopsy study was carried out to check some of the results thus obtained. The kinetics of orally ingested radiocyanocobalamin were also studied.

Chapter 5 reports an in-vitro study of whether vitamin B_{12} bound to the intrinsic factor or in the intestinal wall can be released, under appropriate conditions, from its binding, presumably by an enzyme. In Chapter 6 an ultrafiltration technique is described for the study of the B_{12}-binding capacity of serum, and Chapter 7 describes an attempt to alter the long physiologic half-life of Co^{60}-labeled vitamin B_{12} in the liver.

The methods followed in our studies — the preparation and administration of the oral test dose; the manner of collecting and measuring the radioactivity of samples of feces, urine, and blood; the mode of measuring radioactivity in vivo; and so on — are described below.

The oral test doses of labeled cyanocobalamin were made up in 20 ml. disposable glass vials from stock solutions with water added to make 20 ml. Non-radioactive crystalline vitamin B_{12} was added to make up the desired doses. The vials were inserted in the 20 ml. well-type scintillation counter and their radioactivity measured in counts per minute (cpm). Where the amount of radioactivity administered was too great to be measured directly, aliquots of the test doses, for example one tenth of the dose, were made up for counting purposes. The activity of each test dose was then arrived at by the appropriate multiplication. The test doses were either prepared individually on the afternoon before the day when the tests were to be performed or, more often, in batches of approximately ten. They were then stored in a refrigerator until used, usually within a week or two.

The oral test dose was administered to the patient through a paper straw and the vial rinsed out several times with water to ensure as complete an ingestion of the dose as possible. The straw was thereafter crushed into the vial, the cap replaced, and the residual radioactivity in the vial measured. The difference between the original and the residual count constituted the ingested radioactivity. The tests were generally administered at 8:00 A.M. after an overnight fast, and breakfast was allowed two hours later.

Whenever malabsorption was found, the test was repeated with the addition of intrinsic factor (IF). Hog-stomach intrinsic factor concentrates (IFC) served as a source for this factor. Several batches of IFC have been used during the time these studies have been in progress, all from commercial sources, and their activity per gram has not always been the same. One USP unit of IF contained in these concentrates has therefore been adopted as the standard amount of this factor to be used in the testing procedure for subjects who have shown malabsorption of vitamin B$_{12}$. Intrinsic factor concentrate, when given together with the labeled vitamin, was either mixed with the test dose of the vitamin shortly before the administration of the dose, or it was ingested separately in the form of a gelatin capsule immediately before the radiocyanocobalamin was given. Studies were usually not repeated with less than 4-day intervals in patients with pernicious anemia or malabsorption of vitamin B$_{12}$. In other subjects 7 days or more usually elapsed between repeated tests.

Feces were collected quantitatively in half-gallon, waxed, cardboard containers for 5 to 7 consecutive 24-hour periods. The containers were weighed before they were used. The collection was greatly facilitated by the use of wire baskets which were fitted into the toilet bowl or a bedside commode. These baskets were made to hold the cardboard containers in such a manner that the patients were able to sit down comfortably, and a supply of containers was left with the patient so that one container was used for each bowel movement. This procedure resulted in more laboratory work than if feces had been collected in one box for the entire collection period. Our method was nevertheless preferred because it resulted in better cooperation in the complete collection of the feces. Water was added to the containers and the feces homogenized with a hand pestle. The homogenates were weighed and aliquots were transferred to weighed 20 ml. counting vials in duplicate. The radioactivity of the weighed aliquots was measured in the 20 ml. well-type scintillation counter. The radioactivity of the total stool homogenate was then arrived at by a simple formula:

$$\text{radioactivity of total homogenate} = \frac{\text{activity in aliquot}}{\text{weight of aliquot}} \times \text{weight of total homogenate.}$$

The average of the duplicate radioactivity measurements was used in figuring out the percentage of radioactivity in the fecal homogenate. No tests with incomplete fecal collection were included in this material. Feces were examined for radioactivity until less than 1 per cent of the oral dose was recovered in two consecutive and adequate bowel movements. This usually occurred within 5 to 7 days after the administration of the labeled vitamin, occasionally even earlier. The total fecal radioactivity was always expressed as a percentage of the ingested test dose. The amount of radioactivity not accounted for in the feces was assumed to have been the amount absorbed.

All urine was collected for 24 hours from the time of the parenteral injection of the non-labeled vitamin B_{12} whenever the Schilling test was performed. Sometimes, however, urine was collected beyond this time; in some metabolic studies fractionated urine collections were made. The urine volume was measured and the radioactivity determined on duplicate 20 ml. aliquots. The total urinary radioactivity was then arrived at using the same formula as for the feces, but substituting urinary volume for weight of fecal homogenate. The urinary radioactivity was expressed as a percentage of the orally ingested test dose or, in cases where the fecal activity also was measured, as a percentage of the absorbed radioactivity.

Blood for radioactivity measurements usually was drawn from an antecubital vein at various time intervals following the oral test doses. The radioactivity was measured most commonly in 20 ml. aliquots of plasma and in a few instances also on 20 ml. packed red blood cells. Plasma absorption of vitamin B_{12} has been expressed either as the amount of radioactivity in the plasma, i.e., cpm per 20 ml. volume, or as $\mu\mu g$ of radiocyanocobalamin per ml. plasma. This latter figure was arrived at by using the formula

$$Y = \frac{A}{20B} C,$$

where Y = $\mu\mu$g radiocyanocobalamin per ml. of plasma, A = $\mu\mu$g radio-cyanocobalamin in the oral test dose, B = radioactivity in the oral test dose in cpm, C = observed amount of radioactivity in 20 ml. of plasma.

In-vivo radioactivity measurements following the oral ingestion of radiocyanocobalamin were carried out according to the principle described by Glass and associates (221). The scintillation probe was placed close to the skin over the liver in the right axillary line, over the spleen in the left axillary line, over the various abdominal quadrants, umbilicus, precordium, and the left thigh immediately above the knee. The radioactivity was expressed as cpm above the body background, left thigh.

The radioisotope equipment employed has been described in detail elsewhere (24, 145, 158, 162). For standard use in measuring the radioactivity of urine, feces, tissue, plasma, and packed erythrocytes, a 20 ml. well-type scintillation detector has been employed. An automatic sample changer greatly facilitated the use of this detector (145). For certain studies of plasma radioactivity, a 4 ml. and an 8 ml. well-type scintillation counter have also been used. The scintillation probe used for external body monitoring (158) is the same detector as used for I^{131} uptake studies in our laboratory. The equipment belongs to the Veterans Administration Hospital Radioisotope Service which has a physicist and an electronic technician available for advice, consultation, and help on all matters related to the use of radioactive isotopes and their detection in biological materials. The equipment was used under their supervision and following their instructions. The optimum voltage setting and the over-all efficiency of each detector for the various isotopes were based on assayed material obtained from Merck and Company (Table 1).

Table 1. Over-All Efficiency of 3 Different Well-Type Scintillation Detectors for Various Cobalt Isotopes (efficiency in per cent)

Isotope	4 ml.	8 ml.	20 ml.
Co^{57}	66	57	40
Co^{58}	...	...	18.4
Co^{60}	42	30	24

Regular tap water in disposable counting vials was used as background for the three well-type detectors, since it gave the same result as plasma, urine, or fecal homogenate from a person who had never been subjected to any radioactive isotope studies. The background counts of the empty wells were not used because they were definitely lower than those of the biological materials mentioned. The background of the empty counting vials was found to be intermediate between that of the empty well and that of water or the mentioned biological materials. The counting was always done on duplicate samples of urine or feces. If duplicate aliquots were not obtained (of plasma or tissue, for example), the samples in question were always counted twice. Four unknown samples were preceded and followed by a standard and a background. The average of the background preceding and following the unknowns was used as the true background for the four samples. A preset count of either 12,800 or 32,000 counts was adopted as being ideal for the detection of the low radioactivity we have been working with, especially in the plasma. The background count during the time of these studies varied from about 200 to 300 cpm, most often around 200. The standard deviation of the background counts for preset counts of 12,800 and 32,000 can be seen in Table 2.

Table 2. Standard Deviations of Background Counting (standard deviations in cpm)

Background Count	Preset Count 12,800			Preset Count 32,000		
	1 S.D.	2 S.D.	3 S.D.	1 S.D.	2 S.D.	3 S.D.
200 cpm	1.76	3.52	5.28	1.12	2.24	3.36
250 cpm	2.20	4.40	6.60	1.40	2.80	4.20
300 cpm	2.64	5.28	7.92	1.68	3.36	5.04

In practice the reproducibility of the background counts was found to be slightly inferior to these optimum values. Thus during a period of seven months from November 1954 to May 1955, 95 runs were made on the automatic sample changer altogether, with two or more background counts per run. Out of the 290 individual background counts, 57 per cent were within 1 standard deviation of the mean for each run, 81 per cent within 2, and 93 per cent within 3. It was later found that a slight variation in the high-voltage power supply occurred during the course of a 24-hour period, accounting for the slightly greater than expected variation in the background. The conclusion was, therefore, that any count exceeding the mean background count by 3 standard deviations

Table 3. Percentage of Standard Deviation of Various Counting Rates with a Background Count of 200 cpm

Net cpm in Unknown Sample	Percentage of Standard Deviation, Preset Counts			
	12,800	25,600	32,000	64,000
25	10.8	7.5	6.8	4.8
50	5.6	4.0	3.6	2.6
75	4.0	2.8	2.5	1.8
100	3.2	2.3	2.0	1.4
500	1.3	0.9	0.8	0.6

should be considered significant; i.e., 7 cpm and 5 cpm for preset counts of 12,800 and 32,000 respectively. The standard deviations for counts of 12,800 and 32,000 are 113 and 179; i.e., 0.9 and 0.6 per cent of the respective counts. Table 3 gives the standard deviation in percentages of various counting rates with a background count of 200 cpm, in the neighborhood of which most of our background counts have fallen.

Bioassay was used for the determination of the urine and serum concentrations of vitamin B$_{12}$. For this purpose the method using the green alga *Euglena gracilis* var. *bacillaris* was employed (325, 441, 547, 548). Ultrafiltrates were obtained according to the method of Prasad (505). Identification of vitamin B$_{12}$ was made by paper chromatography using 2,4-lutidine as a solvent (380), or by determining the partition coefficient of radiocyanocobalamin for n-butanol over water. The endogenous creatinine clearance was measured and used as an estimate for the glomerular filtration rate (279). Creatinine determination was carried out according to the method of Hare and Hare (274) and the material was evaluated statistically (35A, 195A, 384A, 507A).

Vitamin B$_{12}$ coenzymes have recently been recognized in bacteria, and coenzyme B$_{12}$ has also been isolated from human and animal livers (22A). Cyanocobalamin apparently can be converted into its coenzyme form both in vitro and in vivo by mammalian tissues and organs (490A). According to Barker, cyanocobalamin and aquocobalamin, which have been previously isolated from liver, appear to be mainly artifacts produced by the chemical or photolytic decomposition of coenzyme B$_{12}$ (22A). The B$_{12}$ coenzymes were unknown when most of the studies in this book were carried out. The radioactivity measured in plasma and organs after ingestion of radioactive B$_{12}$ has been expressed as cyanocobalamin, although it is quite possible that this may not be the true transport or storage form of the vitamin.

The Gastrointestinal Absorption of
Vitamin B₁₂ in Man

1 | A REVIEW OF THE LITERATURE

THE study of the gastrointestinal absorption of vitamin B_{12} was seriously hampered by lack of a suitable technique until radiocyanocobalamin became available for this purpose. Bioassay techniques were tried, but it was found impossible to distinguish patients with pernicious anemia from normal subjects by following the changes in serum and urinary vitamin B_{12} in the first 24 hours after oral doses of the vitamin (122, 632). It is apparent that bioassay techniques were too insensitive to permit the use of oral test doses in the physiologic range. Measurement of the fecal excretion of vitamin B_{12} activity by bioassay also failed to reveal any significant difference between control subjects and patients with pernicious anemia (84, 207). The development of methods using radiocyanocobalamin for the evaluation of the ability to absorb cyanocobalamin, therefore, signified an important step forward both from a scientific and clinical standpoint because it permitted for the first time absorption studies with physiologic test doses of vitamin B_{12}.

The Fecal Excretion Technique: The Heinle Test

Heinle and his colleagues were the first to present a successful study of the absorption of vitamin B_{12} using isotopic technique (289). They administered to two control subjects 0.5 μg cyanocobalamin containing not more than 0.03 μc of Co^{60}. The amount of radioactivity excreted in the feces was determined and found to range between 0 and 42 per cent of the oral test dose. In four patients with pernicious anemia subjected to a similar test, the corresponding excretion figures ranged from 72 to 96 per cent. However, when the same patients were retested with the addition of 90 ml. of normal gastric juice or with 3–100 mg. of hog-stomach IFC, the fecal excretion figures were reduced to 29 per cent or less. This simple test, then, clearly separated the subjects in the control

17

group from the patients with pernicious anemia. The abnormality in the absorption was found to persist also in patients in remission, a finding which made this test even more attractive from a clinical standpoint (289). It was also noted that prior or simultaneous administration of folic acid in daily doses of 50 mg. did not reduce the amount of Co^{60} excreted in the feces. This finding was taken as a refutation of the claim that folic acid promotes the utilization of orally administered vitamin B_{12} (409). Furthermore, it was discovered that when the oral test dose given to the control subjects was increased to 5.5 μg, the fecal excretion figures ranged from a low of 12 per cent all the way to 71 per cent of the ingested dose. This finding emphasized the importance of the size of the oral test dose to be used in the diagnosis of malabsorption of vitamin B_{12} and explained why a previous attempt at using the fecal excretion test had failed in this respect (353, 392). The authors suggested that the method might be of value in diagnosing pernicious anemia and assaying the action of the intrinsic factor.

Many reports have confirmed the original observations of Heinle and his associates (85, 270, 272, 273, 354, 378, 392, 401, 436, 629). The fecal radioactivity has been measured on homogenates of feces (85, 272, 401) or after drying and ashing (270, 378) in scintillation detectors (85, 270, 272, 378, 401) or with Geiger counters (378, 436). There is now general agreement in the literature that patients with pernicious anemia as a group can, with the stool excretion method (85, 270, 272, 273, 354, 378, 401, 436, 629), be separated from control subjects. In some reports overlap has, however, occurred (407, 433, 436) and reservations as to the interpretation of the test have been expressed (407). The fact of overlap might be attributed to the use of oral test doses larger than 0.5 μg as originally recommended (407), or, where it occurs with smaller test doses (434, 436), to inadequate secretion of intrinsic factor in response to the oral test dose of vitamin B_{12} dissolved in water (434). This latter explanation seems attractive, since under appropriate conditions both food (144, 610) and a parasympathicomimetic drug can increase the absorption of vitamin B_{12} (434, 436).

Callender and associates (85), using 0.5 μg oral test doses, found in 13 patients with pernicious anemia a fecal excretion ranging from 76 to 101 per cent of the oral test dose (mean 88.7), while in 10 control subjects the corresponding figures ranged from 14 to 60 per cent (mean 31.0). In 5 control subjects with infections the excretion ranged from 45 to 60 per cent, which is definitely above the average normal value. Infections may therefore interfere with the absorption of cyanocobalamin to some extent. In 8 control subjects the difference between duplicate and triplicate tests ranged from 2 to 36 per cent of the oral dose. In

11 patients with pernicious anemia the corresponding spread ranged from 2 to 22 per cent of the oral dose. Intrinsic factor in the form of neutralized human gastric juice, extract of gastric mucosa, or a precipitate of hog-stomach mucosa, when given together with the radio-labeled cyanocobalamin to patients with pernicious anemia, all effected a decrease in the fecal excretion of radioactivity to a varying degree.

Mollin and associates (436) administered oral test doses of 0.6 μg to 41 control subjects and found the absorption to range from 0.12 to 0.55 μg (mean 0.38 $\pm$ 0.09) while the corresponding figures in 34 subjects with pernicious anemia ranged from zero to 0.21 μg (mean 0.07 $\pm$ 0.03). Thirty-three control subjects and 32 patients with pernicious anemia received 1 μg test doses. The absorption figures in the former group ranged from 0.26 to 0.87 μg (mean 0.56 $\pm$ 0.02) while in the latter they ranged from 0 to 0.28 μg (mean 0.11 $\pm$ 0.08). Overlap occurred in both series. Thus 3 of the control subjects given the 0.6 μg dosage absorbed as little vitamin B_{12} as did 5 patients who received this dose. One control subject given the 1 μg dose absorbed as little as 2 patients given the larger dose. There was, however, no overlap between the absorption of vitamin B_{12} by control subjects and patients with pernicious anemia when the oral dose was given with or shortly after an injection of 0.25 mg. carbamylcholine chloride. Thus, this procedure increased the absorption in control subjects with low absorption values without showing any influence upon the absorption in patients with pernicious anemia. Intrinsic factor concentrate given to 24 subjects with pernicious anemia increased the absorption to an average of 0.32 μg $\pm$ 0.02 μg when the smaller test dose was used and to an average of 0.52 μg $\pm$ 0.03 μg in 21 patients given the larger test dose. Three of 5 subjects with histamine-fast achlorhydria showed as much impairment of vitamin B_{12} absorption as patients with pernicious anemia. In all of these the absorption reverted to normal with the addition of carbamylcholine chloride. Similarly, in 2 of these patients who were given the oral dose with intrinsic factor concentrate the absorption also became normal. Impaired absorption of cyanocobalamin was also observed in 11 of 17 patients with idiopathic steatorrhea, 5 of 6 patients with tropical sprue, and all of 15 subjects with anatomical lesions of the small bowel: 4 with intestinal diverticulosis, 4 with regional ileitis, 3 with intestinal anastomosis or blind loop, and 3 with massive resection of the bowel, and 1 who had gastrocolic fistula. Two patients with enterocolic fistulas and 2 with pancreatic steatorrhea had normal absorption. Thirty patients with intestinal malabsorption showed no improvement in the absorption of cyanocobalamin with the addition of a dose of IFC proved to be effective in Addison's pernicious anemia. Sterilization of the gut with chlortetracycline resulted in a normal absorption of cyano-cobalamin in the 4 patients with intestinal diverticulosis, in 2 of the 4 with regional ileitis, in 2 of the 3 with intestinal anastomosis or blind loop, but no improvement was seen in 3 patients with idiopathic steat-orrhea or in 1 with massive resection of the small bowel. Antibiotic treatment (succinyl sulphathiazole, chlortetracycline, and chloram-phenicol) improved the absorption in 3 of 5 patients with tropical sprue. In 5 subjects a combination of Addison's pernicious anemia and intes-tinal malabsorption occurred.

Halsted and associates (272) have evaluated the fecal recovery meth-od for determining intestinal absorption of Co^{60}-labeled vitamin B_{12}. They found in 21 duplicate or triplicate tests on 14 subjects with in-trinsic factor deficiency a variation in the fecal recovery ranging from 0 to 18 per cent of the oral dose. In 15 repeat tests on 9 subjects with in-testinal disorders the corresponding figures ranged from 3 to 21 per cent and in 27 repeat tests on 19 control patients the range was from 1 to 31 per cent. In these three series as a whole the average variations ranged from 5 to 11 per cent of the oral dose. In 38 tests on 30 control subjects given oral test doses of 0.5 μg vitamin B_{12} the fecal recovery averaged 34 per cent with a range of 5 to 57 per cent, while the corresponding range in 19 tests on 13 patients with pernicious anemia was 78 to 100 per cent. Impaired absorption of vitamin B_{12} was also noted in patients with total and partial gastrectomy, regional enteritis, the blind loop syndrome, sprue, jejunal diverticula, and pancreatic steatorrhea when oral test doses of 0.5 μg were used (271, 272). It is of interest to note that in 3 patients with intestinal stasis, treatment with chlortetracy-cline and tetracycline, but not with neomycin or sulfisoxazole, brought about a great improvement in the absorption of the vitamin (271). In one of these subjects the fecal excretion figure immediately after anti-biotic therapy was 25 per cent. Two weeks after tetracycline was dis-continued the test was repeated with the addition of intrinsic factor, and the fecal recovery of radioactivity was found to be 73 per cent. In the light of the recent discovery that neomycin can cause a malabsorp-tion syndrome including impairment of vitamin B_{12} absorption (328, 329), the fact should be mentioned that this finding was also recorded by Halsted et al. (272) in 1956 in a case of rheumatoid arthritis. This patient excreted in the feces 74 and 75 per cent of the oral test dose in two different tests while on neomycin. The excretion was recorded as 36 and 47 per cent respectively in two separate tests while off this drug. Based on experience, Halsted et al. (273) tabulated the findings of the stool excretion tests in various groups of patients. In normal control subjects no change in fecal radioactivity is noted when intrinsic factor or chlortetracycline is given. In patients with intrinsic factor deficiency, a source of intrinsic factor, but not chlortetracycline, will markedly reduce the excretion of fecal radioactivity. In the blind loop syndrome, treatment with chlortetracycline will reduce the excretion of fecal radioactivity, while intrinsic factor is without effect. In intestinal malabsorption neither intrinsic factor nor chlortetracycline will alter the result of the stool excretion test.

Krevans and associates (354) using 0.5 μg test doses found fecal radioactivity ranging from 9.7 to 49 per cent in 12 normal individuals, and from 3.3 to 45 per cent in 23 tests on 21 patients with a variety of clinical disorders unrelated to vitamin B_{12} deficiency. One control patient with hepatitis and ascariasis excreted 67.2 per cent of the oral test dose in the feces. No correlation was noted between age and the amount of radioactivity recovered in the feces. In 15 patients with pernicious anemia the fecal recovery of radioactivity was 62.1 to 91.7 per cent of the test dose. Subjects with total gastrectomy, sprue, and jejunal diverticulosis with impaired absorption of cyanocobalamin were also reported. In a subject believed to have dietary vitamin B_{12} deficiency fecal radioactivity in the Heinle test was normal on two separate occasions.

MacLean (378), using oral test doses of 0.25 μg Co^{60}-labeled vitamin B_{12}, found the fecal radioactivity in normal individuals to be less than 44.6 per cent of the oral dose. Impaired absorption of cyanocobalamin was recorded in patients with pernicious anemia, with total gastrectomy, and with proximal subtotal gastrectomy, whereas 6 subjects with histamine-fast achlorhydria had normal fecal excretion values.

Leo Meyer (401) used test doses of cyanocobalamin of 1 μg and reported fecal recovery of 12 to 59 per cent in 7 normal subjects, and 89 to 99 per cent in 4 patients with pernicious anemia. Meyer and associates (407) in a different series, also performed with 1 μg test doses, found the fecal excretion to range from 8 to 41 per cent in 6 tests on normal subjects; from 11 to 100 per cent in 33 tests on 18 patients with various illnesses, none of which is known to be associated with impairment of the absorption of vitamin B_{12}; and from 48 to 100 per cent in 14 tests on 10 patients with pernicious anemia. The difference in the fecal radioactivity on repeat tests ranged from 0 to 56 per cent of the oral dose. The poor duplication and the great overlap between control subjects and patients with pernicious anemia are at variance with previously mentioned observations. The larger test dose of 1 μg may explain some of the high excretion figures in control subjects, although even with a test dose of 0.5 μg $Co^{60}B_{12}$ fecal excretion of radioactivity up to 78 per cent of the oral test dose was reported by Meyer et al. in normal subjects (410).

Many investigators have employed the fecal excretion test in subjects with total gastrectomy (86, 270, 272, 278, 354, 366, 378, 611), and found them to behave in a manner similar to patients with pernicious anemia. Two patients with total gastrectomy were, however, unexpectedly found to have a normal vitamin B_{12} absorption (354, 378). As judged by the Heinle test, patients with proximal (378), but rarely subjects with distal (17, 182), subtotal gastrectomy will also lack the ability to secrete intrinsic factor.

The fecal excretion test has revealed normal results in megaloblastic anemia of pregnancy and the puerperium (15, 182) and in epileptics using anticonvulsant drugs (182, 316).

Heinle's fecal excretion test has thus been used to great advantage for testing the ability to absorb cyanocobalamin in megaloblastic anemias and in various diseases of the gastrointestinal tract. A better understanding of the etiology of the megaloblastic anemias has resulted.

Several investigators have shown that in control subjects the fraction of a test dose of labeled cyanocobalamin excreted with the feces increases rapidly with the size of the oral dose from 0.5 to 50 μg (81, 272, 392, 610). The recovery after doses varying from 0.1 to 0.5 μg $Co^{60}B_{12}$ was in the same general range (392). It is interesting to note that even when 0.1 μg is given, a considerable fraction of the ingested radioactivity appears in the feces (392). Swendseid and associates (610) found that normal subjects absorbed on the average a maximum of 1.65 μg vitamin B_{12} from a single oral dose of cyanocobalamin. The absolute average amount absorbed was no greater with 10 μg than with 5 μg test doses. There was no effect on the absorption of a test meal (breakfast without vitamin B_{12}-containing food) when oral doses of 5 μg $Co^{60}B_{12}$ were used, but considerable improvement in absorption occurred in 4 of 7 instances when 0.5 μg test doses were given. The addition of gastric juice or intrinsic factor concentrate to the 5 μg test dose of $Co^{60}B_{12}$ resulted in considerable decrease in the absorption in 3 normal subjects and insignificant increase in 1. This finding indicates that the limited absorption of vitamin B_{12} in control subjects is not due to lack of intrinsic factor, but must have some other cause. It is interesting to note that the maximum absorption values were 1.93 μg and 3.1 μg in 2 patients with total gastrectomy when 5.0 μg $Co^{60}B_{12}$ was given together with intrinsic factor; that is above the average normal absorption when this type of test dose is given to control subjects (610).

Abels and associates (2) administered 1, 5, and 10 μg test doses of radiocyanocobalamin together with human gastric juice to 8 subjects with pernicious anemia and found the average absorption to be 0.65, 2.3, and 3.5 μg respectively. These absorption figures also are higher than the corresponding values observed by Swendseid *et al.* in control subjects (610). Since the maximum absorption of a test dose is higher in pernicious anemia or in the absence of the stomach than in normal subjects, the inference may be made that the stomach or something in the gastric juice inhibits the absorption of vitamin B_{12}. Higher absorption values when the stomach is bypassed have also been observed when the urinary excretion test is used as a measure of B_{12} absorption (115, 333). This phenomenon of apparent inhibition of the absorption of cyanocobalamin by the stomach has been commented on by Citrin and associates (115).

Baker and Mollin (20), investigating the relation between the intrinsic factor and the absorption of vitamin B_{12}, administered increasing amounts of the vitamin to a patient with pernicious anemia but kept the amount of intrinsic factor constant. As the amount of B_{12} was increased, the percentage of absorption decreased but the absolute amount absorbed remained constant. One subject with pernicious anemia was given a constant amount of vitamin B_{12} with differing amounts of pooled gastric juice in seven separate tests. The amount of vitamin B_{12} absorbed increased proportionately with increase in the volume of gastric juice, there being a linear relation between the two; the slope of this line was termed the "B_{12} absorption gradient." In 6 patients with pernicious anemia successive tests were carried out using IFC instead of gastric juice. In each patient a straight-line relation was found between the amount of IF administered and the amount of cyanocobalamin absorbed. However, when larger doses of IFC were given to 2 subjects a point was finally reached where further increases in the amount of IF did not cause any increase in vitamin B_{12} absorption. The level at which further increase in the amount of IF failed to augment the absorption of cyanocobalamin differed in the 2 patients. It was noted that the absorption gradient varied from patient to patient; the authors believed that this suggested that the development of vitamin B_{12} deficiency depends not only on the extent of the failure of IF production but also on the ability of the intestine to absorb the B_{12}-intrinsic factor complex. Thus an individual with a flat absorption gradient is likely to develop vitamin B_{12} deficiency at an earlier stage of failure of IF production than would a similar person with a steeper absorption gradient. The finding of a very flat absorption gradient in one of the patients suggested that an intestinal lesion might be present in addition to the characteristic gastric lesion of pernicious anemia. The findings on gastric biopsy were typical of pernicious anemia, and the fat balance and vitamin A absorption tests were normal. It is therefore unlikely that he suffered from sprue. Baker and Mollin feel that patients with flat absorption gradients are unlikely to respond well to oral therapy with vitamin B_{12} and IFC. They mentioned having seen failure of such therapy in a patient who subsequently responded normally to parenteral injections of vitamin B_{12}. In the light of subsequent knowledge that resistance can develop against heterologous IF in patients with pernicious anemia treated with IFC and vitamin B_{12} orally, and that this resistance can develop very rapidly (after only 3 doses) (1), it would be interesting to know whether patients with flat absorption gradients behave in the same manner when homologous intrinsic factor is employed. Baker and Mollin also noted that preloading with parenteral vitamin B_{12} reduced the amount of the vitamin absorbed from the intestine. The inhibition of the absorption was not marked, however, until very large intramuscular doses were given.

Callender and Evans (82) also compared the fecal excretion of radioactivity with and without parenteral flooding technique and likewise found inhibition of the absorption of the labeled vitamin B_{12} in 16 of 20 subjects; this inhibition was noted whether loading of 1 mg. non-labeled vitamin B_{12} was given simultaneously with or 2 hours after the oral test dose.

Callender and Evans (81) confirmed the findings of Baker and Mollin that within limits a stoichiometric relation exists between the amount of vitamin B_{12} absorbed and the quantity of IF administered to patients with pernicious anemia. Furthermore, in control subjects as well as in patients with pernicious anemia an upper limit of absorption was noted. The addition of large amounts of IFC seemed to inhibit the absorption of $Co^{60}B_{12}$ from the gastrointestinal tract both in control subjects and in patients with pernicious anemia. This inhibition of the absorption of cyanocobalamin by large amounts of IFC was thought to be caused by the inert vitamin B_{12}, 0.4 μg, present in the concentrate and thus giving rise to an isotopic dilution of the test dose. A patient with a flat absorption gradient similar to the patient described by Baker and Mollin was also observed. Patients with steatorrhea and malabsorption of cyanocobalamin showed in general no response to a quantity of IFC which was found effective in patients with pernicious anemia. However, some response was noted when massive doses of IFC were employed.

It has since been shown that large quantities of hog IFC and even human gastric juice may inhibit the absorption of cyanocobalamin in normal subjects as well as patients with pernicious anemia (81, 113, 227, 610). Taylor and associates (616) studied this phenomenon in greater detail employing the Heinle technique. Using an impure pig IFC, they were able to confirm the inhibitory effect of excessive amounts of this substance in control subjects and patients with pernicious anemia. They showed that the inhibition was not a function of the vitamin B_{12} content in the preparation. The inhibition persisted after heat treatment of the IFC, which destroys IF activity but does not affect its capacity to bind cyanocobalamin. It appeared to them that the inhibition might be due to oversaturation of some intestinal acceptor mechanism or to the presence of vitamin B_{12}-binding material contaminating the IF, or to both.

Recently the Heinle test has been used to investigate the intestinal absorption of liver-bound radiocyanocobalamin (472, 526). In patients with pernicious anemia the average absorption from single oral doses of 3–35 μg vitamin B_{12} was 36 per cent of the liver-bound radioactivity and 7 per cent of 4–50 μg non-bound crystalline radiocyanocobalamin. The corresponding figures in control subjects were 29 and 17 per cent, respectively. In one patient with pernicious anemia as much as 32 μg B_{12} was retained of an oral dose of 35 μg liver-bound cyanocobalamin given orally. The clinical responses were far less impressive than would be expected from the estimated amount of vitamin B_{12} absorbed. According to the findings of Reizenstein and Nyberg the oral ingestion of 40 grams of beef liver once a week should suffice to keep patients with pernicious anemia in remission. It is very difficult to reconcile these figures with the experience with oral liver therapy in patients with pernicious anemia (428–430). The reason for the discrepancy is not entirely clear, but it is quite possible that not all of the liver radioactivity absorbed represented vitamin B_{12} (526). The problem in question is an important one and relates to the absorption of cyanocobalamin in the absence of the gastric intrinsic factor. In this respect it should be mentioned that it has been claimed recently that vitamin B_{12} in the form of a polypeptide complex is readily absorbed by patients with pernicious anemia and that intrinsic factor probably does not exist (285, 286, 447–450). Because of inadequacy in the experimental design, the work of Heathcote and Mooney has not been accepted (93, 215, 256, 311B, 357, 359). The question of the vitamin B_{12} polypeptide complexes and their gastrointestinal absorption may not have been completely settled yet (281, 413, 446, 450, 580). A continuous search is going on for extragastric substances capable of promoting the absorption of cyanocobalamin (53, 54, 103, 110–112, 125, 174, 257, 291, 299, 303, 309, 474, 476, 529), but none has yet been found that can substitute for the gastric intrinsic factor of Castle.

The Urinary Excretion Technique: The Schilling Test

Schilling (557) observed that when an injection of a large dose of non-radioactive vitamin B$_{12}$ was administered shortly after the oral test dose of labeled cyanocobalamin a considerable amount of radio-activity was excreted in the subsequent 24-hour urine collection. No or negligible activity was found in the urine of patients with pernicious anemia subjected to the same procedure unless a source of intrinsic factor such as human gastric juice or a hog intrinsic factor preparation was administered together with the labeled vitamin. When the gastric juice was boiled, its effect on the urinary radioactivity disappeared. Oxytetracycline therapy did not improve the recovery of radioactivity in the urine of patients with pernicious anemia given the labeled vitamin alone, thus refuting the theory that intestinal bacteria deprive the host of dietary vitamin B$_{12}$. No radioactivity was detected in the urine in normal subjects or patients with pernicious anemia given labeled vitamin B$_{12}$ and IF when the parenteral injection of the large dose of non-labeled cyanocobalamin was omitted. This observation was suggested as a new method for the study of intrinsic factor activity, since it could be used in patients with pernicious anemia in remission. Schilling et al. (558–560) have since reported on the quantitative 24-hour urinary radioactivity obtained in various control subjects and patients with achlorhydria, pernicious anemia, or gastrectomy (Tables 4 and 5). The latter two groups were examined both without and with the addition of a source of IF. Patients with pernicious anemia were readily separated from control subjects. Patients with total gastrectomy behaved in a manner similar to those with pernicious anemia. Both of these groups showed great improvement in the excretion of urinary radioactivity when IF was supplied. Subjects with achlorhydria showed a wide range of urinary radioactivity. Most revealed excretion figures within the normal range, but some were below normal or even in the range found in patients with pernicious anemia. The reproducibility of the urinary excretion test was investigated by Schilling (560) in repeat tests in 11 subjects. The difference between duplicate tests varied from 0 to 8.5 per cent of the oral test dose. There was no correlation between the urinary radioactivity and the urinary volume or age of the patients (559).

Schilling administered the oral test doses of 1–2 μg cyanocobalamin containing approximately 0.5 μc Co^{60} in 100 ml. of water on a fasting stomach and served a light breakfast without vitamin B$_{12}$-containing food 1 hour later. The parenteral injection of non-labeled vitamin B$_{12}$ was administered 2 hours after the ingestion of the labeled test dose. Urine was collected quantitatively for 24 hours from the time the oral

Table 4. Results of the Schilling Test in Some of the Larger Series in the Literature: 24-Hour Urinary Radioactivity, Expressed as a Percentage of Oral Dose

Author	Size of Oral Dose (μg)	Control Subjects			Pernicious Anemia			Total Gastrectomy			Achlorhydria		
		No.	Average	Range	No.	Average	Range	No.	Average	Range	No.	Average	Range
Schilling (558)	1-2	5	11.0	3.3-19.9	17	0.6	0-2.5	4	0.3	0-0.7	16	11.4	4.6-20.3
Schilling et al. (560)	1-2	18	14.2	7.0-22.2	34	0.6	0-2.3	13	0.2	0-1.0	31	11.6	2.2-29.5
Schilling (559)	1-2	9	14.7	7.0-21.0	23	0.6	0-2.3	8	0.2	0-1.0	26	13.0	3.2-29.6
Callender and Evans (82)	0.5	32	25.9	15.8-39.6	23	2.3	0-7.5						
Goldberg et al. (234)	0.46	14	17.4	6.2-33.4	7	1.4	0.2-3.7						
Rabiner et al. (509)	2.0	24	13.3	5.0-34.2	36	0.85	0.5-3.0						
Maslow et al. (388)	0.66	26	20.8	10.7-35.5	60	2.24	0-6.9						
Gräsbeck et al. (252) ...	1-2	11	18.2	12.6-26.8	18	0.5	0-2.1						
MacLean (379)	0.37-0.9	10	10.0	6.7-31.0	5		<1.0	10		<1.0			<1.0-32.0
Oxenhorn et al. (485) ...	0.4-0.5	20	17.9	9.0-36.0	15	0.5	0-1.2						

Table 5. Effect of Intrinsic Factor (IF) on the Schilling Test in Pernicious Anemia and Total Gastrectomy: 24-Hour Urinary Radioactivity, Expressed as a Percentage of Oral Dose

Author	Size of Oral Dose (μg)	Pernicious Anemia						Total Gastrectomy					
		Without IF			With IF			Without IF			With IF		
		No.	Average	Range	No.	Average	Range	No.	Average	Range	No.	Average	Range
Schilling (558)	1-2	17	0.6	0-2.5	17	8.0	3.1-15.0	4	0.3	0-0.7			
Schilling et al. (560) ..	1-2	34	0.6	0-2.3	34	10.1	3.1-30.0	13	0.2	0-1.0	12	7.6	3.3-18.2
Schilling (559)	1-2	23	0.6	0-2.3	19	9.5	3.4-15.0						
Rabiner et al. (509) ...	2	36	0.85	0.5-3.0	33	8.2	1.8-19.2						
Maslow et al. (388)	0.66	60	2.24	0-6.9	60	15.0	8.0-27.2						
Gräsbeck et al. (252) ..	1-2	18	0.5	0-2.1	9	10.7	4.4-26.0						
MacLean (379)	0.37-0.9	5	<1.0		5	10.6	5.2-17.2	10	<1		10	10.3	6.0-15.0
Oxenhorn et al. (485) ..	0.4-0.5	15	0.5	0-1.2	15	12.9	6.3-30.5						

27

vitamin was given. The radioactivity was determined on aliquots of urine with a Geiger counter, later in a well-type scintillation counter. The urinary radioactivity was expressed as percentage of the ingested radioactivity.

Many smaller variations of this test have been made. The oral test dose of the vitamin (30, 234, 349, 379, 388, 415, 501, 509), the amount of radioactivity given (349, 379, 501, 509), the timing of the parenteral injection (82, 115, 234, 415, 560), the mode of administering the injection (42, 234, 379, 388), the amount of cyanocobalamin injected (177), and the number of injections and the collection periods (177, 294, 365, 415, 657) have varied. The urinary radioactivity has been measured in various ways — in aliquots (379, 415, 509), directly (234, 379, 501), or after elaborate procedures such as evaporation (42, 557), concentration (333, 349, 655), or precipitation (348) of the radioactivity or absorption to activated carbon (72). The radioactivity has been measured with Geiger counters (42, 415, 557) or more often with scintillation detectors (72, 82, 115, 177, 234, 348, 349, 379, 388, 501, 509). The test has been used extensively for research as well as for clinical purposes. The results of some of the larger series are found in Tables 4 and 5, where they can be compared with those obtained by Schilling. They all confirm the observations of the originator of the test. Subjects with total gastrectomy behave like patients with pernicious anemia and can easily be separated from control subjects. The group of achlorhydric patients is a heterogeneous one, because, as Table 4 shows, it contains people with normal, borderline, and definitely abnormal absorption of vitamin B_{12}. Latent pernicious anemia is a term that can be used for achlorhydric subjects with below-normal results in the Schilling test. They may also show low serum vitamin B_{12} concentration (482) even in the absence of anemia, and they may have total achylia gastrica similar to that found in Addison's pernicious anemia (379).

Because of its simplicity, the urinary excretion test has found great clinical application in the diagnosis of macrocytic anemias and subacute combined degeneration of the spinal cord without anemia (415, 609). It is only a semiquantitative test of the absorption of vitamin B_{12}, but this fact does not detract from its usefulness.

The value of the Schilling test, as well as of all methods for the measurement of the absorption of radiocyanocobalamin, is enhanced by the fact that the test can be applied whether the patients with pernicious anemia are in relapse or remission. In addition to patients with pernicious anemia, total gastrectomy, or histamine-fast achlorhydria, the Schilling test has revealed malabsorption of cyanocobalamin in various conditions and diseases such as after gastric resection (44, 68, 349, 372,

372A, 507), in gastritis (584, 586), after resection of the small bowel (6, 127, 200, 352, 354, 392, 485), in idiopathic sprue (200, 485, 519), tropical sprue (537, 574), after pancreatectomy (392), in cystic fibrosis of pancreas (200), regional ileitis (354), diverticula of the small bowel (500, 568), blind loop of the small intestine (157, 200, 392, 485), in agammaglobulinemia (132, 200), in myxedema (365), in patients harboring fish tapeworms (66, 337, 468, 471), in familial selective vitamin B_{12} malabsorption with proteinuria (120, 246), in patients with juvenile pernicious anemia without achylia gastrica (118, 275, 392, 601), and in patients with pernicious anemia who have developed resistance against heterologous intrinsic factor (31, 197, 492, 565–567, 587, 602, 608). The rapid development of knowledge in this field of medicine has been greatly facilitated by the availability of this simple testing procedure.

Since the urinary excretion method is a semiquantitative test for the absorption of cyanocobalamin, the relationship between the results of this test and those of the more quantitative fecal excretion test has been evaluated. Callender and Evans (82) observed in 113 combined tests a good correlation between the urinary excretion of radioactivity and the absorption of the cyanocobalamin as measured by the recovery of radioactivity in feces. The correlation coefficient between these two methods of estimating the absorption of vitamin B_{12} was 0.909. In 84 tests in which the absorption as measured by the Heinle test exceeded 15 per cent of the oral test dose an average of 34 per cent of the absorbed radioactivity was excreted in the 24-hour urine collection. Because of the large experimental error this ratio of 1:3 did not apply when the absorption, according to the fecal excretion method, was below 15 per cent of the oral dose. Correlation between the results of the Heinle and the Schilling tests has also been made by other investigators (73, 380). Bull found the average urinary excretion to be 40 per cent of the absorbed radioactivity (73), while MacLean and Bloch observed 33.9 to 38.8 per cent in 3 subjects studied (380). Though these figures confirm the work of Callender and Evans, none of them explains why only such a limited amount of the labeled vitamin is excreted in the urine during a period when most of a large parenteral dose is excreted (107, 122, 355, 442, 595). It is apparent that there is a fundamental difference in the handling of the injected and the ingested vitamin B_{12}, since so much less of the labeled cyanocobalamin can be accounted for in the urine. MacLean and Bloch showed that the radioactivity recovered in the urine really represents unaltered cyanocobalamin and not a breakdown product of the vitamin (380).

The reproducibility of the Schilling test was investigated by Chow and associates (109), by Citrin et al. (115) and by Adams and Seaton

(5). The variations between repeated tests were found to range from 0 to 8.8 per cent of the oral test dose (109, 115). The effect of age on the excretion values was investigated by several groups (106, 109, 201). The results confirmed the observations of Schilling and failed to reveal any significant variation in the absorption by age, although in some older people below-normal excretion values were observed (106, 109). The excretion figures in these isolated instances usually improved with the addition of IF (106, 109). These people should be watched for vitamin B_{12} deficiency as evidenced by a low serum B_{12} concentration (106, 482). With low serum B_{12} levels and low absorption values they should be regarded as cases of latent pernicious anemia and treated accordingly even if their hemoglobin values are normal (80, 482). Normal urinary excretion values are usually not improved by adding an exogenous source of IF to the labeled cyanocobalamin (106). Some impure IFC may even inhibit the absorption of vitamin B_{12} (113, 655), and an inhibitory factor has been detected in certain crude IF preparations derived from hog duodenum (427). Recently preparations have been made which apparently do not inhibit the absorption and may even increase it in control subjects (113, 173, 655).

It is important to know that kidney disease and uremia may impair the urinary excretion of radioactivity (73, 169, 234, 356, 371, 415, 516, 517). In uremia the urinary excretion values in the Schilling test may be as low as in patients with pernicious anemia. In contrast to normal subjects, patients with impaired kidney function wil continue to excrete radioactivity for several days after the oral ingestion of the labeled cyanocobalamin. Normal total excretion values may be obtained if the collection period is extended over several days. The low 24-hour urinary excretion values are not due to lack of intrinsic factor, since the addition of this factor did not improve the absorption (517). The urinary excretion of parenterally administered vitamin B_{12} in renal failure has also been found to be delayed and decreased (355) and it is believed that the low excretion values found in uremia are the result of decreased glomerular filtration rate more than of decreased intestinal absorption of vitamin B_{12} (355, 517).

For clinical purposes it is also important to know that infections may be associated with abnormally low urinary excretion values (415), while the values will return to normal during the convalescence. Unless the excretion values observed during an infection are within the normal range, the test must be repeated weeks later. The diagnosis of malabsorption of cyanocobalamin from a test during an acute infection can therefore not be considered reliable.

In a large series of patients with partial gastrectomy, the urinary excretion of radioactivity was found to be below 10 per cent of the oral dose, the lower limit of normal, in 37 of 119 patients (372), i.e., in approximately 30 per cent. Absorption was greatly improved or corrected by the addition of an exogenous source of intrinsic factor. Reduction of the absorption to values observed in pernicious anemia (0 to 5 per cent) was not observed in any of the group operated on for duodenal ulcer. However, 18 of 78 patients who underwent resection for ulcer or carcinoma of the stomach showed excretion values in this range. These findings are in accordance with clinical and laboratory data collected by other investigators (17, 68, 144, 372A, 377). Badenoch and associates (17) observed defective absorption of vitamin B_{12} in 5 patients with megaloblastic anemia following gastric resection for ulcer of the stomach. Furthermore, they found that these patients had gastric atrophy comparable in severity to that seen in pernicious anemia. MacLean (377) observed that megaloblastic anemia did not develop in patients with gastric resection for duodenal ulcer, but only after operation for ulcer or carcinoma of the stomach. MacLean found further that histological examination of the stomach from patients who later developed pernicious anemia showed extensive gastritis, and from his experience he thinks it is possible to predict from the histological picture of the resected portion of the stomach which patient will develop pernicious anemia after gastric resection.

Proximal subtotal gastrectomy does not always give rise to impaired vitamin B_{12} absorption (372A), as was at first believed (378). The amount of fundus and corpus resected undoubtedly plays a large role (44). The work of Brodine and associates (68) suggests that only persons with gastric resections and gastrojejunostomies, and not those with gastroduodenostomies, develop impaired vitamin B_{12} absorption. Apparently food intake can stimulate the absorption of cyanocobalamin in patients with gastric resections, but not in normal subjects or in patients with pernicious anemia (144). When testing patients with gastric resections it is therefore recommended that the labeled vitamin B_{12} be administered with a B_{12}-free meal.

Some interesting observations have been made by Siurala and associates regarding the absorption of cyanocobalamin in atrophic gastritis and the relation between this condition and pernicious anemia (584). These investigators examined 78 patients with various degrees of gastritis and compared the results with those from 50 patients with pernicious anemia and 35 control subjects. The Schilling test showed results below 5 per cent in 49 of the patients with pernicious anemia and below 10 per cent in all of them. In severe atrophic gastritis the excretion values were below 5 per cent in 10, below 10 per cent in 17, and above 10 per cent in 7 patients. In moderate atrophic gastritis the figures were above 10 per cent in 38 of 40 patients, below 10 per cent in 2, and below 5 per cent in 1. In 14 subjects with superficial gastritis and in the control subjects with normal gastric mucosa all excretion values were above 10 per cent. Repeated tests with the addition of carbamylcholine chloride usually failed to show improvement in the urinary excretion of radioactivity in subjects with severe atrophic gastritis when the baseline excretion was below 5 per cent, although intrinsic factor effectively improved the absorption. In subjects with borderline excretion values, carbamylcholine chloride as a rule raised the urinary recovery of radioactivity to above the 10 per cent level. Furthermore, it was found that hydrochloric acid secretion and uropepsin excretion tended to decrease as the mucosal lesion progressed and that the absorption of cyanocobalamin and serum B$_{12}$ concentration revealed the same tendency. Three cases were presented which might be considered intermediate stages between non-specific atrophic gastritis and actual pernicious anemia. Of great interest was the observation that with progression of the gastritis the hydrochloric acid secretion appeared to fail first, and the ability to secrete pepsin next, while the ability to produce intrinsic factor was maintained longest and was not lost until in the end stages of atrophic gastritis. Poliner and Spiro (502) and Glass et al. (233) have recently made similar observations. The excellent study by Siurala et al. leaves the impression that there is no real difference between the gastric lesion in pernicious anemia and severe gastritis, and that the latter may show transition into pernicious anemia. Doig and Wood (152) also subscribe to the hypothesis that the gastric lesion in pernicious anemia is the end stage of chronic gastritis. Magnus now feels that atrophic gastritis and gastric atrophy represent stages in the same pathological process (382), a point of view which is altered from his earlier one (383).

These findings are very interesting because many years ago Knud Faber very succinctly pointed out that patients dying from Addison's pernicious anemia might show the typical histological picture of diffuse chronic gastritis (185, 186, 189, 189A) instead of gastric atrophy as would be expected according to the theory of Fenwick (194, 195). The gastric lesion in pernicious anemia has since been carefully studied by many observers either in autopsy material or from gastric biopsy samples obtained in vivo or by gastroscopy (12, 18, 71, 129, 151, 383, 384, 386, 398, 454, 487, 579, 583, 665). These studies have not resulted in complete unanimity as to the basic anatomic defect in the stomach. Some authors have stressed the findings of gastric atrophy (151, 194, 383, 384, 454), while others have put more emphasis on atrophic gastritis (71, 323, 324, 398, 487). Some investigators have found both types of change in patients with pernicious anemia (12, 129, 148, 335, 386, 654). It is not unlikely that the gastric atrophy is the final end stage in a long and chronic process of gastritis (152, 186, 323, 324, 382, 584), although the final proof for this contention is yet to come (613). Siurala and associates (584) think that a decrease of IF production resulting in pernicious anemia may develop in at least two different ways: it may sometimes be due to a specific lack of IF independent of the pathologic-anatomic condition of the gastric mucosa, and in other instances may result from a chronic atrophic gastritis. The possibility that the basic anatomic lesion in pernicious anemia arises on the basis of autoimmunity should be given serious considerations (386A, 480, 564, 615, 618A). In line with the modern theory of immunology as propounded by Burnet (77, 78), the finding of chronic lymphocytic infiltration with plasma cells in the gastric mucosa (71, 129, 398) strengthens the hypothesis that the gastric lesion in pernicious anemia arises on the basis of autoimmunity. Future work may shed more light on the pathogenesis of the anatomic lesion in the stomach of patients with Addison's pernicious anemia.

Aided by the Schilling test, observers have found out some interesting things about the influence of steroids on the absorption of vitamin B_{12}. Several investigators (199, 239) have observed that steroids were capable of increasing the urinary excretion of radioactivity in patients with pernicious anemia. Since no improvement in vitamin B_{12} absorption occurred after total gastrectomy, Gordin (239) thought the improvement seen in patients with pernicious anemia must be due to increased secretion of intrinsic factor. Frost and Goldwein (199) found, however, no such increase in the intrinsic factor production in the patient with pernicious anemia they examined. The fact that improvement in the absorption of cyanocobalamin is possible with steroid therapy (199, 239, 478, 479) and that vitamin B_{12} serum concentration can increase considerably in some (239) but not all patients (147B) during such treatment may explain why some patients with pernicious anemia have been observed to go into remission when such drugs have been administered (147B, 239). Recently Østergaard Kristensen has given conclusive proof for the contention that steroids can increase the secretion of intrinsic factor in patients with pernicious anemia (479, 480).

Extensive observations have been made regarding the urinary excretion test in pernicious tapeworm anemia (55, 66, 337, 468, 469, 471). On the basis of this test it has been confirmed that patients with pernicious tapeworm anemia have absorption values in the pernicious anemia range, and that non-symptomatic carriers of the fish tapeworm have urinary excretion values below normal. In both groups the absorption returned to normal following the worm cure. An interesting observation was made in non-anemic carriers of *Diphyllobothrium latum*. Although these patients showed a return of their absorption test to normal in 1 to 6 weeks, only partial correction of the absorption values was observed during the first week after the expulsion of the worms (471). It is not unlikely that this gradual improvement in the absorption figures results from the improvement in the gastritis that has been observed in a great number of subjects with fish-tapeworm anemia after worm expulsion (582). The findings by Kaipainen and Ohela (337) that intrinsic factor can increase the urinary radioactivity in the Schilling test and by Kaipainen and Tötterman (338) that intrinsic factor can induce a reticulocyte response in pernicious tapeworm anemia naturally raise the question whether there is in reality a decreased production of intrinsic factor in subjects with fish-tapeworm anemia. While previous investigations (55, 314, 315) seemed to confirm the presence of this substance in the gastric juice of persons with fish tapeworm, recent observations may be interpreted to indicate some relative insufficiency of intrinsic factor in this condition (57, 66, 337, 338). Nyberg (469) thinks that the tapeworm influences the B$_{12}$-IF complex and/or has a blocking effect on the intestinal mucosa resulting in impaired absorption of vitamin B$_{12}$. It is generally believed that the fish tapeworm competes with the organism for the available supply of cyanocobalamin in the intestinal tract (55). The worm's ability to take up radiolabeled B$_{12}$ in situ in the human intestine may vary from strain to strain. After the oral ingestion of radiocyanocobalamin lower contents of radioactivity in the expelled worms have been recorded in the United States than usually observed in Finland (467, 569). This finding may explain the rarity of pernicious tapeworm anemia in this country in subjects harboring the tapeworm.

Besides testing quantitative differences between control subjects and patients with various diseases the Schilling test has also been used to gain basic information on the mode of absorption of vitamin B$_{12}$. Gaffney *et al.* (201) administered labeled vitamin B$_{12}$ in oral doses of 2, 8, 50, and 250 μg to control subjects. Following "flushing" injections given two hours later they regained in 24-hour urine on the average 0.24, 0.37, 0.55, and 1.35 μg of labeled B$_{12}$ in the respective groups. Thus, although the absolute urine values increased, the percentage of the oral dose excreted decreased from 12 per cent to a mere 0.54 per cent. The absorption of this vitamin must therefore be very inefficient at very high dosage levels. These findings confirm the observations made by the fecal excretion method. Best and associates (42) studied the absorption of radiocyanocobalamin in patients with pernicious anemia with oral doses of 2 and 15 μg together with intrinsic factor. Their figures seemed to indicate a urinary excretion of radioactivity proportional to the logarithm of IF dosage at low to moderate dosage levels, but they did not exclude the possibility of a linear approach to a plateau.

With the help of the Schilling test the fundamental question of the site of the absorption of vitamin B_{12} has been approached. Citrin and associates (115) introduced the labeled vitamin through polyvinyl tubes passed down to various portions of the intestine. Good absorption was usually found when the test dose was delivered into the ileum, indicating that this part of the intestine has the ability to absorb cyanocobalamin. Good absorption was also noted when the material was introduced into the duodenum and jejunum. This result was interpreted to mean that the whole small intestine was capable of absorbing the vitamin. Though this interpretation may be correct, it cannot be considered proven because it may be possible that the labeled vitamin was carried down into the lower part of the small bowel before it was absorbed. No absorption of the vitamin occurred from the large bowel or rectum even with the addition of intrinsic factor or following sterilization of the gut with antibiotics. It is interesting to note that the absorption was greater in 6 of 7 subjects when the test dose was inserted into the duodenum as compared with oral ingestion. An inhibitory role of the stomach on the absorption was suggested. With the help of enteric-coated release capsules of radiocyanocobalamin for use in the Schilling test a similar inhibitory effect of the stomach was found (333). Best and associates (39) also studied the absorption by the Schilling method after placing the labeled cyanocobalamin by tube in various parts of the gastrointestinal tract. When the upper jejunum was blocked off by a balloon and the test dose delivered to the intestine above the obstruction, practically no urinary radioactivity was recovered, not even after release of the balloon 12 hours later. The deduction was made that vitamin B_{12} cannot be absorbed by the upper small bowel, and, furthermore that intrinsic factor concentrate was destroyed by too long a sojourn there. Because the conditions of the experiments are so unphysiologic and because stasis of the intestinal contents can in some still unknown way impair the absorption of vitamin B_{12}, one should interpret these findings with great caution.

After the basic discovery was made that calcium ions are needed for the uptake of vitamin B_{12} by liver slices and isolated rat small intestines (305–308) it was soon learned that calcium ions are apparently also necessary for the absorption of cyanocobalamin from the gastrointestinal tract of man. Gräsbeck and Nyberg (249) showed that EDTA could greatly reduce the urinary excretion of radioactivity in the Schilling test in control subjects even down to levels found in patients with pernicious anemia and that, furthermore, the addition of calcium resulted in a reversal of the excretion figures to normal levels. In sprue the effect may be analogous to that seen in control subjects given EDTA. Loss of calcium from the intestinal contents in the form of calcium soaps may explain the low urinary excretion figures in some (248) but not all (301, 537) patients with steatorrhea. Some investigators did not find inhibition of vitamin B_{12} absorption by EDTA (3, 528).

When fractionated urine collections are made in the Schilling test, no or negligible amounts of radioactivity are found in the urine until approximately 4–6 hours after the ingestion of the test dose (40, 60, 557) and the maximum excretion is usually delayed until the 6–12 hour interval (40, 60, 557) or even later (40). It was postulated that the delayed peak was related to the time it takes for vitamin B_{12} to be transported in the intestine to the point of absorption or to the duration of the intracellular metabolic processes of absorption (40). Since the same kind of delay occurred when the labeled vitamin was introduced into the proximal ileum, it was believed that the transit time could be excluded and thus that the delay in the excretion of urinary radioactivity was related to mucosal cell processes (39).

An interesting phenomenon was described by Schwartz et al. (567) using the Schilling test. These and other investigators (31, 400, 443, 492, 566, 567, 602, 608) noted that patients with pernicious anemia treated orally with vitamin B_{12} and hog-stomach IFC showed a good response initially but after varying lengths of time they went into relapse. Under these circumstances the patients responded quickly to vitamin B_{12} or liver preparations given parenterally (567). With the aid of the Schilling test a considerable number of patients with pernicious anemia treated with B_{12} together with heterologous IFC orally was found to have developed a block against the action of the IF, so that ordinary doses of this factor no longer promoted the absorption of the vitamin (31, 492, 565–567, 587, 602, 608). This was believed to be the reason for the frequent relapses in these patients. Both human (31, 566, 567, 602, 608) and rat (566) IF were found effective in these patients who developed resistance against hog IFC. Furthermore, it was learned that the block could be overcome by the administration of massive doses of hog IFC (33, 587, 608). The exact cause for the development of resistance against the heterologous IFC is still under debate. It has been postulated that it is caused by a phenomenon of immunity since blocking antibodies against IF have been found in the blood of patients treated with these preparations (564–566), but not all observations can be explained on this basis (565). Some investigators have found no evidence of circulating antibodies in patients with resistance against IF (4, 602). The older stomach preparations were successful in the long-term oral treatment of patients with pernicious anemia, while it appears to be the newer more potent IFC that are responsible for the development of the resistance phenomenon (565, 566). The reason for this discrepancy is not known. The practical implication from all these studies is that it is very hazardous to treat patients with pernicious anemia with oral preparations containing small doses of vitamin B_{12} together with hog stomach IFC.

The mechanism of action of the IF is still not well understood. From recent papers on the subject (29, 30A, 126, 213, 245, 358, 465, 651) it appears that vitamin B_{12} binding is essential for intrinsic factor activity, although it should be pointed out that very active IF preparations with low B_{12}-binding capacity have been described (193, 358, 656). The work by Bishop and his associates (46) has helped in clarifying the relation between binding power and intrinsic factor activity. These investigators used the urinary excretion test as a measure of absorption of cyanocobalamin from the gastrointestinal tract. In one test an oral dose of $Co^{60}B_{12}$ was followed immediately by an oral dose of normal human gastric juice which had been incubated at room temperature with an equivalent amount of non-radioactive vitamin B_{12}. In the second part of the experiment, the $B_{12}Co^{60}$ was bound to the IF in the gastric juice and the non-radioactive B_{12} was free. The resulting data suggested that the B_{12} already bound by the gastric juice, presumably to the IF, was preferentially absorbed. Preferential absorption of B_{12} bound to IF has been confirmed by other investigators (561, 626). Bunge and associates (75) found the in-vitro binding of cyanocobalamin by gastric juice to be a selective process with a distinct preference for cyanocobalamin over pseudovitamin B_{12} or 5,6-dimethylbenzimidazole. At the same time, neither pseudovitamin B_{12} nor 5,6-dimethylbenzimidazole competed with radiocyanocobalamin for the physiologic mechanism effective in the absorption of cyanocobalamin. Similar preferential binding of vitamin B_{12} by IF from hog-stomach mucosa has been found by Gregory and Holdsworth (258). Thus, binding of vitamin B_{12} by IF is probably necessary for the intrinsic factor activity, but the reverse is not true, since many substances capable of binding vitamin B_{12} lack the ability to promote the absorption of this vitamin (282, 651).

Katz and his associates (340A) have recently made practical use of the finding that in the presence of free cyanocobalamin vitamin B_{12} bound to IF is preferentially absorbed in patients with pernicious anemia. These investigators administered orally $Co^{60}B_{12}$ bound to gastric juice and free $Co^{57}B_{12}$ simultaneously to 20 control subjects, 10 patients with pernicious anemia, and 4 patients with ileal resection. After a "flushing" injection of "cold" B$_{12}$, urinary radioactivity was measured with a differential counting technique. The three groups of subjects were easily separated: the control subjects showed good and equal absorption of the two B$_{12}$ isotopes, patients with pernicious anemia showed reduced absorption of the free B$_{12}$ but good absorption of the B$_{12}$ bound to gastric juice, and patients with ileal resection showed reduced and equal absorption of the two isotopes.

The urinary excretion test has been used extensively for the evaluation of the activity of various intrinsic factor preparations (29, 42, 175, 519, 541, 627, 657). Comparison has been made between the activity as measured by the urinary excretion method and the conventional hematologic assay method. In general a good correlation has been observed between assay by hematologic response compared with the urinary excretion tests (42, 519, 541, 627, 657), although this correlation is far from complete (42, 657). The reason for the discrepancy in some instances is not altogether clear. Best (42) has pointed out that variable and seemingly inconsistent clinical responses have also been noted when patients with pernicious anemia in relapse were treated parenterally with preparations having various B$_{12}$ activities, and this phenomenon has also been well recognized and elaborated on by the USP Anti-Anemia Preparations Advisory Board (287). Best (42) thinks that this represents part of the biologic variability seen in the disease. Another factor to be considered is the testing procedure. There are several variables in the performance of the Schilling test and a uniform and universally accepted procedure for the quantitative evaluation of intrinsic factor activity has not been worked out. Thus oral test doses ranging from 0.5 to 15 μg have been in use (42, 82), and both gastric juice (627) and hog-stomach concentrates (177, 657) have been used as reference standards. Furthermore, there is disagreement as to how much intrinsic factor concentrate should be employed in the Schilling test. Williams and associates (657) suggested that the samples to be tested should be given in amounts 2–3 times the minimum daily oral dose. On the other hand, the work by Toporek et al. (627) suggests more consistent response with the use of one minimum daily oral dose, since inhibition of absorption was seen when larger amounts were employed. Because inhibitory substances may be found in intrinsic factor preparations and because of the possibility of the existence of an optimum ratio of intrinsic factor to vitamin B$_{12}$ (627), a series of as many as four Schilling tests with varying doses of IFC and the same dose of $Co^{60}B_{12}$ on the same patient with pernicious anemia may be required for complete evaluation of the potency of experimental IF preparations (627).

The absorption from the gastrointestinal tract of various vitamin B_{12} analogues has also been investigated by Rosenblum and associates (539, 540, 542). Using the Schilling test these investigators observed the absorption in young healthy males of the following analogues: Chloro-, sulfato-, nitro-, and thiocyanatocobalamins, and in addition the following analogues with altered substituents in the benzimidazole moiety of the vitamin: 5,6-dichlorobenzimidazole, 5-hydroxybenzimidazole, and 5,6-desdimethylbenzimidazole analogues. Common for all of these analogues was a decreased absorption as compared with cyanocobalamin. Parenterally they seemed to have a flushing effect much similar to cyanocobalamin. Of all the mentioned substituted compounds, dichlorobenzimidazole had the best absorption, approximately half that of cyanocobalamin. In this case, maximal excretion was attained after flushing injections with unlabeled homologous compound. The superior absorption of cyanocobalamin over the other compounds was attributed to either the chemical specificity of the substituted cyano-group or the tightness of its binding in the cobalt coordination sphere (542).

Callender and Denborough (80) and McIntyre and associates (390) studied relatives of patients with Addison's pernicious anemia. As compared with control subjects an increased number of relatives had low vitamin B_{12} absorption values, low serum vitamin B_{12} levels, and achlorhydria. Two relatives were unsuspectingly found to have pernicious anemia in relapse (80).

In-Vivo Measurements of Hepatic Uptake of Radioactivity: The Glass Test

Glass and associates (221) discovered that following an oral test dose of Co^{60}-labeled vitamin B_{12} normal subjects accumulated a considerable amount of radioactivity over the liver region, while patients with pernicious anemia revealed no or negligible activity unless a source of intrinsic factor was administered simultaneously. They suggested this simple procedure of in-vivo measurement of hepatic uptake of radioactivity as a test for the absorption of vitamin B_{12} and for the evaluation of intrinsic factor activity. The value of this method has been confirmed in subsequent works by the same group (214, 216–219, 222, 224–229, 231, 232) as well as by many other investigators (9, 60, 74, 105, 503, 504). Because the radioactivity of the unabsorbed vitamin B_{12} in the colon may interfere with the measurements of activity over the liver region and because the activity in the liver accumulates gradually, a waiting period of approximately 6–10 days after the ingestion of the test dose is necessary before the measurements can be performed. An accelerated modification of the test has, however, been described (218, 232) in which the patient is given a laxative 24 hours and a cleansing enema 48 hours after the administration of the tracer dose. The hepatic radioactivity measurement is made immediately after the enema is given. Although this measurement is taken before the peak of the hepatic radioactivity curve is reached, it has allowed separation of control subjects from patients with pernicious anemia or malabsorption of cyanocobalamin in 48 hours (218). If impaired absorption of the vitamin is discovered, the test is repeated with the addition of a source of intrinsic factor. For a complete test in such instances, four days are required (218). If one injects intramuscularly an amount of $Co^{60}B_{12}$ similar to the oral dose and then determines the increment in hepatic radioactivity 6–7 days later, one is afforded a better comparative measurement of the intestinal assimilation of vitamin B_{12} (229). It is not known whether an oral dose of radiocyanocobalamin is deposited in the liver to the same extent as a similar dose administered intramuscularly. The method therefore doesn't quantitate the intestinal absorption of the vitamin, but it provides a way to express the efficiency of absorption of B_{12} in terms of parenteral equivalents of the intestinal assimilation of cyanocobalamin (229). The hepatic uptake method appears just as valuable as the Heinle or the Schilling test (60, 74, 218, 503). Good correlation has been found between the hepatic radioactivity and the amount of labeled vitamin B_{12} absorbed (60, 196, 503). Results similar to those found with the stool and urinary excretion tests have been recorded. Thus, impaired absorption was found in patients with pernicious anemia (9, 74, 196, 214, 218, 221, 229, 231, 503), sprue (214, 218, 229), and total gastrectomy (196, 214, 229, 231); some patients with partial gastrectomy (196, 214, 231), regional ileitis (214, 229), liver disease (219, 229, 230), resection of ileum (196), some patients with histamine-fast achlorhydria (214, 218, 229); and patients with subacute combined degeneration of the spinal cord without anemia (9). Improvement in the absorption with the addition of intrinsic factor was found in patients with pernicious anemia, partial and total gastrectomy, or achlorhydria and impaired absorption values, but not in patients with sprue or regional ileitis. No increase in hepatic radioactivity was found in normal subjects with the addition of IF to the test dose of labeled vitamin B_{12} (214). No evidence of a general impairment in the absorption of cyanocobalamin was found as a function of advancing age (228). However, more older people had impaired intestinal assimilation of the vitamin because of the more frequent occurrence of hypo- and anacidity in elderly people (228).

It is interesting to note that more or less pronounced impairment of the uptake of vitamin B_{12} by the liver was observed after the oral inges- tion of the labeled test dose in some patients with liver disease such as hepatitis, cirrhosis, primary and secondary liver malignancy, leukemic infiltration of the liver, and obstructive jaundice (219). In 4 out of 5 tests the addition of intrinsic factor did not increase the hepatic uptake of radioactivity. It was believed that the impaired deposition of radio- activity in liver disease was not owing to a decreased production of the intrinsic factor, but rather to impairment in the ability of the diseased liver cells to take up vitamin B_{12} from the portal circulation. Such an impairment of the uptake of cyanocobalamin could account for the ele- vated serum vitamin B_{12} concentration frequently found in liver dis- ease. However, since most of the cases with severe liver disease showed normal hepatic radioactivity after parenterally administered cyanoco- balamin, it is possible that the absorption of vitamin B_{12} from the gas- trointestinal tract really was decreased in those instances. Subjects with liver disease or gastrointestinal malignancies may have steatorrhea or intestinal stasis, both of which tend to impair the absorption of cyano- cobalamin; this kind of impairment of the assimilation of vitamin B_{12} cannot be corrected by the addition of intrinsic factor. Since the stool excretion of radioactivity was not recorded in these subjects with liver disease and decreased hepatic radioactivity, the possibility of impaired absorption from the gastrointestinal tract can certainly not be excluded.

Glass and associates (224) made the interesting observations that the percentage of hepatic uptake of radioactivity decreased when in- creasing amounts of labeled vitamin B_{12} were ingested by control sub- jects. It became clear to them that an inverse relation existed between the amount of vitamin B_{12} ingested and the efficiency of its absorption in the intestine. For example, these studies showed that the oral dose of 0.5 μg resulted in a hepatic uptake of radioactivity equivalent to that observed after intramuscular injection of 90.5 per cent of this dose, but that this equivalent rapidly decreased on increase of the intake to 3 per cent of the dose of 50 μg (224). Thus, the increment in the amount of B_{12} ingested from 0.5 to 50 μg resulted in an average increase of vita- min B_{12} absorbed from about 0.45 μg to 1.5 μg. The efficiency of absorp- tion was found best in the physiologic dosage range of 0.5 to 1.0 μg. The addition of intrinsic factor did not result in improvement in this effi- ciency of absorption in normal subjects. From these observations Glass and associates inferred that there exists in the intestine a partial muco- sal block against the absorption of cyanocobalamin. To them these observations also suggested the presence of an "intestinal B$_{12}$-acceptor" with a function like that of apoferritin in iron metabolism. Later work has confirmed Glass's observation regarding the decreasing efficiency of B$_{12}$ absorption with increasing oral test doses (2, 42, 431, 610). Findings have also been presented to support the contention that an acceptor mechanism exists in the intestinal mucosal cells (2, 126, 305, 306).

The relation between intrinsic factor and vitamin B$_{12}$ absorption has also been investigated with the Glass test (227). When increasing doses of intrinsic factor, together with a constant oral dose of labeled vitamin B$_{12}$, were administered to subjects with total gastrectomy or pernicious anemia, hepatic uptake of radioactivity also increased up to a certain point. However, further increment in the amount of intrinsic factor concentrate or gastric juice had no enhancing effect and might even result in decreased intestinal absorption of the vitamin (227). This is in agreement with previously mentioned studies (20, 81). Clinical assays of IFC have also been compared with the results of the Glass test (222). In general a good agreement was recorded between the results of the hepatic uptake method and the hematopoietic responses in patients with pernicious anemia in relapse. This was always true if the results of the hepatic uptake method were strictly positive or negative. If, however, the results of the isotope test were equivocal, the correlation was not reliable and the results of the hematologic assay could be negative, moderately positive, or optimally positive. Glass thinks that there are three possibilities for this discrepancy in a small number of the tests. The first is a lack of an optimal ratio between the labeled vitamin and the intrinsic factor, the second is the presence of non-radioactive B$_{12}$ in the IFC, which may result in isotopic dilution of the test dose, and the third is excessive binding of B$_{12}$ by inert materials present in some crude IFC.

Plasma Absorption of Radiocyanocobalamin: Doscherholmen and Hagen, Booth and Mollin

Booth and Mollin (60), using Co^{56}B$_{12}$ with a very high specific activity, succeeded in measuring the plasma radioactivity of 10 ml. plasma samples in a scintillation counter. They administered 1 μg oral test doses and determined the plasma absorption curves in 7 control subjects and 5 patients with pernicious anemia and were able to separate the two groups. They found that in the control subjects there was no or negligible activity in the plasma until about 4 hours after the ingestion of the test dose. The peak radioactivity was found in the 8–12 hour interval. The falling off of the curve was slow, and even after one week radioactivity was usually still present in measurable amounts. In subjects with pernicious anemia, no or negligible activity was observed in the plasma unless a source of intrinsic factor was supplied together with the labeled vitamin. In repeated tests on the same persons there was a good correlation between plasma radioactivity and the amount of vitamin B_{12} absorbed as judged by the fecal excretion test.

Doscherholmen and Hagen (161–163), using Co^{60}-labeled vitamin B_{12} with specific activity of about 1 $\mu c/\mu g$, succeeded in measuring the radioactivity of 20 ml. plasma samples in a scintillation well counter. They found plasma absorption curves identical with those described by Booth and Mollin. Furthermore, a high correlation between the results of the plasma absorption and those obtained by the Schilling method was observed. This method was used with various-sized test doses for the study of the absorption of cyanocobalamin in control subjects and patients with pernicious anemia (158). It was established that subjects with pernicious anemia can absorb vitamin B_{12} when it is given in large doses without the addition of intrinsic factor. When the vitamin was given in physiologic amounts, no or negligible absorption took place unless a source of intrinsic factor was supplied. The shape of the two absorption curves differed, leading to the conclusion that a dual mechanism exists for the absorption of cyanocobalamin. Portal vein blood showed an absorption curve similar to that from blood of a peripheral vein (160), suggesting that the delay in the absorption of cyanocobalamin must be caused by the small intestine (160). This is similar to the findings described in rats (59). The use of radiocyanocobalamin allowed the study of the kinetics of the vitamin after its oral ingestion (165A). Aided by scintillation spectrometry and Co^{57}-labeled vitamin B_{12} it was possible to distinguish between control subjects and patients with malabsorption of vitamin B_{12} using only 4 ml. of plasma and 0.5 μc Co^{57} (154).

Goldberg and associates (234) have also measured the radioactivity in the plasma following the oral administration of radio-labeled cyanocobalamin. They have confirmed the findings of the delayed plasma absorption described above and they were also able to separate control subjects from patients with pernicious anemia.

Total Body Counting

Recently a total body counter has been used successfully in the study of the gastrointestinal absorption and the body turnover rate of vitamin B_{12} (293, 374A, 525A). The method can successfully differentiate between patients with pernicious anemia and control subjects. Because a total body counter is very expensive, this method of measuring the absorption of cyanocobalamin is still out of reach for most laboratories.

Recently several articles have appeared in which the absorption of vitamin B$_{12}$ as well as the various absorption tests have been discussed (217A, 218, 244, 293, 433).

2 | URINARY EXCRETION TESTS

SHORTLY after the urinary excretion test had been described, it was decided to investigate the value of this test in order to learn whether one could satisfactorily separate control subjects from patients with pernicious anemia by this simple method. The test was performed on two groups of patients, the first group consisting of patients with various illnesses, none of which was known to be associated with abnormalities in the absorption or metabolism of vitamin B_{12}. The second group was expected to show abnormally low absorption of cyanocobalamin because it consisted of patients diagnosed as having pernicious anemia on clinical grounds—that is, they exhibited macrocytic anemia, megaloblastic bone marrow, and histamine-fast achlorhydria, and showed a good response to parenteral administration of vitamin B_{12}. The fecal and urinary radioactivities of the two groups were determined, making it possible to estimate the absorption of vitamin B_{12} quantitatively by subtracting the fecal radioactivity from the oral test dose, and to express the urinary excretion either as a percentage of the oral test dose or as a percentage of the absorbed amount of radiocyanocobalamin. Since the oral test dose originally used by Schilling, 2.0 μg vitamin B_{12}, was considerably larger than the dose recommended by Heinle, 0.5 μg B_{12}, it was decided to measure the absorption with various-sized doses in order to discover the optimum dose for this particular test. The amounts chosen were 0.1, 0.5, and 1.0 μg vitamin B_{12} containing 0.02–0.07 μc Co^{60}. The test was started at 8 A.M. after an overnight fast, and a light breakfast was served two hours later. The intramuscular injection of 1 mg. non-labeled cyanocobalamin was given two hours after the oral dose, and urine was collected quantitatively for 24 hours from the time of the injection of the "cold" vitamin.

Results in Control Patients *

Ten tests were performed on 9 control subjects using 0.1 μg test doses (Table 6). The average fecal excretion was 28.9 per cent of the oral dose with a range from 14.4 to 73.9. The average urinary radioactivity was 26.1 per cent of the ingested test dose with a range from 13.1 to 47.9. In only one of the ten tests was a stool excretion value over 33 per cent encountered, subject J.C., who suffered from psoriatric arthritis. He had the highest fecal and the lowest urinary excretion of radioactivity.

Sixty-two tests were performed on 52 control subjects employing the test dose of 0.5 μg vitamin B$_{12}$ (Table 7). The average fecal excretion of radioactivity amounted to 38.7 per cent of the oral test dose with a range from 8.3 to 84.5 per cent. The average urinary radioactivity was 23.2 per cent of the oral dose with a range from 0 to 46.5 per cent. In 5 tests the urinary radioactivity was below 10 per cent. The fecal excretion values were above 50 per cent in 11 instances, whereas in the same tests the urinary excretion figures were below 10 per cent in only one subject, J.B., who suffered from diabetes mellitus and rheumatoid arthritis. There was a discrepancy between the results of the fecal and urinary radioactivity in subject F.N. on two different occasions. Both times the fecal radioactivity indicated normal absorption, but no radioactivity was detected in the urine. The patient was suffering from diabetes, inactive tuberculosis, and had had resection of the lower part of the small intestine for regional ileitis. His kidney function was normal. There was nothing to indicate that feces or urine had been lost or that the injection of "cold" vitamin B$_{12}$ was omitted. While it is well known that infestation with fish tapeworm may give a result similar to the one in question (66), there was nothing in the history to indicate the presence of intestinal parasites. Furthermore, the feces were negative for ova and parasites. Though it is quite possible that this man should not be included in a list of control subjects because patients with resection of ileum (6, 61, 133) and regional ileitis may have impaired absorption of cyanocobalamin (214, 354, 436), and some patients with diabetes may also have low vitamin B$_{12}$ absorption (603), it was not deemed advisable to exclude him on these grounds, since the fecal excretion figures showed normal absorption. His urine was collected for three consecutive days after the injection of the B$_{12}$ in each of the two tests, and delayed urinary excretion of radioactivity, if present, should have been

---

* Brief abstracts by Doscherholmen and Hagen of the material covered by pages 46–58 appeared in Clin. Res., 4: 83, 1956, Grune & Stratton, New York (157A); and in Proc. 6th Congr. Internat. Soc. Hemat., Boston, 1956, Grune & Stratton, New York, 328, 1958 (159B).

Table 6. Fecal and 24-Hour Urinary Radioactivity in Control Subjects after Ingestion of 0.1 μg B_{12} Containing 0.02–0.07 μc Co^{60}, with 1 mg. "Cold" B_{12} Given Intramuscularly 2 Hours after Oral Dose

Patient	Age	Date of Examination	Diagnosis	Radioactivity, % of Oral Dose	
				Feces	Urine
P.H.	61	7-11-54	myocardial infarction	26.5	18.1
P.H.	61	7-19-54	myocardial infarction	24.9	30.2
J.K.	41	7-12-54	spontaneous pneumothorax	22.8	32.0
M.L.	34	8-15-54	erysipelas	14.4	47.9
E.M.	40	8-2-54	peptic ulcer	25.7	32.0
N.S.	40	7-11-54	coronary disease	15.4	23.6
F.U.	57	7-12-54	heart failure	32.8	30.1
H.B.	67	2-20-56	coronary disease	31.5	18.3
J.C.	40	2-20-56	psoriatric arthritis	73.9	13.1
J.N.	69	2-20-56	coronary disease	21.5	15.7
Average				28.9	26.1
Range				14.4–73.9	13.1–47.9

Table 7. Fecal and 24-Hour Urinary Radioactivity in Control Subjects after Oral Dose of 0.5 μg B_{12} Containing 0.02–0.07 μc Co^{60}, with 1 mg. "Cold" B_{12} Given Intramuscularly 2 Hours after Oral Dose

Patient	Age	Date of Examination	Diagnosis	Radioactivity, % of Oral Dose	
				Feces	Urine
S.B.	56	8-27-54	arteriosclerosis	56.4	35.6
S.B.	56	9-3-54	arteriosclerosis	22.4	25.9
D.B.	21	1-12-54	hilar lymphadenopathy	35.7	29.3
H.C.	60	7-28-54	myocardial infarction	43.0	20.2
H.C.	60	8-4-54	myocardial infarction	40.2	20.9
H.C.	60	8-12-54	myocardial infarction	13.2	22.2
R.C.	30	2-9-55	obesity, hypertension	56.8	21.1
R.C.	30	2-23-55	obesity, hypertension	77.7	13.3
W.C.	64	10-29-54	emphysema	47.0	20.2
C.D.	63	11-24-54	arteriosclerosis	65.9	12.6
C.D.	63	12-3-54	arteriosclerosis	43.9	18.1
J.D.	36	2-9-55	hepatitis	33.5	20.8
J.D.	36	12-3-54	hepatitis	44.6	21.9
A.D.	26	1-5-55	psychoneurosis	45.5	32.8
J.E.	65	1-6-55	duodenal ulcer	49.3	28.1
E.A.	77	9-29-54	hiatus hernia	44.9	12.6
E.F.	59	2-7-55	duodenal ulcer	51.6	10.9
J.G.	65	10-28-54	duodenal ulcer	49.8	34.7
H.H.	65	1-12-55	arteriosclerosis	58.7	17.2
G.H.	42	2-11-55	pulmonary tuberculosis	44.8	28.9
J.J.	62	2-7-55	hypertension	44.2	17.1
R.K.	39	2-7-55	duodenal ulcer	55.8	20.8
E.M.	57	11-23-54	coronary disease	84.5	10.8
A.M.	31	2-11-55	pulmonary tuberculosis	63.4	24.0

Table 7. (Continued)

Patient	Age	Date of Examination	Diagnosis	Radioactivity, % of Oral Dose	
				Feces	Urine
W.M.	59	8-27-54	duodenal ulcer, hypertension arteriosclerosis, myocardial infarction	17.1	27.2
W.M.	59	9-3-54	duodenal ulcer, hypertension arteriosclerosis, myocardial infarction	8.3	27.8
W.M.	59	9-20-54	duodenal ulcer, hypertension arteriosclerosis. myocardial infarction	25.3	25.7
I.N.	59	2-13-54	peptic ulcer	46.2	32.5
D.O.	62	1-6-55	myocardial infarction	35.5	32.5
W.L.	45	1-5-54	duodenal ulcer	18.4	29.6
C.P.	29	9-13-54	tuberculosis	36.3	14.5
R.P.	34	1-5-55	duodenal ulcer	31.3	44.5
M.P.	62	1-6-55	duodenal ulcer, gout	44.7	14.6
R.R.	32	2-11-55	pulmonary tuberculosis	67.6	14.2
F.S.	44	1-5-55	psychoneurosis	34.1	29.4
C.S.	58	2-7-55	myocardial infarction	43.1	16.7
R.S.	47	2-14-54	duodenal ulcer	46.6	28.6
R.T.	27	10-28-54	coronary disease	36.6	37.7
F.T.	33	1-5-54	duodenal ulcer	10.6	46.5
R.W.	60	3-16-54	cirrhosis of the liver	32.1	30.0
E.W.	21	11-24-54	subacute lymphoid leukemia	34.3	13.2
W.B.	49	10-3-55	rheumatoid arthritis	28.2	9.5
C.G.	60	10-3-55	hernia	15.2	29.5
E.C.	39	10-17-55	tuberculosis	17.7	19.8
J.H.	58	10-17-55	rheumatoid arthritis	21.3	28.3
R.N.	28	10-17-55	rheumatoid spondylitis	40.1	9.1
R.N.	28	10-24-55	rheumatoid spondylitis	18.1	21.9
E.H.	46	10-31-55	bronchial carcinoma	34.2	30.5
A.T.	43	10-31-55	coronary disease	22.6	33.3
W.B.	60	11-14-55	coronary disease	28.7	23.0
W.B.	30	11-14-55	Hodgkin's disease	27.6	35.5
G.P.	36	11-14-55	psychoneurosis	32.3	31.6
J.W.	37	11-28-55	rheumatoid arthritis	29.6	22.8
F.K.	57	1-9-56	duodenal ulcer, silicosis	44.8	12.4
R.U.	47	12-5-55	pericarditis	46.5	30.2
E.Y.	57	2-20-56	rheumatoid arthritis	23.0	26.0
J.B.	25	1-23-56	rheumatoid arthritis, diabetes mellitus	65.7	6.8
N.B.	60	1-23-56	coronary disease	17.2	27.6
H.B.	67	1-23-56	coronary disease	31.4	39.4
E.K.	57	1-23-56	duodenal ulcer	38.3	18.6
F.N.	36	9-4-54	pulmonary tuberculosis, regional ileitis, diabetes mellitus	24.9	0
F.N.	36	9-13-54	pulmonary tuberculosis, regional ileitis, diabetes mellitus	49.7	0
Average				38.7	23.2
Range				8.3–84.5	0–46.5

discovered. The 24-hour urinary volume was 1,730 and 2,224 ml. on the first day of the two tests, respectively. These volumes are larger than the average 1,425 ml. 24-hour volume for the entire 62 control tests, but not so large as to interfere with the radioactivity measurements. A laboratory error, although not excluded, was thought unlikely. This is especially true for the second test which was done because of the discrepancy in the results of the first test. The most likely explanations for the discrepancy are that some feces were lost (though this was not admitted by the patient) or that the urine was in reality borrowed from someone else. Unless excreta are collected under 24-hour supervision (113), errors in collection may happen, especially if the patients are aware of the investigative nature of the tests and know that the tests are without benefit to themselves.

The urine was collected for a second 24-hour period in all 62 tests. In 44 of these urine collections no radioactivity was detected. In 18 of them the radioactivity ranged from 1.3 to 11.1 per cent of the oral test dose, average of all 62 collections was 1.7 per cent. Fourteen of the 18 patients who revealed activity in the second-day urine collection also collected the urine for a third 24-hour period. In only 2 of these was there any detectable urinary radioactivity present (3.6 and 11.9 per cent of the oral dose, respectively).

Eight tests were performed on 8 control subjects employing a test dose of 1.0 μg radiocyanocobalamin. The average fecal excretion of radioactivity in these tests was 53.0 per cent of the oral dose with a range from 22.6 to 90.9 per cent (Table 8). The average urinary radioactivity amounted to 15.2 per cent of the oral test dose with a range from 2.2 to 26.2 per cent. It is of interest to note that in 5 of the tests the fecal

Table 8. Fecal and 24-Hour Urinary Radioactivity in Control Subjects after Oral Dose of 1.0 μg B$_{12}$ Containing 0.04–0.07 μc Co^{60}, with 1 mg. "Cold" B$_{12}$ Given Intramuscularly 2 Hours after Oral Dose

Patient	Age	Date of Examination	Diagnosis	Radioactivity, % of Oral Dose	
				Feces	Urine
C.A.	61	1-26-54	duodenal ulcer	55.6	12.0
C.J.	37	2-2-54	diverticulosis of colon	22.6	17.2
I.N.	59	2-23-54	peptic ulcer	67.0	23.7
R.S.	47	2-2-54	duodenal ulcer	25.0	17.9
C.T.	67	2-6-56	diaphragmatic hernia	71.1	10.7
J.K.	41	2-6-54	mitral stenosis	59.9	11.9
W.G.	29	2-6-56	mitral stenosis	32.2	26.2
C.W.	61	2-6-56	coronary disease	90.9	2.2
Average				53.0	15.2
Range				22.6–90.9	2.2–26.2

Table 9. Comparative Absorption Values in Control Subjects and Patients with Pernicious Anemia

	Oral Dose of Co⁶⁰-Labeled Cyanocobalamin					
	0.1 µg		0.5 µg		1.0 µg	
	Average	Range	Average	Range	Average	Range
Control Subjects						
Fecal radioactivity, percentage of oral dose	28.9	14.4–73.9	38.7	8.3–84.5	53.0	22.6–90.9
Urinary radioactivity, percentage of oral dose	26.1	13.1–47.9	23.2	0–46.5	15.2	2.2–26.2
Absorbed vitamin B_{12}, percentage of oral dose	71.1	26.1–85.6	61.3	15.5–91.7	47.0	9.1–77.4
Urinary vitamin B_{12}, percentage of absorbed vitamin	37.5	20–56.0	39.4	0–81.7	34.3	22.2–71.8
Patients with Pernicious Anemia						
Fecal radioactivity, percentage of oral dose	84.5	64.5–107.4	80.0	60.0–92.3	75.5	48.6–89.8
Urinary radioactivity, percentage of oral dose	0.8	0–5.2	0.1	0–1.5	0.5	0–2.4
Absorbed vitamin B_{12}, percentage of oral dose	16.2	0–35.5	20.0	8.3–40.0	24.5	10.2–51.4
Urinary vitamin B_{12}, percentage of absorbed vitamin	3.3	0–25.4	0.5	0–6.7	1.4	0–6.8

radioactivity was above 50 per cent of the dose ingested, but in only one subject, C.W., was the urinary radioactivity below 10 per cent. This same subject had also the highest fecal excretion of radioactivity.

In Table 9 a tabulation has been made of the averages and ranges for the fecal and urinary excretion of radioactivities at the three dosage levels. The amount of vitamin B_{12} absorbed has also been calculated. When the test dose is increased from 0.1 to 1.0 μg the percentage of the dose excreted in the feces increases from an average of 28.9 to 53.0 per cent, while at the same time the absorbed amount of the test dose decreases from an average of 71.1 to 47.0 per cent. The average urinary excretion of radioactivity expressed as percentage of the oral test dose at the same time decreased from 26.1 to 15.2 per cent. However, the average urinary radioactivity expressed as percentage of the absorbed vitamin showed no consistent change, varying only between 34.3 and 39.4 per cent.

The amount of radioactivity excreted in the urine has been correlated with the quantity of absorbed radiocyanocobalamin. The correlation coefficient was 0.39 and 0.65 for the groups that received the 0.5 and 1.0 μg test doses, respectively. Both of these values are significant. The corresponding value for the group that received the 0.1 μg test dose was 0.53. For the number of tests performed in this group, this figure is not completely significant at the 95 per cent confidence level. It is felt that if more tests had been included the correlation coefficient in this group also would have become significant.

In the subjects who received 0.5 μg test doses the 24-hour urinary excretion of radioactivity was correlated with the age of the patients (r = 0.025) and with the 24-hour urine volume (r = 0.084). In both instances a positive correlation was ruled out.

Results in Patients with Addison's Pernicious Anemia

Ten absorption tests were carried out on 9 patients with pernicious anemia using the 0.1 μg oral test dose of labeled B_{12} (Table 10). The average fecal excretion of radioactivity was 84.5 per cent of the ingested dose with a range from 64.5 to 107.4 per cent. The average urinary excretion of radioactivity in the same tests was 0.8 per cent of the oral test dose with a range from 0 to 5.2 per cent.

Fourteen tests were performed on 14 patients with pernicious anemia, employing 0.5 μg radiocyanocobalamin as a test dose (Table 11). The average fecal excretion of radioactivity in these tests amounted to 80.0 per cent of the oral test dose with a range from 60.0 to 92.3 per cent. The average urinary radioactivity in the same tests was 0.1 per cent of the oral dose with a range from 0 to 1.5 per cent.

Table 10. Fecal and 24-Hour Urinary Radioactivity in Patients with Addison's Pernicious Anemia after Oral Dose of 0.1 µg Co⁶⁰B₁₂ (0.02 µc), with 1 mg. "Cold" B₁₂ Given Intramuscularly 2 Hours after Oral Dose

Patient	Age	Date of Examination	Radioactivity, % of Oral Dose	
			Feces	Urine
F.S.	67	6-4-54	66.4	0
E.L.	57	5-10-54	64.5	2.8
E.L.	57	5-31-54	79.1	0
O.M.	60	5-13-54	95.3	0
T.B.	68	6-3-54	88.6	0
B.B.	55	7-7-54	80.3	0
P.C.	57	5-29-54	107.4	0
A.C.	59	8-19-54	91.5	0
A.G.	65	5-22-54	92.7	0
C.J.	54	5-13-54	79.5	5.2
Average			84.5	0.8
Range			64.5–107.4	0–5.2

Table 11. Fecal and 24-Hour Urinary Radioactivity in Patients with Addison's Pernicious Anemia after Oral Dose of 0.5 µg Co⁶⁰B₁₂ (0.02 µc), with 1 mg. "Cold" B₁₂ Given Intramuscularly 2 Hours after Oral Dose

Patient	Age	Date of Examination	Radioactivity, % of Oral Dose	
			Feces	Urine
A.A.	63	7-16-54	77.7	1.5
A.C.	59	8-19-54	91.5	0
C.J.	54	3-11-54	82.2	0
O.J.	57	2-13-54	90.0	0
F.K.	65	9-30-54	60.0	0
P.L.	66	11-11-54	60.6	0
A.L.	66	10-30-54	85.5	0
E.L.	57	4-19-54	86.2	0
J.M.	48	9-7-54	81.7	0
N.N.	58	8-20-54	74.5	0
A.S.	60	10-1-54	74.9	0
I.Z.	59	9-2-54	90.0	0
P.W.	80	1-10-55	73.2	0
O.M.	60	4-24-54	92.3	0
Average			80.0	0.1
Range			60.0–92.3	0–1.5

Five tests were performed on 4 subjects with pernicious anemia with the 1.0 µg oral test dose. The average fecal excretion of radioactivity in this series amounted to 75.5 per cent of the oral test dose with a range from 48.6 to 89.8 per cent (Table 12). The average urinary radioactivity in the same tests was 0.5 per cent with a range from 0 to 2.4 per cent.

In Table 9 the various excretion or absorption figures in the three groups of pernicious anemia patients can be compared with each other and with the corresponding values in the three control series. Patients with pernicious anemia have very high average fecal excretion values, and conversely very low urinary excretion figures. The amount of vitamin B_{12} calculated to have been absorbed in these patients was on the average two ninths to half as much as that in the control groups. In patients with pernicious anemia the urinary radioactivities expressed as percentages of the absorbed cyanocobalamin were much smaller than the corresponding figures in the control groups. It is not clear why patients with pernicious anemia should excrete with the urine less of the absorbed radioactivity than the control subjects. An erroneously high estimate of the absorption in pernicious anemia might explain this phenomenon. It is, therefore, possible that the Heinle method gives too high values for the absorption of cyanocobalamin in this disease. Recent experiments on rat intestine (664) may explain why the fecal excretion method might conceivably result in too high an estimate for the absorption of vitamin B_{12} in pernicious anemia. These studies showed that intrinsic factor did not interfere with the intestinal uptake of the vitamin, but that it was essential for the retention of the absorbed cyanocobalamin in the gut. According to this finding, then, in the absence of IF the intestine would no longer be able to retain the vitamin and it would flow back into the intestinal lumen and gradually be lost with

Table 12. Fecal and 24-Hour Urinary Radioactivity in Patients with Addison's Pernicious Anemia after Oral Dose of 1.0 µg B_{12} Containing 0.02–0.04 µc Co⁶⁰, with 1 mg. "Cold" B_{12} Given Intramuscularly 2 Hours after Oral Dose

Patient	Age	Date of Examination	Radioactivity, % of Oral Dose	
			Feces	Urine
W.E.	44	2-1-54	48.6	0
W.E.	44	1-25-54	64.6	2.4
O.J.	57	2-5-54	86.5	0
E.L.	57	5-24-54	89.8	0
V.S.	57	2-11-54	87.8	0
Average			75.5	0.5
Range			48.6–89.8	0–2.4

the feces. If this point of view is correct, the loss of radioactivity from the intestinal mucosal cells in patients with pernicious anemia might conceivably take place over many days and continue beyond the period of stool collection.

If the parenteral dose of cyanocobalamin had a smaller "flushing" effect in patients with pernicious anemia than in control subjects, this might also conceivably explain the observed discrepancy between the two groups of patients. After parenteral loading doses of cyanocobalamin some (107, 631, 632) but not all (122, 437, 442, 595) investigators have detected lower urinary excretion of the vitamin in patients with pernicious anemia as compared with control subjects. The differences in the handling of parenterally injected vitamin B_{12}, if they really exist, are so small that it is unlikely that they can account for the discrepancy in the urinary radioactivities, expressed as percentages of the absorbed vitamin, observed between control subjects and patients with pernicious anemia.

A complete quantitative fecal collection is difficult to obtain. From Table 9 it can be seen that if an average loss of approximately 15 to 20 per cent of feces occurred in patients with pernicious anemia, the percentage of absorbed radioactivity excreted in the urine would equal the average amount found in the control groups. There is, however, no reason to believe that loss of feces occurred only in patients with pernicious anemia. Granted that the loss of feces may be equally large in the control groups, one will still be left with a great discrepancy in the percentage of absorbed radioactivity excreted in the urine in the two groups. It is therefore doubtful that incomplete fecal collection can explain the discrepancy.

Perusal of the literature regarding the Heinle test and the Schilling test, referred to in the introduction, also leads to the conclusion that a discrepancy exists between the percentage of the absorbed radioactivity excreted in the urine in patients with pernicious anemia and control subjects. An artifact as the cause for this phenomenon is unlikely, but its true significance is yet unknown.

The phenomenon under discussion might conceivably be related to the bacterial flora in the small intestine. It has been known for many years that patients with Addison's pernicious anemia have a rich coliform flora in their small bowels (135) and that suppression of this flora by various means (147, 367, 571, 572) may induce remission or at least partial remission in some of them. Since coliform bacteria have the ability to take up B_{12} in vitro (76, 137A, 142, 209) they might conceivably do so also in vivo, and thus compete with the organism for available cyanocobalamin in the intestinal tract. If bacteria compete with the organism for vitamin B_{12} in the small intestine, thus depriving it of this vitamin, intrinsic factor apparently prevents the bacteria from taking up the vitamin in vivo since a normal urinary excretion of radioactivity (expressed as a percentage of the "absorbed" amount) was observed whenever this factor was administered together with the labeled vitamin. Intrinsic factor in vitro may not always be capable of preventing coliform bacteria from taking up cyanocobalamin (209), but in-vitro experiments may not always duplicate in-vivo phenomena and they certainly do not rule out some bacterial interference with the absorption of vitamin B_{12} in vivo. It should, however, be noted that whenever the absorption of cyanocobalamin has been tested after pretreatment with oral antibiotics no significant improvement over and above the control values has been reported in patients with Addison's pernicious anemia (273, 354, 401, 557). The bacteria found in the small intestine can therefore not play any significant role in the malabsorption of cyanocobalamin in pernicious anemia. It is not known whether bacterial uptake of vitamin B_{12} in the small bowel can account for the fact that these patients excrete in their urine a lower than normal amount of the "absorbed" radioactivity, but this possibility should be kept in mind.

Comparing the fecal excretion figures it is evident that there was overlap at all three dosage levels between the control groups and those with pernicious anemia. In the groups which received the smallest oral test dose, 1 control subject had higher fecal excretion value than 2 patients with pernicious anemia. In the groups which received the 0.5 µg test dose 8 patients with pernicious anemia had lower fecal excretion values than that of the highest in the control subjects. In the groups with the largest oral test dose, all the patients with pernicious anemia showed lower fecal excretion figures than that of the highest in the control series.

Comparing the urinary excretion values it is evident that there was no overlap in the two groups which received the smallest oral dose. If one is allowed to exclude the patient F.N. who showed inconsistent results of the urinary and the fecal excretion tests, there was likewise no overlap in the two groups which received 0.5 µg radiocyanocobalamin in the oral test dose. However, in the two groups with the largest oral test dose, one definite instance of overlap occurred.

A hundred nine urinary excretion tests were performed. It is of great significance that the test revealed very low excretion values in all of 29 tests in 21 patients with a clinical diagnosis of pernicious anemia. The averages and ranges in our material correspond closely to those observed by other investigators (Table 4). In 80 tests on 69 control subjects, 2 patients revealed urinary excretion values in the range found in pernicious anemia. One of these showed normal, the other very high fecal excretion values. While an undefined error is possible to account for the findings in the first patient, it is likely that low absorption existed in the second patient. One should not be surprised at all to find an occasional patient with low vitamin B_{12} absorption among people who have never shown evidence of pernicious anemia. In control subjects chosen at random, it is bound to happen once in a while by chance alone. The control subjects did not have a gastrointestinal diagnostic workup before being included in our control series. Since most of them are in the middle or older age group, it is quite possible that some of them had gastric achlorhydria, although this was not investigated, and achlorhydric individuals have been found to have vitamin B_{12} absorption from normal levels down to the pernicious anemia range. It was not our intention to choose normal subjects as controls, but rather to use a cross-section of a hospital population. In so doing, we may well have included people with diseases which on occasions will reveal lowered urinary excretion values in the Schilling test such as patients with gastritis, gastric achlorhydria, infections, arteriosclerosis, or hypertension with kidney changes, diabetes, etc. With all the subsequent knowledge in mind, it is quite possible that we later would have been much more rigid in our requirements for choosing the subjects in our control series. It should, however, be remembered that a laboratory test that can successfully separate sick people without and with pernicious anemia is of much greater value than one that cannot be used on sick patients at all for various reasons. It was therefore gratifying to find that the test was so successful and reliable in patients with many and various diseases, some of which were even very serious.

The percentage of the oral test doses recovered in the urine declined as these doses were increased. The average decrease was not significant until the test doses were increased from 0.5 to 1 μg vitamin B_{12}. The same tendency to lowered urinary excretion values with increasing test doses is evident from Table 4. In diagnostic work both 0.1 and 0.5 μg test doses seem superior to the 1.0 μg dose. Since there is such a small difference between the excretion values with the two smaller doses, and because it has become a widespread custom to use the 0.5 μg test dose, most of our later absorption studies have been performed with doses of this magnitude.

When the oral test doses were increased from 0.1 to 1.0 μg cyanocobalamin the total average amount of vitamin B_{12} that was absorbed increased from 0.071 to 0.47 μg in control subjects. With a ten-fold increase in the oral test dose the absorption rose only 6.5 times. The phenomenon of decreased efficiency of the intestinal assimilation of vitamin B_{12} with increasing oral test doses has been observed and commented upon by other investigators (2, 20, 42, 81, 224, 229, 610). It is of interest that even with the smallest test doses there never was a hundred per cent absorption of the ingested vitamin, although the intestine had the capacity to absorb many times this amount when larger oral doses were administered. The reason for this is not entirely clear. It may be that some of the vitamin is taken up by bacteria in the lower small intestine, and thus escapes from the host.

The fecal excretion test as a means for the separation of control subjects from patients with pernicious anemia was not satisfactory in these series. Although the average fecal excretion of radioactivity was always much greater in patients with pernicious anemia than in the control groups, there was overlap in too many individual instances. Overlap has been found in the Heinle test before (407, 436). We should remember that the test as performed here is in its strictest sense not a Heinle test, because we subjected our patients to the injection of a large "flushing" dose of non-labeled vitamin B_{12}. In order to determine whether the parenteral "flushing" dose had any influence upon the fecal excretion of radioactivity 18 stool excretion tests (test dose 0.5 μg B_{12} 0.02 μc Co^{60}) were performed on 17 different control subjects without any "flushing"

Table 13. Fecal Excretion of Radioactivity in Control Subjects after Oral Dose of 0.5 μg $Co^{60}B_{12}$ (0.02 μc) When No Parenteral B_{12} Was Given

Patient	Age	Date of Examination	Diagnosis	Fecal Radioactivity, % of Oral Dose
W.M.	44	3-3-54	fractured femur	23.8
W.M.	44	3-10-54	fractured femur	19.5
P.A.	52	4-19-55	chronic lymphatic leukemia	34.4
W.B.	33	12-28-53	psychoneurosis	24.7
B.B.	25	3-8-55	pulmonary tuberculosis	23.9
N.F.	56	4-19-55	chronic myeloid leukemia	22.8
R.H.	25	4-6-55	rheumatoid spondylitis	15.9
F.H.	71	4-7-55	carcinoma of stomach	43.8
W.J.	38	3-8-55	coronary disease	44.7
K.N.	26	3-7-55	lupus erythematosus	19.4
C.O.	65	4-6-55	emphysema	18.1
R.P.	25	4-7-55	rheumatic heart disease	18.9
L.P.	25	4-19-55	regional ileitis	31.8
E.O.	52	4-6-55	cirrhosis of the liver	39.5
H.R.	41	2-25-54	fractured femur	10.4
G.S.	43	3-7-55	cirrhosis of the liver	42.0
E.N.	30	2-11-54	peptic ulcer	41.0
J.Z.	34	8-15-54	peptic ulcer	17.2

Average 27.3
Range 10.4–44.7

injection (Table 13). The average fecal excretion of radioactivity in these 18 tests was 27.3 per cent of the oral dose, with a range from 10.4 to 44.7 per cent. The difference between the average value of 38.7 per cent with, and 27.3 per cent without "flushing" is statistically significant ($p < 0.01$). From this comparison it appears that the large parenteral injection of vitamin B_{12} inhibits the absorption of the labeled cyanocobalamin from the gastrointestinal tract. Similar observations have been made by other investigators (20, 82). The most likely explanation for this inhibition of the absorption of the tracer dose is that isotopic dilution of the ingested vitamin took place in the gastrointestinal tract. Recently an enterohepatic circulation of cyanocobalamin has been described (250, 253, 475, 523, 525) which readily explains why isotopic dilution of the test dose may occur when a large parenteral dose of non-labeled cyanocobalamin is administered.

Reproducibility of the Results of the Urinary and Fecal Excretion Tests Performed Simultaneously

Laboratory tests must be shown to be reproducible before they are universally accepted as being of value in clinical medicine. It was therefore decided to investigate the reproducibility of these absorption tests. A tabulation of the results has been made of the simultaneously performed fecal and urinary excretion tests in 10 of the control subjects (Table 14). One week or more elapsed between repeat tests. The average variation in the urinary excretion test was 5.7 per cent with a range from 0 to 12.8 per cent. These figures are in close agreement with those reported previously (115, 162, 560). They show a satisfactory reproduc-

Table 14. Reproducibility of the Fecal and Urinary Excretion Tests Carried out Simultaneously, with 1 mg. "Cold" B_{12} Given Intramuscularly 2 Hours after Oral Dose

Patient	Dose of $Co^{60}B_{12}$		Radioactivity, % of Oral Dose					
			Feces			Urine		
	μg	μc	1st Test	2nd Test	3rd Test	1st Test	2nd Test	3rd Test
S.B.	0.5	0.02	56.4	22.4		35.6	25.9	
H.C.	0.5	0.02	43.0	40.2	13.2	20.2	20.9	22.2
R.C.	0.5	0.02	56.8	77.7		21.1	13.3	
W.M.	0.5	0.02	17.1	8.3	25.3	27.2	27.8	25.7
G.L.	0.5	0.02	22.8	27.2		22.0	19.6	
F.N.	0.5	0.02	24.9	49.7		0	0	
C.D.	0.5	0.02	65.9	43.9		12.6	18.1	
J.D.	0.5	0.02	33.5	44.6		20.8	21.9	
P.H.	0.1	0.02	26.5	24.9		18.1	30.2	
R.N.	0.5	0.07	40.1	18.1		9.1	21.9	
Average variation			18.8			5.7		
Range of variation			1.6–34.0			0–12.8		

ibility. The average variation in the fecal excretion values was 18.8 per cent with a range from 1.6 to 34.0 per cent. These figures reveal a wider range as well as a higher average variation than those observed in the Schilling test. Thus, a better reproducibility was found in the urinary excretion test. The range of variation in the fecal excretion values reported here is in close agreement with those previously reported (85, 272). Halsted *et al.* found a range between 1 and 31 per cent in their miscellaneous group and Callender *et al.* between 2 and 36 per cent in their control series. Their averages for the variation in the fecal excretion values are somewhat lower, 8 per cent and 13.6 per cent, respectively. Neither Halsted nor Callender used the "flushing" procedure in their series, which may account for the difference in the average values, if it is not caused by chance alone.

Response to Intrinsic Factor in Patients with Pernicious Anemia

The poor absorption of vitamin B_{12} in patients with pernicious anemia is caused by a deficient gastric secretion of intrinsic factor. The absorption will be restored to normal when an exogenous source of this substance is supplied. The intrinsic factor can be of homologous or heterologous origin. In our experiments we have most commonly used commercially available hog stomach intrinsic factor concentrates. The amount of these concentrates most commonly used has been one USP unit, although in some instances the response has also been tested with fractions or multiples of this dose. Table 15 shows the effect of the intrinsic factor on the fecal and urinary excretion of radioactivity in 5 patients with pernicious anemia. It is evident that in each instance the fecal activity decreased when this factor was added while at the same time the urinary radioactivity increased. The fecal activity declined to below 50 per cent in 7 of the 10 tests. The urinary radioactivity increased to above 10 per cent in 8 and was in the borderline range between 5 and 10 per cent in 2 of the 10 tests. The average urinary excretion figure is slightly lower than that obtained in the comparable control series examined with the same dose of labeled vitamin B_{12}. The comparative values are 18.2 and 23.2 per cent respectively. Similar observations have been recorded by other investigators as seen from Tables 4 and 5. This phenomenon may be due to the presence of inhibitory substances in the crude intrinsic factor concentrates or to the fact that the optimum amount of IFC has not been employed, or that some of the concentrates have too high contents of vitamin B_{12} causing isotopic dilution of the tracer dose, or that some patients have developed resistance against the heterologous intrinsic factor. The average fecal excretion figure after the addition of intrinsic factor also indicates

Table 15. Effect of Intrinsic Factor Concentrate (IFC) on Fecal and 24-Hour Urinary Radioactivity in Patients with Pernicious Anemia

Patient	Date of Examination	Dose of Co⁶⁰B₁₂ μg	μc	IFC Units	Radioactivity, % of Oral Dose			
					Without IFC		With IFC	
					Feces	Urine	Feces	Urine
A.C. 8-19-54		0.5	0.02	0	91.5	0		
A.C. 8-26-54		0.5	0.02	2			31.8	7.0
A.C. 9-1-54		0.5	0.02	5			38.7	17.6
V.S. 2-11-54		1.0	0.04	0	87.8	0		
V.S. 4-2-54		0.5	0.02	1			62.6	6.5
V.S. 2-21-54		0.5	0.02	1			73.1	13.7
E.L. 4-19-54		0.5	0.02	0	86.2	0		
E.L. 5-3-54		0.5	0.02	0.5			31.8	20.3
E.L. 6-7-54		0.5	0.02	1			44.9	12.1
E.L. 6-14-54		0.5	0.02	1			75.2	10.7
O.J. 2-13-54		0.5	0.02	0	90.0	0		
O.J. 2-25-54		0.5	0.02	1			32.7	28.5
O.J. 3-4-54		0.5	0.02	1			27.7	28.3
C.J. 3-11-54		0.5	0.02	0	82.2	0		
C.J. 3-18-54		0.5	0.02	1			21.6	37.1
Average					87.5	0	44.0	18.2
Range					82.2–91.5		21.6–75.2	6.5–37.1

slightly lower absorption than in the comparable control series. The two values to be compared are 44.0 per cent and 38.7 per cent, respectively. Perusal of the fecal excretion figures shows that the average absorption of radioactivity with IFC was 56.0 per cent with a range from 24.8 to 78.4 per cent. The average excretion of radioactivity in the urine was 33.1 per cent of the absorbed activity with a range from 10.3 to 50.9 per cent. This figure compares favorably with the urinary excretion of radioactivity, likewise expressed as percentage of absorbed vitamin B_{12}, in control subjects.

The effect of various dosages of IFC on the 24-hour urinary radioactivity was investigated in 4 patients with pernicious anemia (Table 16). The oral dose of radiocyanocobalamin was kept constant. The urinary radioactivity increased when the amount of IFC was raised from a quarter to a half of a USP unit. In each instance, however, there was a decline in the radioactivity excreted when the amount was raised from a half to three quarters of a unit. When unknown samples of IFC were tested on these patients, the maximum urinary activity obtained exceeded only slightly that seen after the administration of half a USP unit. Inhibition of absorption of vitamin B_{12} by large doses of IF or IFC is by now a well-known phenomenon (81, 113, 227, 610, 616, 655), although some preparations free of inhibitory action have been prepared

Table 16. Effect of Various Dosages of Intrinsic Factor Concentrate (IFC) on 24-Hour Urinary Radioactivity in Pernicious Anemia; Oral Dose 0.5 µg B_{12} Containing 0.05–0.07 µc Co^{60}, 1 mg. "Cold" B_{12} Given Intramuscularly 2 Hours after Oral Dose

Patient	IFC Units	Urinary Radioactivity, % of Oral Dose	Patient	IFC Units	Urinary Radioactivity, % of Oral Dose
L.M.	0	1.7	O.J.	0	1.1
L.M.	0.5	19.0	O.J.	0.5	28.0
L.M.	0.75	8.5	O.J.	0.75	25.4
L.M.	0.75	11.5	O.J.	Xmax*	33.1
L.M.	Xmax*	25.5	D.L.	0	2.3
W.H.	0	3.8	D.L.	0.25	15.7
W.H.	0.5	25.9	D.L.	0.5	21.1
W.H.	0.75	16.7	D.L.	0.75	14.6
W.H.	0.75	21.3	D.L.	Xmax*	27.3
W.H.	Xmax*	26.1			

* Maximum excretion of radioactivity with an unknown IFC.

(113, 655). Since vitamin B_{12} and IF apparently must be present in an optimum concentration in order to avoid inhibitory action (627), it has been recommended to test unknown samples of IFC at differing dosage levels before judgment is passed as to their activity (627). This advice seems to be well supported by our studies.

Results in Patients with Total Gastrectomy

If the contention is true that the stomach is the only site for the production of the intrinsic factor (270, 490), then total gastrectomy should lead to loss of this factor and inability to absorb vitamin B_{12}. And this is in fact what has been found by many investigators (86, 214, 229, 231, 270, 272, 278, 354, 366, 378, 611) (Table 4). The addition of a potent intrinsic factor will correct the defective absorption in patients with total gastrectomy as well as in patients with pernicious anemia. In other words, patients with total gastrectomy behave just like subjects with pernicious anemia. Clinically they will all develop pernicious anemia if they are left untreated and live long enough to exhaust their body stores of cyanocobalamin. The time interval from the operation to the development of frank megaloblastic anemia may vary from months to several years (278, 381) in untreated patients, mainly due to varying body stores of cyanocobalamin. Four subjects with total gastrectomy have been found to absorb some (86) or a normal amount of radiocyanocobalamin (169, 354, 378). This unusual finding, if not a laboratory error, may mean that intrinsic factor can be produced outside the stomach by a few persons. It has long been known that ectopic gastric mucosa can be found in the small intestine, especially in association with Meckel's diverticulum (326, 594), and, if these four observations are

Table 17. Fecal and/or 24-Hour Urinary Radioactivity in Patients with Total Gastrectomy after Oral Dose of $Co^{60}B_{12}$, with 1 mg. "Cold" B_{12} Given Intramuscularly 2 Hours after Oral Dose

Patient	Age	Date of Examination	Dose of $Co^{60}B_{12}$ µg	µc	IFC Units	Without IFC Feces	Without IFC Urine	With IFC Feces	With IFC Urine
C.C.	67	1-18-54	1.0	0.04	0	103.5	0		
C.C.	67	3-24-54	0.5	0.02	0	84.6	0		
C.C.	67	2-21-55	0.5	0.02	1			56.9	22.5
C.C.	67	3-7-55	0.5	0.02	1			64.7	13.9
C.C.	67	3-15-55	0.5	0.02	1			57.6	18.5
H.L.	64	3-14-54	0.5	0.02	0	90.6*			
H.L.	64	3-27-54	0.5	0.02	0		0		
H.L.	64	4-3-54	0.5	0.02	1			49.3	4.2
L.M.	35	1-25-54	1.0	0.04	0	84.0	0		
L.M.	35	3-1-54	0.5	0.02	0	95.5	0		
L.M.	35	3-8-54	0.5	0.02	1			81.9	5.7
L.M.	35	5-23-55	0.5	0.07	1				14.2
W.W.	58	5-17-55	0.5	0.07	0		2.1		
W.W.	58	5-24-55	0.5	0.07	1				13.0
J.S.	61	12-13-55	0.5	0.08	0		2.2		
J.S.	61	12-20-55	0.5	0.08	1				24.3
H.H.	68	11-7-55	0.5	0.05	0		1.1		
H.H.	68	11-11-55	0.5	0.05	0.5				17.9
Average						91.6	0.7	62.1	14.9
Range						84.0–103.5	0–2.2	49.3–81.9	4.2–24.3

* No parenteral B_{12} given.

correct, it is even possible that intrinsic factor can be produced ectopically as well.

In 6 patients who had undergone total gastrectomy, the B_{12} absorption was investigated with the Schilling test both with and without intrinsic factor. In ten tests the fecal radioactivity was also determined. The results (Table 17) showed that without intrinsic factor the fecal and urinary excretion values were indeed in the same general range as found in patients with Addison's pernicious anemia. In all 6 subjects the absorption figures improved with the addition of intrinsic factor concentrates. Four patients showed good, two (H.L. and L.M.) only modest response in their urinary excretion values with intrinsic factor. Minor improvement in the absorption values on the addition of intrinsic factor has also been described previously in some patients with total gastrectomy (231, 270, 560) as well as in individual patients with pernicious anemia (20, 81, 560). The impaired absorption after the addition of intrinsic factor found in some patients with total gastrectomy may be caused by a relative resistance to the heterologous IF or by the diarrhea or steatorrhea which some of these patients may suffer from.

Subject L.M. was one such patient. She had a surgical revision made of her esophago-jejunostomy in order to improve this condition. The result of her urinary excretion test with IFC was 5.7 per cent before and 14.2 per cent after this repair operation. At the same time improvement was noted in her diarrhea.

Results in Patients with Partial Gastrectomy

The development of megaloblastic anemia in patients who have undergone partial gastrectomy is a rare occurrence. In a series of 1,550 patients MacLean *et al.* (377) found the incidence to be less than 1 per cent. The high incidence of low or borderline absorption of cyanocobalamin in patients with partial gastrectomy (372) came, therefore, as a great surprise. The question naturally may be raised whether patients with subclinical vitamin B_{12} deficiency are being overlooked among subjects who have had gastric resections.

The fecal and/or the urinary excretion tests were performed on 35 patients after partial gastric resection (Table 18). In 12 with low or borderline absorption values the tests were repeated with the addition of a source of intrinsic factor. The fecal excretion values ranged from 51.4 to 93.1 per cent, which is higher than in control subjects. The urinary excretion values ranged from 0 to 27.2 per cent — that is, from definitely abnormal values to within the normal range.

Twelve patients (34.3 per cent) had values below 10 per cent at one time or another and 3 (8.6 per cent) below 5 per cent. This experience is thus in close agreement with that of Lous and Schwartz (372). The absorption of cyanocobalamin improved to within the normal range when IFC was added to the radio-labeled vitamin B_{12} test dose except in subjects C.H. and C.P. One of these patients, C.P., had intestinal malabsorption which could account for the lack of response to IFC, the other subject, C.H., was not investigated for this possibility and his lack of response to IFC is, therefore, unexplained.

Serum concentrations of cyanocobalamin were determined in 8 patients with low or borderline low absorption of cyanocobalamin. In four instances values were below the lower normal range, namely 100 $\mu\mu$g/ml. In two instances borderline low values were found (between 100 and 150 $\mu\mu$g/ml.), while in two patients the values were entirely normal. One of the subjects with the abnormally low values had a macrocytic anemia which responded to parenteral vitamin B_{12} therapy.

Comments are needed on 6 patients who developed macrocytic or megaloblastic anemia after their gastric resections. Patient C.M. had undergone a 75 per cent gastric resection in 1951 for a gastric ulcer. He

Table 18. Fecal and/or 24-Hour Urinary Radioactivity in Patients with Partial Gastrectomy after Oral Dose of $Co^{60}B_{12}$, with 1 mg. "Cold" B_{12} Given Intramuscularly 2 Hours after Oral Dose

Patient	Age	Date of Examination	Dose of $Co^{60}B_{12}$		IFC Unit	Radioactivity, % of Oral Dose			Comments
			μg	μc		Without IFC		With IFC	
						Feces	Urine	Urine	
A.G.	66	7-21-54	0.5	0.02	0	53.3	11.7		75% g.r., B I for d.u. in 1952.
J.C.	60	2-19-55	0.5	0.02	0	51.4	10.0		75% g.r., B II for d.u. in 1951.
C.M.	62	5-27-54	0.1	0.02	0	59.6	7.1		75% g.r., B I for g.u. in 1951. Megaloblastic anemia 1954, active pulm. Tbc., no definite response to B_{12} or folic acid.
M.M.	68	11-8-54	0.5	0.02	0	93.1	0		75% g.r., B II for d.u. in 1949. Megaloblastic anemia 1954, good response to B_{12}.
J.W.	63	2-3-55	0.5	0.02	0	87.9	2.1		75% g.r., B II for g.u. and d.u. in 1944.
J.W.	63	11-2-55	0.5	0.05	1			15.2	Macrocytic anemia and subacute combined degeneration of the spinal cord 1954. No response to B_{12}.
Z.J.	60	4-22-57	0.5	0.07	0		1.0		90% g.r., B II for carcinoma in 1956.
Z.J.	60	5-1-57	0.5	0.07	0.75			17.3	
C.H.	71	12-3-57	0.5	0.07	0		5.8		90% g.r., B II for carcinoma of stomach in 1957. Posterior column disease before operation, possible luetic.
C.H.	71	12-11-57	0.5	0.05	1			5.8	
C.P.	56	4-21-60	0.5	0.07	0		9.5		85% g.r., B II for g.u. in 1956. Secondary steatorrhea. Serum B_{12} concentration 293 μμg/ml. in 1960.
C.P.	56	4-26-60	0.5	0.07	1			8.4	
A.H.	72	4-11-60	0.5	0.07	0		6.8		g.r., B I for carcinoma of stomach in 1956. Macrocytic anemia with serum B_{12} concentration of 41 μμg/ml. in 1960.
A.H.	72	4-14-60	0.5	0.07	1			23.0	
P.H.	48	8-19-57	0.5	0.07	0		7.2		80% g.r., B II for g.u. in 1947.
P.H.	48	8-27-57	0.5	0.07	0.75			24.3	
R.R.	52	3-13-58	0.5	0.07	0		8.6		75% g.r., B I for d.u. in 1951.
R.R.	52	3-24-58	0.5	0.07	0.5			28.9	
D.B.	71	4-20-60	0.5	0.07	0		9.5		75% g.r., B II for g.u. in 1956. Serum B_{12} 88 μμg/ml. in 1960.
D.B.	71	5-24-60	0.5	0.07	1			17.0	

Initials	Age	Date						Notes
A.M.	42	3-18-59	0.5	0.07	0	9.7		80% g.r., B II for g.u. in 1949. Steatorrhea, malabsorption. Serum B₁₂ 88 μμg/ml. in 1959.
A.M.	42	3-31-59	0.5	0.07	0	10.1		
A.M.	42	3-18-59	0.5	0.07	1	10.9	20.8	75% g.r., B I for d.u. in 1951. Serum B₁₂ 192 μμg/ml. in 1959.
M.S.	50	9-22-55	0.5	0.10	0	8.1		g.r., B II for g.u. in 1957. Chronic pancreatitis. Serum B₁₂ 115 μμg/ml. in 1960.
M.S.	50	9-4-58	0.5	0.07	0	7.5		
M.S.	50	10-3-58	0.5	0.07	1	10.2	18.2	
V.C.	66	3-28-60	0.5	0.07	0	11.4		g.r., B II for d.u. in 1945. Vagotomy 1947. Steatorrhea.
V.C.	66	3-31-60	0.5	0.07	1	10.7	20.1	
H.R.	36	9-2-55	0.5	0.05	0	15.1		75% g.r., B II for d.u. in 1948. Serum B₁₂ 88 μμg/ml. in 1959.
H.R.	36	10-3-55	0.5	0.05	1	12.4	15.6	
L.D.	65	11-4-59	0.5	0.07	0	14.0		85% g.r., B I for g.u. 1955. Cirrhosis of the liver.
A.R.	58	9-23-57	0.5	0.07	0	15.0		g.r., for d.u. years ago. Serum B₁₂ 346 μμg/ml. in 1960.
A.R.	58	6-19-58	0.5	0.07	0	15.2		
R.H.	63	4-6-60	0.5	0.05	0	16.8		75% g.r., B II for g.u. in 1949.
L.M.	66	2-15-60	0.5	0.07	0	16.6		g.r., B II for d.u. in 1945.
S.M.	67	9-22-55	0.5	0.08	0	16.8		Subtotal g.r., B II for d.u. in 1950.
R.H.	45	5-4-60	0.5	0.07	0	17.0		g.r., B II for d.u. in 1950.
K.F.	39	7-25-59	0.5	0.07	0	17.1		g.r., B II for peptic ulcer in 1949.
C.A.	56	1-12-59	0.5	0.07	0	17.3		80% g.r., B II for peptic ulcer in 1946.
A.S.	40	1-25-56	0.5	0.07	0	17.4		80% g.r., B II for g.u. in 1947. Active pulm. Tbc. and megaloblastic anemia in 1955. Serum B₁₂ 275 μμg/ml. in 1959.
B.J.	55	1-4-56	0.5	0.05	0	17.5		75% g.r., B II for d.u. in 1956.
K.A.	35	6-26-56	0.5	0.07	0	22.2		80% g.r., B II for d.u. in 1948.
H.W.	55	12-7-55	0.5	0.07	0	24.0		75% g.r., B II for d.u. in 1947.
F.M.	57	8-26-57	0.5	0.07	0	24.2		g.r., B II for d.u. in 1948.
F.H.	63	9-23-57	0.5	0.07	0	26.8		g.r., B II for carcinoma of stomach in 1947. g.r. in 1948.
O.F.	70	12-16-58	0.5	0.07	0	26.5		g.r., B I for d.u. in 1956.
R.A.	64	4-25-59	0.5	0.07	0	27.2		50% g.r. for d.u. in 1943.
D.S.	44	2-14-58	0.5	0.07	0			g.r., B II for d.u. in 1951.
R.M.	49	3-11-58	0.5	0.07	0			
J.S.	55	2-26-58	0.5	0.07	0			

d.u. = duodenal ulcer.
g.r. = gastric resection.
g.u. = gastric ulcer.

B I = Billroth I anastomosis.
B II = Billroth II anastomosis.

was admitted with active pulmonary tuberculosis and a hemoglobin of 9.8 grams per 100 ml. of blood in 1954. Bone marrow examination showed a megaloblastic anemia in partial remission. There was no definite reticulocyte response or improvement in the hemoglobin values with parenteral vitamin B$_{12}$ treatment or a subsequent course of folic acid therapy. M.M. was subjected to a 75 per cent gastric resection for duodenal ulcer in 1949. He was admitted with a hemoglobin of 11.6 grams per 100 ml. of blood in 1954. Bone marrow at that time was megaloblastic. Parenteral vitamin B$_{12}$ therapy was followed by a satisfactory response in reticulocyte count and hemoglobin.

Subject J.W. had undergone a 75 per cent gastric resection for gastric and duodenal ulcers in 1944. He was admitted with a macrocytic anemia, a hemoglobin of 12.2 grams per 100 ml. of blood, and a subacute combined degeneration of the spinal cord in 1954. Bone marrow examination at that time revealed a normoblastic anemia, although it should be mentioned that he had taken brewer's yeast daily for one week before this examination was performed. There was no response in the neurological picture, reticulocyte count, or the hemoglobin upon treatment with vitamin B$_{12}$ parenterally. Patient C.H. was admitted with a carcinoma of the stomach with a secondary hypochromic microcytic anemia in 1957. Free hydrochloric acid was present in the gastric juice. Evidence of posterior column disease was present, possibly related to an old luetic infection. A 90 per cent gastric resection was performed and chemotherapy was given (68 mg. of triethylene thiophosphoramide in divided doses). Five months later he was found to have a macrocytic anemia with a hypoplasia of the bone marrow, probably related to the chemotherapy for cancer. Patient A.H. had undergone a gastric resection for carcinoma of the stomach in 1956. In 1960 while being treated for a traumatic fracture he developed a macrocytic anemia with a hemoglobin of 8.9 grams per 100 ml. of blood. There was no bone marrow examination, but the serum concentration of vitamin B$_{12}$ was found to be 41 $\mu\mu$g/ml. at that time. Parenteral vitamin B$_{12}$ treatment resulted in a satisfactory response in reticulocyte count and hemoglobin. Subject B.J. had an 80 per cent gastric resection for gastric ulcer in 1947. He was admitted with active pulmonary tuberculosis in 1955. While on chemotherapy for this disease he developed a megaloblastic anemia with a hemoglobin of 10.8 grams per 100 ml. of blood. Vitamin B$_{12}$ absorption was within the normal range. There was a maximum reticulocyte response of 4.6 per cent three days after the administration of the parenteral test dose of vitamin B$_{12}$ used in the Schilling test. Without further therapy, the hemoglobin rose gradually and reached a normal level 8 months later. This patient was an alcoholic with evidence of cirrhosis of the liver and intestinal malabsorption. He was believed to suffer from multiple deficiencies due to his malabsorption syndrome.

From these observations it is evident that an occasional patient with partial gastric resection will show an abnormally low absorption of cyanocobalamin, low serum vitamin B_{12} level, as well as macrocytic anemia responding to vitamin B_{12} therapy. It is also evident that some patients have low absorption values and low serum vitamin B_{12} concentrations without signs of macrocytic anemia. If a low serum vitamin B_{12} level is accepted as an index of the body's store of cyanocobalamin, these patients are deficient in this vitamin, but their deficiency is on a subclinical level. Whether they will develop overt megaloblastic anemia without proper therapy cannot be stated at this time, but this possibility should always be kept in mind. The typical megaloblastic anemia of vitamin B_{12} deficiency does not develop until vitamin B_{12} concentration has fallen to a level below 90 to 120 $\mu\mu g$ of cyanocobalamin per ml. of serum (443, 443B). In some patients with low serum vitamin B_{12} levels the blood picture may, however, be normal or almost normal for periods of at least one to two years (443). Thus, subclinical vitamin B_{12} deficiency may exist for a long period of time before overt megaloblastosis is recognized. Mild pernicious anemia, very difficult to diagnose, has been reported to be present for at least six years before the condition was recognized (435). It is important to recognize subclinical deficiency of vitamin B_{12} (481) because sometimes damage to the nervous system may occur with no or little change in the blood picture (9, 301, 443). All patients with gastric resection having low absorption of cyanocobalamin and low concentrations of serum vitamin B_{12} should be treated with parenteral vitamin B_{12} in a manner similar to those having pernicious anemia or total gastrectomy. Patients with low absorption values and borderline or normal serum B_{12} concentrations should be followed with serum B_{12} determinations as well as clinically. If it is impossible to obtain serum determinations, less harm is done to the patients by giving them vitamin B_{12} parenterally than to wait for clinical deficiency to develop.

Results in Patients with Histamine-Fast Achlorhydria

Fourteen combined urinary and fecal excretion tests were performed on eleven patients with various diseases (Table 19). All of them had histamine-fast achlorhydria. In the first ten patients the urinary radioactivity was within the normal range and in only one of them was the fecal radioactivity above 50 per cent. One subject, F.S., is of special interest. He showed a high fecal and no urinary radioactivity on one occasion, indicating inability to absorb cyanocobalamin. When IFC

Table 19. Fecal and/or Urinary 24-Hour Radioactivity in Patients with Histamine-Fast Achlorhydria after Oral Dose of 0.1–0.5 μg B_{12} Containing 0.02–0.08 μc Co^{60}, with 1 mg. "Cold" B_{12} Given Intramuscularly 2 Hours after Oral Dose

Patient	Age	Date of Examination	Dose of $Co^{60}B_{12}$ μg	μc	Diagnosis	Radioactivity, % of Oral Dose Feces	Urine
R.S. 55		7-1-54	0.5	0.02	Hodgkin's disease	27.1	11.7
G.P. 61		9-28-54	0.5	0.02	Laennec's cirrhosis	36.0	26.2
C.B. 59		8-12-54	0.5	0.02	osteoporosis	26.3	24.1
J.B. 58		3-31-54	0.5	0.02	cholelithiasis	31.9	12.0
H.G. 63		8-5-54	0.1	0.02	multiple sclerosis	38.1	24.7
L.F. 63		3-27-54	0.5	0.02	cholelithiasis	27.7	22.3
G.L. 73		3-31-54	0.5	0.02	osteitis deformans	22.8	23.6
G.L. 73		8-19-54	0.5	0.02	osteitis deformans	27.2	19.6
R.S. 60		10-14-54	0.5	0.02	diarrhea	25.4	20.1
A.S. 57		4-16-54	0.5	0.02	peripheral neuritis	71.3	15.5
J.W. 67		7-8-54	0.1	0.02	pulmonary emphysema	27.8	30.8
F.S. 60		7-24-54	0.5	0.02	cancer of pancreas	93.7	0
F.S. 60		8-3-54	0.5	0.02	cancer of pancreas	60.0	10.6*
F.S. 60		8-11-54	0.5	0.02	cancer of pancreas	54.3	9.3
M.E. 53		9-9-55	0.5	0.02	peripheral neuritis		31.1
T.M. 46		2-14-56	0.5	0.06	pneumonia, diabetes		12.2
E.L. 62		12-13-56	0.5	0.07	cholelithiasis		27.2
W.M. 44		3-16-54	0.5	0.02	fractured femur		20.8
A.O. 66		7-2-56	0.5	0.07	polyposis of colon		27.3
E.T. 73		7-27-56	0.5	0.07	tuberculosis		21.4
C.H. 64		9-8-55	0.5	0.08	peripheral neuritis		23.7
Average †							20.2
Range							0–31.1

* With 1 USP unit intrinsic factor concentrate.
† Excluding test with IFC.

was supplied, the radioactivity measurements revealed great improvement in the absorption of this vitamin. It would be tempting to regard this patient as being deficient in intrinsic-factor production; but when the study was repeated without IFC, both the fecal and the urinary excretion tests showed that absorption of vitamin B_{12} did occur, although probably in a subnormal range. The most likely explanation for the varying absorption of cyanocobalamin in the absence of any source of exogenous intrinsic factor is that the endogenous secretion of this factor varied from time to time. Another, but less likely, explanation is that he had intermittent intestinal malfunction which on occasion interfered with the absorption of vitamin B_{12}. The urinary excretion of radioactivity in the twenty tests performed without the addition of IFC ranged from 0 to 31.1 per cent, with an average of 20.2 per cent, of the oral test dose. This latter figure is slightly below the corresponding value observed in the control series in Table 7.

The findings in these patients are much in agreement with previous reports (379, 559, 560), which all show that most patients with histamine-fast achlorhydria have a normal vitamin B_{12} absorption and, presumably, intrinsic-factor production. It is to be expected that a few patients will be found with impaired absorption in this group (349, 379, 482, 501, 560), since many of them will have a varying degree of gastritis, which so often is associated with lowered vitamin B_{12} absorption (586, 586A). Some of the subjects with gastric achlorhydria may indeed be suffering from latent pernicious anemia with a relative vitamin B_{12} deficiency (482). If not treated, they may develop overt pernicious anemia as soon as their body stores of the vitamin have become completely depleted.

Results in Patients with Posterolateral Column Disease of the Spinal Cord

The urinary excretion test was performed in eleven subjects with posterolateral column disease (Table 20). Vitamin B_{12} deficiency was considered at one time or another a possible etiologic factor in the development of the disease. Anemia was, however, not a major problem in any of them. The absorption of cyanocobalamin was abnormally low in three of the patients, reverting to normal or nearly normal with the addition of IFC. In the other eight the absorption values were in the normal range. The first three subjects in this series were regarded as having Addison's pernicious anemia. With vitamin B_{12} therapy only one subject (J.M.), who had had the disease for a short time, improved. It is well known that subacute combined degeneration of the spinal cord can exist in pernicious anemia in the absence of overt anemia (9, 25, 121, 288, 332, 346, 551A, 639). While this is true especially for patients brought into hematologic remission with folic acid therapy (121, 288, 551A, 653), it can be seen even in the absence of such treatment (25, 346). It is apparent then that in some instances, for unknown reasons, the central nervous system is more sensitive to the deficiency of vitamin B_{12} than the blood-forming organ (653). One of our patients had taken

Table 20. 24-Hour Urinary Radioactivity in Patients with Posterolateral Column Disease of the Spinal Cord after Oral Dose of $Co^{60}B_{12}$, with 1 mg. "Cold" B_{12} Given Intramuscularly 2 Hours after Oral Dose

Patient	Age	Date of Examination	Dose of $Co^{60}B_{12}$		IFC Unit	Radioactivity, % of Oral Dose		Comments
			μg	μc		Without IFC	With IFC	
M.L.	54	5-18-60	0.5	0.07	0	0		s.c.d. for 3 years. Normal hgb. Serum B_{12} 16 μμg/ml. No appreciable response to B_{12} administered parenterally.
M.L.	54	5-23-60	0.5	0.07	1		9.5	
J.M.	65	3-4-55	0.5	0.02	0	0		s.c.d. for a few weeks time. Normal hgb.
J.M.	65	3-31-55	0.5	0.02	1		16.6	Good response to parenteral B_{12} therapy.
O.H.	67	9-2-59	0.5	0.07	0	4.4		s.c.d. for 10 years. Normal hgb. No appreciable response to parenteral B_{12} therapy.
O.H.	67	9-10-59	0.5	0.07	1		20.8	
J.T.	47	10-29-58	0.5	0.07	0	12.7		degenerative disease of the nervous system, cause unknown
W.N.	48	10-22-58	0.5	0.07	0	15.4		multiple sclerosis
P.B.	64	10-8-58	0.56	0.5	0	18.0		myeloneuropathy, alcoholism
F.B.	60	5-11-59	0.5	0.05	0	19.0		spastic paraparesis
J.S.	69	9-24-59	0.5	0.07	0	19.6		myeloneuropathy, herniated cervical disc
U.S.	65	12-23-57	0.5	0.07	0	20.0		s.c.d. of unknown etiology
J.K.	70	10-29-58	0.5	0.07	0	23.0		taboparesis, Guillain-Barré syndrome
G.C.	44	4-16-58	0.5	0.07	0	25.0		multiple sclerosis, chronic brain syndrome

s.c.d. = subacute combined degeneration of the spinal cord.

vitamin capsules containing folic acid before entering the hospital, which may explain why his anemia was not overt.

The normal urinary excretion tests in eight of the subjects ruled out malabsorption of cyanocobalamin. Because of their dietary histories, lack of response to vitamin B_{12}, and subsequent clinical findings, they were not believed to have vitamin B_{12} deficiency. It should be remembered, though, that normal vitamin B_{12} absorption in itself doesn't rule out vitamin B_{12} deficiency. In fact, subacute combined degeneration of the spinal cord with low serum vitamin B_{12} concentration and good response to vitamin B_{12} therapy have been observed in dietary vitamin B_{12} deficiency (12). Vegetarians may conceivably ingest so much folic acid in their diet that a megaloblastic anemia caused by vitamin B_{12} deficiency will be masked, at least for some time, while the nervous system may be the first to show overt signs of the deficiency. Although pure nutritional vitamin B_{12} deficiency is very rare, attention should nevertheless be paid to the nutritional history in any obscure case of posterolateral column disease as well as to the serum level of cyanocobalamin, and the vitamin B_{12} absorption test.

Results in Patients with Faber's Pernicious Anemia

In 1893 Knud Faber observed a 27-year-old woman who suffered and subsequently died from pernicious anemia. This patient had clinical signs of incomplete small bowel obstruction and at postmortem examination was found to have two strictures of the small intestine with stasis of the bowel contents above (182A, 182B). Faber expressed the opinion that there was a connection between the development of pernicious anemia and the diseased bowel in this patient. He thought that the stasis of the bowel contents above the strictures might have led to the formation of bacterial toxins which were absorbed and destroyed the red blood cells. In the subsequent years many papers confirmed the existence of pernicious anemia in patients with various intestinal diseases such as strictures, anastomoses, and blind loops of the small bowel. Several excellent reviews on the subject have appeared (11, 23, 88, 271, 331, 399, 645). Whereas a connection between the stomach and pernicious anemia was suggested by Fenwick's work (194, 195), the observations of Faber and others indicated that the intestine rather than the stomach, at least in some cases, might be responsible for the development of the anemia. Faber's work did not in any way refute the observations of Fenwick, but it added new information and clearly showed that pernicious anemia could occur in association with a diseased bowel. The observed cases of intestinal pernicious anemia, pernicious tapeworm anemia (554), and the results from animal experimentation (572, 573) lent support to the old Hunterian theory (322, 367) of intestinal disease with intestinal autointoxication as the cause of Addison's pernicious anemia. Enterostomy with intestinal lavage was even proposed and tried in order to relieve patients with Addison's pernicious anemia of the presumed intoxication (147, 570–572). The theory of intestinal autointoxication in pernicious anemia lost ground after the discovery of the extrinsic and the intrinsic factors of Castle. Papers on the subject of intestinal pernicious anemia did, however, continue to appear also after 1929 (23, 67, 79, 88, 136, 271, 284, 458, 491, 499, 530, 531, 556, 562, 585, 607, 620, 638), and it became evident that lack of intrinsic factor was not always the cause of pernicious anemia (147A, 562, 596, 638). Measurement of serum concentration of vitamin B$_{12}$ (412) has shown that subjects with chronic intestinal diseases which often lead to intestinal pernicious anemia may have a deficiency of vitamin B$_{12}$ comparable to that found in patients with Addison's pernicious anemia. Absorption studies with radio-labeled cyanocobalamin have helped to clarify the pathogenic mechanism responsible for the development of the vitamin deficiency in subjects with intestinal pernicious anemia. In deference to a most outstanding physician, gastroenterologist, medical teacher, and clinical investigator, the term Faber's pernicious anemia is used in this chapter for the macrocytic, megaloblastic, vitamin B$_{12}$–responsive anemia that develops secondary to a diseased bowel.

There is a controversy regarding the use of the name pernicious anemia (55, 267, 301, 504). In the Anglo-American literature the name is used synonymously with the term Addison's pernicious anemia. In other countries pernicious anemia is given a wider interpretation and corresponds to what are today recognized as pure vitamin B$_{12}$–deficiency states. This latter concept seems to be historically more correct (55) and modern American writers have also used the term in this wider sense (368, 504). As far back as 1887, Lichtheim was aware that "pernicious anemia is not an etiological entity, but a syndrome which may be due to variety of etiologic factors" (55), and Knud Faber in 1895 talked about the genuine pernicious anemia (that is, the Addisonian type) as opposed to the pernicious tapeworm anemia and the pernicious anemia associated with intestinal disease (182A). Faber emphasized the similarity in the clinical picture in these conditions and from his work one has the impression that he was searching for a common denominator for them all. It was not until 1948, however, that such a denominator, vitamin B$_{12}$, was discovered. It is also a fact that is so frequently overlooked that the first type of pernicious anemia to be cured was that seen in patients with fish tapeworm (554). The cure was very simple: expulsion of the worm. Furthermore, it should be remembered that a cure for the intestinal pernicious anemia was observed in 1924 (573) — that is, before Minot and Murphy made their famous discovery of the beneficial effect of liver treatment in Addison's pernicious anemia (429). The last few years have taught us a little about the great role the intestine plays in the development of vitamin B_{12} deficiency and pernicious anemia; it has become clear that for a number of years we have placed too much emphasis upon the role of the stomach in the development of this disease, just as some older clinicians especially on the European continent perhaps put too much emphasis upon the intestine (322, 368, 396, 397, 571, 573). From the standpoint of therapy there is one more good reason why the anemias caused by vitamin B_{12} deficiency all should be labeled "pernicious." It might conceivably happen that folic acid therapy, instead of vitamin B_{12}, might be administered to patients with Faber's pernicious anemia if the disease was given the more "neutral" term intestinal megaloblastic anemia. Such a calamity is unthinkable if the term intestinal pernicious anemia or Faber's pernicious anemia is adopted, because of the universally accepted knowledge that vitamin B_{12} is the correct therapy for pernicious anemia.

Five patients with the Faberian type of pernicious anemia have been examined (Table 21); all had anatomical lesions of the small intestine with stasis of the bowel contents. A brief summary of the case histories will be given since most of them created problems in diagnosis and therapy when they were first seen.

J.R. was a 32-year-old male who developed megaloblastic anemia in 1952 with a hemoglobin of 7.5 grams per 100 ml. of blood.* A diagnosis of regional ileitis was made in 1943. Because of failure to improve on medical therapy, ileocolostomy was performed in April 1944 and in August of the same year a surgical closure of the ileal loop distal to the anastomosis was undertaken. Barium enema revealed an ileocolostomy just distal to the hepatic flexure with well-functioning stoma. The terminal ileum was constricted and had the appearance of regional ileitis. Just distal to the anastomosis there was a blind loop of small intestine filled with contrast material. Gastric acidity was normal. A three-week trial with vitamin C therapy given parenterally resulted in a maximum reticulocyte response of 13.6 per cent and an improvement in hemoglobin to 11.2 grams per 100 ml. of blood. Bone marrow was, however, still megaloblastic. One week's trial with oral vitamin B_{12} treatment, 90 μg per day, had no effect on the reticulocyte count or the hemoglobin, but subsequent parenteral injections of vitamin B_{12} led to a

* An abstract about this case by Doscherholmen and Hagen appeared in J. Lab. Clin. Med., 44:790, 1954, published by the C. V. Mosby Company, St. Louis (157).

Table 21. Fecal and/or 24-Hour Urinary Radioactivity in Patients with Intestinal (Faber's) Pernicious Anemia after Oral Dose of $Co^{60}B_{12}$ with 1 mg. "Cold" B_{12} Administered Intramuscularly 2 Hours after Oral Dose (in all patients the anemia responded satisfactorily to parenteral B_{12} therapy)

Patient	Age	Date of Examination	Dose of $Co^{60}B_{12}$ μg	μc	Diagnosis	IFC Units	Radioactivity, % of Oral Dose			
							Without IFC Feces	Urine	With IFC Feces	Urine
J.R.	34	3-16-54	0.5	0.02	regional ileitis,	0	80.5	0		
J.R.	34	3-22-54	0.5	0.02	ileocolostomy, blind	1			84.8	0
J.R.	34	3-31-54	0.5	0.02	loop	3			100.2	0
J.R.	34	4-19-54	0.5	0.02		1			103.3*	0*
W.M.	30	2-12-55	0.5	0.02	regional ileitis, small	0	84.1	0		
W.M.	30	2-26-55	0.5	0.02	bowel resection, jejunocolostomy, dilated loops of small bowel	3			88.8	0
A.U.	35	1-12-55	0.5	0.02	regional ileitis, ileocolostomy	0	93.9	0		
A.U.	35	2-19-55	0.5	0.02		1			100.6	0
J.D.	34	7-8-58	0.56	0.25	regional ileitis, small	0		0.9		
J.D.	34	7-25-58	0.56	0.25	bowel resection, stric-	1				0.6
J.D.	34	7-29-58	0.56	0.25	tures, and ileocolostomy,	0		0.5*		
E.T.	70	4-4-57	0.56	0.05	small bowel diverticula,	0		2.1		
E.T.	70	4-10-57	0.56	0.05	steatorrhea	0.75				6.2
E.T.	70	5-6-57	0.56	0.05		0		15.9†		

* Pretreatment with neomycin.
† Pretreatment with Achromycin.

74

maximum reticulocyte response of 5.8 per cent and to a complete hematologic remission. On maintenance therapy with parenteral vitamin B_{12} his hemoglobin was found to be 15.9 grams per cent in 1954. Vitamin B_{12} absorption studies employing the urinary and fecal excretion methods at that time revealed no absorption of cyanocobalamin even after the addition of a potent source of intrinsic factor. Pretreatment with neomycin, 2 grams daily for four days, did not improve the absorption of the vitamin. While he was in complete remission his serum concentration of cyanocobalamin was found to be 341 $\mu\mu$g per ml.

W.M. was a 25-year-old male who developed a severe anemia in 1950 with a hemoglobin of 5.2 grams per 100 ml. of blood. After a long illness, regional ileitis was diagnosed in 1946 and an enteroanastomosis was performed. Later in the same year resection of part of the small bowel was undertaken. His bone marrow was megaloblastic. Gastric acidity was normal. X-ray examination of the gastrointestinal tract showed moderately dilated loops of the small intestine. The nutritional status was poor and peripheral edema was present. Folic acid therapy, 15 mg. q.i.d., was followed by a peak reticulocyte count of 15.2 per cent eight days after the initiation of treatment. Several injections of cyanocobalamin were then given without any definite secondary reticulocyte response being observed. Iron therapy was added because hypochromasia of the red blood cells was also present. His hemoglobin rose gradually to normal values. He was maintained on folic acid treatment (20 mg. daily) until his hemoglobin started to decrease in the latter part of 1952. Despite increase in the intake of folic acid to 30 and later 40 mg. daily, his hemoglobin continued to decline until a value of 10.2 grams per cent was reached in March 1953. Bone marrow at this time was again megaloblastic. No neurological signs were present. Folic acid treatment was discontinued and large doses of vitamin B_{12} were given parenterally. A maximum reticulocyte response of 8.4 per cent was noted. A course of intravenous iron was also administered because a hypochromic anemia was present as well. His hemoglobin has since been maintained at a normal level on parenteral vitamin B_{12} and oral iron therapy. Vitamin B_{12} absorption studies in 1955 revealed no absorption of cyanocobalamin even after the addition of IFC (Table 21). While in complete hematologic remission his serum concentration of vitamin B_{12} was 430 $\mu\mu$g/ml.

A.U. was a 30-year-old male who was found to have a severe megaloblastic anemia and a hemoglobin of 4.7 grams per 100 ml. of blood in April 1950. He had developed terminal ileitis in 1935 and had resection of the last two feet of ileum together with the first part of the colon. He was completely well for seven years before he was noted to have recurrence of the disease. In 1949 he developed abscess formation with a fistula in the lower right quadrant. In March 1950 at laparotomy he was found to have extensive regional ileitis with skip areas in between and with markedly dilated and thickened terminal ileum. An ileotransverse colostomy was performed. Three weeks later he was found to have a severe dimorphic anemia. Gastric acidity was normal. Ankle reflexes were absent and the vibration sense was questionably reduced in the lower extremities. He was treated for one week with 60 μg vitamin B_{12} orally daily without any response in reticulocyte counts or hemoglobin. Folic acid therapy, 30 mg. daily, was then instituted and the reticulocyte count rose to a maximum of 46.8 per cent on the eighth day of treatment. On this therapy his hemoglobin rose to 11.7 grams per cent. His hypochromic anemia was treated with iron tablets given orally. A fulminating posterior column degeneration of the spinal cord developed within two months after the institution of the folic acid therapy. This drug was therefore discontinued and vitamin B_{12} and crude liver extract were given intramuscularly daily. Signs and symptoms of the nervous complication disappeared almost completely within four weeks. He has since been maintained in neurologic and hematologic remission on parenteral vitamin B_{12} and liver extract and an occasional course of iron therapy for iron deficiency. His vitamin B_{12} absorption was investigated in 1955 and it was discovered that he was unable to absorb cyanocobalamin from the gastrointestinal tract even in the presence of a potent intrinsic factor (Table 21). While he was in complete remission his serum concentration of cyanocobalamin was 125 $\mu\mu$g/ml.

J.D. was a 34-year-old male who was found to have a macrocytic anemia with a hemoglobin of 9.7 grams per 100 ml. of blood in 1958. He had had periods of crampy abdominal pains since 1944. A diagnosis of regional ileitis was made by X-ray examination in 1956. Medical therapy was unsuccessful and in 1957 resection of the distal four and a half feet of ileum and the first half foot of colon was performed with an end-to-end anastomosis. He developed diarrhea with frequent watery stools after the operation and within nine months X-ray examination showed recurrent regional ileitis with skip areas in the terminal ileum and mild obstruction. His bone marrow was found to be megaloblastic and the serum concentration of vitamin B_{12} was 58 $\mu\mu$g/ml. Gastric juice contained a normal amount of hydrochloric acid. He received vitamin B_{12} parenterally and showed a maximum reticulocyte response of 14.0 per cent. His hemoglobin subsequently rose to normal levels. The Schilling test showed urinary excretion of radioactivity in the range usually found in patients with Addison's pernicious anemia, but no improvement of the absorption value was noted after the addition of IFC

(Table 21). Pretreatment with 8 grams of neomycin given in divided doses over a 24-hour period likewise had no effect on the absorption of cyanocobalamin. While he was in complete remission his serum vitamin B_{12} concentration was 117 $\mu\mu g/ml$.

E.T. was a 67-year-old male who was studied for anemia in 1954. He had noted swelling of the legs for about six weeks and had had diarrhea alternating with constipation for twenty-five or thirty years. He was found to have a macrocytic anemia with hemoglobin of 6.6 grams per cent and a megaloblastic bone marrow. There was histamine-fast achlorhydria. X-ray examination showed multiple small bowel diverticula. Treatment with parenteral vitamin B_{12} brought about a complete hematologic remission, which has been maintained with vitamin B_{12} injections. He was readmitted for his diarrhea in 1957, and examination revealed steatorrhea. He was treated with Achromycin orally and his diarrhea improved greatly while this drug was being administered, but recurrence was noted shortly after the drug was discontinued. Subsequently separate courses of sulfaguanidine and neomycin were given with no effect on the diarrhea. A course of diiodohydroxyquin, 650 mg. t.i.d., was followed by cessation of diarrhea within 24 hours. When the drug was discontinued after a short course of therapy the diarrhea recurred within 36 hours. With reinstatement of the diiodohydroxyquin therapy, prompt cessation of the diarrhea was again noted. A 5-week course of this drug was then given. During and after this course of treatment he passed one solid stool daily. His weight increased nineteen pounds and he felt better and stronger than previously. After the drug was discontinued there was an interval of several months before a mild diarrhea recurred. His weight has, however, been maintained. In 1957 vitamin B_{12} absorption was studied (Table 21). Without intrinsic factor the urinary excretion of radioactivity in the Schilling test was found to be in the range observed in patients with pernicious anemia. After the addition of a potent source of intrinsic factor a slight increase in the excretion value was noted. After pretreatment with Achromycin the Schilling test was within the normal range without any intrinsic factor being administered. This finding showed that the endogenous production of intrinsic factor was intact. While he was in complete remission his serum vitamin B_{12} concentration was 194 $\mu\mu g/ml$.

These five patients are believed to have suffered from overt vitamin B_{12} deficiency at the time of their megaloblastic anemia. In subject J.D., serum vitamin B_{12} was, in fact, measured and found to be below normal before the therapy was started. The other patients had no determination of their serum cyanocobalamin activity before therapy and while being treated with parenteral vitamin B_{12} they all exhibited serum concentrations of this vitamin in the normal or borderline normal range, which also is the usual finding in patients with Addison's pernicious anemia on parenteral treatment (442A). Two of the patients were originally believed to have nutritional megaloblastic anemia but treatment with folic acid was unsuccessful because of the rapid appearance of posterior column disease in one (A.U.) and the development of megaloblastic anemia after a temporary remission in the other (W.M.). They both showed excellent response to parenteral vitamin B_{12} therapy, indicating the true nature of their deficiency. The development of neurological signs and symptoms in patients with pernicious anemia treated with folic acid is by now a well-known phenomenon (288, 551A, 640, 653). The fact that folic acid in pharmacologic but not in physiologic amounts (387) can bring about a complete hematologic remission in pernicious anemia is also well known. These remissions are often just temporary (653), as exemplified by subject W.M. It is not known why subject A.U. so rapidly developed posterior column disease on folic acid therapy while patient W.M. was treated with this drug for two and a half years and then went into hematologic relapse without any neurological signs being present. Such a difference in the response to folic acid in pernicious anemia is, however, a familiar phenomenon (653). Patient E.T. was, on clinical grounds, first believed to have Addison's pernicious anemia, but the diagnosis was altered on the second admission. By this time the syndrome of multiple small bowel diverticula, megaloblastic anemia, and steatorrhea had become well known (13, 14, 47, 146, 205, 271, 354, 489, 596, 628, 652) and our patient was found to belong to this group. The results of the vitamin B_{12} absorption studies clearly showed that his endogenous intrinsic factor production was intact despite his histamine-fast achlorhydria. However, to prove this point the absorption of cyanocobalamin had to be carried out after oral pretreatment with Achromycin (tetracycline).

The fact that parenteral but not oral B_{12} therapy was effective in subjects J.R. and A.U. indicated defective absorption of cyanocobalamin, later confirmed by the combined urinary and fecal excretion methods. Patient J.R. was treated correctly from the first time he was seen with his megaloblastic anemia; folic acid was never administered to him. The partial response to ascorbic acid noted in this patient is of great interest, since similar response has been observed previously in Addison's pernicious anemia (456). There was no dietary deficiency in patient J.R. and no overt signs of vitamin C deficiency. Because complete conversion of the megaloblastic anemia did not take place, it is apparent that vitamin C deficiency was not the primary defect in this patient. Vitamin C augments the production of folinic acid from folic acid (460), and since folinic acid is believed to be the more active substance in the body, it is possible that through some mass action of vitamin C more folinic acid was made available in the organism. The mechanism of the action of vitamin C may, however, be more complex (456).

The reason for the vitamin B_{12} deficiency in patients with Faber's pernicious anemia is apparently a defect in the absorption of cyanocobalamin (157, 200, 271, 392, 436, 485, 568). In contrast to what is seen in Addison's pernicious anemia, this defect is not corrected by the addition of intrinsic factor (157, 200, 271, 392, 436, 485, 568). The lack of response to heterologous intrinsic factor was not caused by acquired resistance to this factor, because none of our patients had ever been in contact with hog-stomach intrinsic factor preparations before the absorption tests were performed. The gastric juice in Faber's pernicious anemia has been found to contain intrinsic factor by bioassay technique (94, 147A, 457, 562, 596, 638), and the absorption of radiocyanocobalamin may return to normal when the gut is sterilized with a broad-spectrum antibiotic of the tetracycline group (271, 392, 436, 485, 568), but not with neomycin (147A, 157, 271) or chloramphenicol (147A), indicating adequate secretion of intrinsic factor. It is not clear why there should be such a difference between these antibiotics (271). Certainly neomycin is a very effective drug for the sterilization of the intestine; but this drug is in itself capable of inducing gastrointestinal malabsorption including that of vitamin B_{12} (328, 329) and maybe this phenomenon is connected with the inability of neomycin to restore the absorption of vitamin B_{12} to normal in these instances. It is also quite possible that the action of the tetracycline-type drugs is more complex and not only due to the sterilization of the gut. Thus, it should be noted that sulfisoxazole and chloramphenicol, which also are quite effective against gram negative bacteria, likewise both failed to restore the absorption of cyanocobalamin to normal in patients with Faber's pernicious anemia (147A, 271).

Achromycin but not sulfaguanidine or neomycin led to improvement in the diarrhea of patient E.T. The use of diiodohydroxyquin was suggested by Dr. R. D. Woodson, because of its beneficial effect in amoebic dysentery. A striking improvement in the diarrhea and the general nutritional status of the patient ensued. After a prolonged course the effect lasted for several months. There was no evidence of amoebic dysentery and the effect must be explained in some other way. It will be interesting to see whether the dramatic benefit exhibited by this one patient can be duplicated in other subjects with similar afflictions.

In this chapter the term Faber's pernicious anemia has been used in its widest sense to mean a malady that develops secondary to intestinal disease ("som följe av tarmlidelse"– 182A). It might be argued that only those patients with an intact intestine showing stasis of the small bowel contents should be included, since Faber's case had strictures with stasis of the bowel content. This would then exclude certain patients with small bowel disease, primarily those with resection and by-passing of the ileum. It is not clear why inability to absorb vitamin B_{12} develops in patients with Faber's pernicious anemia. It has been suggested, among other things, that stasis of the intestinal contents gives rise to a fecal flora and that the bacteria may compete with the organism for the available cyanocobalamin (11, 271, 645) in the same way as a fish tapeworm lodged in the small intestine will (55, 56, 58, 65). Such an explanation seems logical because coliform bacteria (76, 137A, 142, 209, 330) as well as bacteria obtained from stagnant small intestinal loops (147A) have the ability to take up vitamin B_{12} from a solution. Experiments on animals with surgically induced strictures of the small intestine (572, 573) or blind loops (89, 319, 320, 518, 553, 622–625, 645) point toward the stasis as a very important factor in the development of the anemia. Although the exact mechanism whereby the intestinal stasis prevents the absorption of vitamin B_{12} is unknown (271), removal of the stasis by surgical intervention may result in normal absorption of vitamin B_{12} (147A) and permanent cure of Faber's pernicious anemia in humans (7, 573, 643, 652) as well as cure of the anemia that develops in animals after the creation of intestinal blind loops (320, 623). Since broad-spectrum antibiotics can improve the absorption of vitamin B_{12} in patients with Faber's pernicious anemia it was to be expected that they also will induce hematologic remissions in patients with this disease, and such is also the case (198, 457, 585). The anemia in animals with artificially created small intestinal stasis may not necessarily be identical with Faber's pernicious anemia in humans (11). Thus, it has been pointed out that although the anemia often was macrocytic and hyperchromic it was impossible to demonstrate unequivocal megaloblastic changes in the bone marrow of the experimental animals in contrast to the usual findings in patients with Faber's pernicious anemia (11). Despite this, the link between the experimental anemia in animals and the disease in man is close, and it is generally believed that bacterial invasion of the upper bowel can explain most, if not all, of the manifestations of the blind-loop syndrome (11). Another factor to be considered in certain operated cases is the bypass of or surgical excision of ileum, the most important site for the absorption of vitamin B_{12} (61). The fact that the anemia in experimental animals can be alleviated (645) or prevented (625) by broad-spectrum antibiotics as in man (198, 457, 585) strengthens the hypothesis that bacterial invasion of the small bowel is responsible for the anemia in the blind-loop syndrome. Vitamin B_{12} is usually (11, 271) but not invariably (209) curative in the anemia of the blind-loop syndrome in man. Likewise, liver extract or vitamin B_{12} may (318) or may not (645) be of great value in the anemia of animals with artificially created intestinal blind loops. Therapy with folic acid may produce excellent results in the experimental anemia in animals (645) and in the disease in man (11). In recent years there has, therefore, been a tendency to regard the intestinal megaloblastic anemia as being due primarily to a deficiency of folic acid rather than to a lack of vitamin B_{12} (11). This opinion may not be correct. In the blind-loop syndrome multiple deficiencies may frequently be present (11). In our own experience, deficiency of vitamin B_{12} seemed to be the single etiologic factor responsible for the development of the megaloblastic anemia. If the metabolism of cyanocobalamin cannot be adequately studied in patients with the blind-loop syndrome, parenteral vitamin B_{12} therapy should always be included in the routine treatment of these cases. Otherwise disastrous results may ensue in the subjects who are primarily deficient in cyanocobalamin.

Results in Patients with Various Intestinal Diseases: Regional Ileitis, Non-Tropical Sprue, and Secondary Steatorrhea

Two subjects with regional ileitis were examined with the Schilling test (Table 22). One had a normal, the other an impaired absorption of cyanocobalamin. The latter showed no improvement in the absorption figure after the addition of IFC. This patient, E.F., also suffered from steatorrhea. He had a serum vitamin B_{12} concentration of 263 $\mu\mu g/ml.$, indicating that, although his absorption of cyanocobalamin was abnormally low, he still had not exhausted his body stores of this vitamin. Apparently not all patients with regional ileitis are unable to absorb vitamin B_{12} (200), although sooner or later they may show this defect in the gastrointestinal function (157, 214, 354, 436) and some may even develop megaloblastic anemia (79, 436, 499). They may then often be found to have strictures, anastomoses, or blind loops of the small intestine or secondary steatorrhea. When serum vitamin B_{12} determinations are carried out in patients with regional ileitis low values are frequently observed (123, 412). Low absorption values may be restored to normal by steroid therapy (123) or antibiotic therapy (436).

Three patients with idiopathic steatorrhea were examined with the urinary excretion test. One of them, L.P., showed an abnormally low urinary excretion value with submaximal response to IFC. One pa-

Table 22. 24-Hour Radioactivity in Patients with Intestinal Disease, Primary and Secondary Steatorrhea, after Oral Dose of $Co^{60}B_{12}$, with 1 mg. "Cold" B_{12} Given Intramuscularly 2 Hours after Oral Dose

Patient	Age	Date of Examination	Dose of $Co^{60}B_{12}$ μg	μc	IFC Unit	Diagnosis	Urinary Radioactivity, % of Oral Dose Without IFC	With IFC
C.K.	23	10-3-56	0.56	0.5	0	regional ileitis	17.1	
E.F.	41	3-16-60	0.5	0.07	0	regional ileitis, steatorrhea	2.6	
E.F.	41	3-21-60	0.5	0.07	1			1.9
L.P.	41	3-18-60	0.5	0.07	0	non-tropical sprue	2.4	
L.P.	41	3-29-60	0.5	0.07	1			5.2
A.H.	42	2-9-54	1.0	0.04	0	non-tropical sprue	10.4	
L.A.	64	7-11-58	0.5	0.07	0	non-tropical sprue	23.5	
C.L.	60	4-29-58	0.5	0.07	0	cancer of pancreas, Whipple's procedure, steatorrhea	5.2	
C.L.	60	5-12-58	0.5	0.07	1	chronic pancreatitis,		8.6
S.W.	41	4-16-58	0.5	0.07	0	steatorrhea	5.5	
S.W.	41	4-30-58	0.5	0.07	1			7.0
A.O.	72	4-3-58	0.5	0.07	0	cancer of pancreas, steatorrhea	7.2	
A.O.	72	4-10-58	0.5	0.07	1			1.0
F.S.	73	5-19-60	0.5	0.07	0	75% gastric resection, Billroth II, steatorrhea	7.9	
F.S.	73	5-24-60	0.5	0.07	1			3.7
C.E.	59	12-1-58	0.5	0.07	0	recurrent pancreatitis	14.8	
H.O.	43	4-2-58	0.5	0.07	0	chronic pancreatitis	15.9	
C.H.	63	2-24-60	0.5	0.07	0	gastric resection, Billroth II, steatorrhea	19.2	
A.T.	65	1-12-60	0.5	0.07	0	gastric resection, Billroth II, diarrhea, steatorrhea	24.8	

tient, A.H., had a borderline excretion figure, and one, L.A., a completely normal figure. This variable absorption of cyanocobalamin in primary sprue is consistent with findings previously reported (81, 182, 229, 231, 436, 485, 568).

Eight patients with secondary steatorrhea were examined with the urinary excretion test. The steatorrhea was associated with chronic pancreatitis in three, gastric resection in three, with gastric resection plus pancreatitis following Whipple's procedure for carcinoma of pancreas in one, and with carcinoma of pancreas, unoperated, in one. In four of the patients the urinary excretion values were abnormally low, in four they were within the normal range. With the addition of IFC one subject with low absorption of cyanocobalamin (C.L.) showed some improvement in the absorption value, while the other three showed either lower or essentially unchanged absorption values. The results from the absorption studies in these patients confirm previous work (200, 392, 485). The conclusion has previously been made that the vitamin B_{12} absorption test is not a reliable diagnostic test for the malabsorption syndrome (200). The results reported here are in agreement with this conclusion.

Recently it has been shown that sodium bicarbonate given orally can correct the malabsorption of vitamin B_{12} associated with pancreatic insufficiency (462). This very important observation indicates that there is a pH optimum for the absorption of vitamin B_{12} in the gut, a finding which is in agreement with earlier experiments conducted by Castle and his associates (95). Pancreatin also will correct the malabsorption of cyanocobalamin seen in patients with pancreatic insufficiency (462). The reason for this finding is, however, not understood.

Results in Patients with Miscellaneous Diseases

The Schilling test was carried out in 27 patients with various diseases (Table 23). One patient, M.T., who suffered from megaloblastic anemia of pregnancy, was found to have a normal absorption of cyanocobalamin, which is the usual finding in this disease (15, 395). Patients with this type of anemia can secrete intrinsic factor (15, 262). Their response to parenteral liver or vitamin B_{12} therapy is usually disappointing (15, 43, 143, 262, 621, 634), whereas good response almost always results when folic acid is administered (15, 204, 621, 634). It is therefore believed that megaloblastic anemia of pregnancy results primarily from a folic acid deficiency. During pregnancy, vitamin B_{12} serum concentrations may be lower than normal (292) and in some cases of megaloblastic anemia of pregnancy and the puerperium the level of cyanocobalamin in the serum may be abnormally low (327). In the tropics,

Table 23. 24-Hour Urinary Radioactivity in Subjects with Miscellaneous Diseases after Oral Dose of $Co^{60}B_{12}$, with 1 mg. "Cold" B_{12} Given Intramuscularly 2 Hours after Oral Dose

Patient	Age	Date of Examination	Dose of $Co^{60}B_{12}$ μg	Dose of $Co^{60}B_{12}$ μc	Diagnosis	Urinary Radioactivity, % of Oral Dose
M.T.	41	3-10-56	0.5	0.05	megaloblastic anemia of pregnancy	18.3
D.J.	40	6-4-54	0.5	0.02	megaloblastic anemia, folic acid deficiency	17.1
F.S.	64	7-22-54	0.5	0.02	megaloblastic anemia in a vegetarian	17.9
F.S.	64	7-28-54	0.5	0.02	megaloblastic anemia in a vegetarian	26.2
P.N.	65	11-16-59	0.5	0.07	subacute myeloid leukemia	27.7
S.J.	69	1-28-59	0.5	0.07	subacute myeloid leukemia	13.4
W.W.	41	10-7-59	0.5	0.05	acute myeloid leukemia	28.1
E.M.	61	11-5-56	0.56	0.50	acute myeloid leukemia	24.5
J.M.	61	7-11-58	0.5	0.07	chronic myeloid leukemia	25.0
C.L.	68	4-18-60	0.5	0.07	chronic lymphoid leukemia	21.0
C.P.	82	10-9-56	0.56	0.50	chronic lymphoid leukemia	25.3
N.L.	65	2-16-60	0.5	0.07	myelofibrosis	6.7
N.L.	65	2-23-60	0.5	0.07	myelofibrosis	5.4*
R.S.	53	5-18-59	0.5	0.07	myelofibrosis	20.3
M.W.	43	2-12-59	0.5	0.07	cirrhosis of liver	14.3
O.L.	59	12-11-58	0.5	0.07	cirrhosis of liver	22.5
E.P.	38	9-24-57	0.5	0.07	cirrhosis of liver	24.7
H.A.	67	6-18-59	0.5	0.07	cirrhosis of liver	26.7
D.F.	36	2-4-59	0.5	0.07	cirrhosis of liver	31.0
D.H.	65	10-2-57	0.5	0.07	cirrhosis of liver	31.7
R.M.	42	2-29-60	0.5	0.07	peripheral neuritis	6.1†
R.M.	42	3-8-60	0.5	0.07	peripheral neuritis	9.7*†
R.M.	42	5-24-60	0.5	0.07	peripheral neuritis	14.8
H.T.	56	1-13-59	0.5	0.07	peripheral neuritis	15.4
C.J.	36	10-15-59	0.5	0.07	peripheral neuritis	16.4
C.J.	57	6-4-57	0.5	0.07	peripheral neuritis	17.2
E.H.	31	12-16-57	0.5	0.07	peripheral neuritis	20.1
D.H.	41	8-5-59	0.5	0.07	peripheral neuritis	20.3
O.S.	36	10-27-58	0.5	0.07	peripheral neuritis	21.8
L.H.	38	1-14-60	0.5	0.07	diabetic neuropathy, nocturnal diarrhea	6.0
L.H.	38	1-20-60	0.5	0.07	diabetic neuropathy, nocturnal diarrhea	6.4*
G.D.	38	4-24-58	0.5	0.07	diabetes mellitus, nocturnal diarrhea	4.3
G.D.	38	5-12-58	0.5	0.07	diabetes mellitus, nocturnal diarrhea	12.8*

* With 1 USP unit intrinsic factor concentrate.

† On parenteral B_{12} therapy.

vitamin B_{12} is commonly effective in treating the megaloblastic anemia associated with pregnancy and the puerperium (105A, 134, 488). Although patients with the disease outside the tropics rarely respond satisfactorily to liver extract or vitamin B_{12} therapy (172, 637), exceptions occur (374, 461, 604, 636, 637). Massive doses of this vitamin may induce good response in some cases (343, 452), and this may even happen with a normal serum vitamin B_{12} concentration (343). Such a phenomenon may be ascribed to a mass action, but it is poorly understood. If vitamin B_{12} influences the folic acid metabolism as has been suggested (666), it is quite possible that the increased serum B_{12} concentrations which follow large injections of this vitamin may facilitate the mobilization and/or utilization of folic acid or its derivatives (653, 666).

One patient, D.J., had subsisted on milk and other liquids for three months because of sore gums after the extraction of some teeth. He was admitted with a severe megaloblastic anemia which did not respond to parenteral vitamin B_{12} therapy. Because of the dietary history, normal vitamin B_{12} absorption, and subsequent excellent response to folic acid, it is believed that he suffered from a deficiency of folic acid.

A vegetarian, F.S., developed a megaloblastic anemia and was found on two different occasions to have a normal absorption of cyanocobalamin. He responded to parenteral treatment with vitamin B_{12}. Gastric analysis showed that the hydrochloric acid secretion was intact. It is possible that this patient suffered from a pure nutritional vitamin B_{12} deficiency, but this may be difficult to prove, because serum concentration of vitamin B_{12} was not measured.

Seven patients with various kinds of leukemia showed a normal absorption of cyanocobalamin. One subject, R.S., with myelofibrosis revealed a normal, another, N.L., an abnormally low urinary excretion value. In this latter patient there was no improvement in the recovery of urinary radioactivity on the addition of IFC. X-ray examination of the small bowel in this patient showed a deficiency pattern and he may be suffering from a sprue syndrome.

Six patients with cirrhosis of the liver showed urinary excretion values within the normal range, indicating that their secretion of IF was intact.

Seven of eight patients with neuritis of various types showed absorption values within the normal range. One patient, L.H., revealed an abnormally low urinary excretion value with no improvement on the addition of IFC. He suffered from diabetic neuropathy and also from nocturnal diarrhea with a malabsorption syndrome. The last patient, G.D., also suffered from diabetic nocturnal diarrhea. He showed an abnormally low urinary excretion value, but there was a considerable improvement when IFC was administered simultaneously with the labeled cyanocobalamin.

False Positive and Negative Urinary Excretion Tests

If the Schilling test results in no or negligible excretion of urinary radioactivity the test is positive — that is, it indicates malabsorption of cyanocobalamin. The test can be falsely positive for several reasons. It is apparent that incomplete urinary collection will reduce the quantity of radioactivity regained and a low normal figure may thus conceivably drop below the lower normal limit. This, then, emphasizes the most commonly encountered difficulty with the Schilling test, the quantitative collection of the 24-hour urine. If the result of the test is unequivocally within the normal range and no other radioactive isotopes have been administered, one can be fairly certain that a normal absorption of cyanocobalamin is present. On the other hand, if a low or borderline value is obtained, there is always the question of whether the urine collection was complete.

In uremia or in patients with impaired kidney function a low 24-hour urinary excretion value is often encountered (73, 169, 234, 516, 517). This may falsely be reported as a positive test. When the kidney function is impaired, radioactivity continues to be excreted for several days following the single "flushing" injection (415, 517), whereas in control subjects most of the radioactivity is excreted during the first day (415, 517). To avoid false positive tests in patients with impaired kidney function, we have adopted a three-day urinary collection period (Table 24). By adding up the radioactivity excreted over the three-day period, it should be possible to tell patients with uremia apart from patients with pernicious anemia. One patient with pernicious anemia and uremia has even been used for the purpose of testing unknown preparations of IFC in this way (Table 24). In some uremic patients we have preferred to use the plasma absorption technique instead of the Schilling test. In one instance a false positive urinary excretion test was encountered because the test material was lost through an emesis immediately after the dose was given. We have confirmed the findings of others (20, 82) that excessive treatment with parenteral vitamin B$_{12}$ may reduce the absorption of radiocyanocobalamin administered orally (subject R.M., Table 23). In order to learn more about the interference of the gastrointestinal absorption of cyanocobalamin by pretreatment with massive doses of "cold" vitamin B$_{12}$ given parenterally, an experimental study was carried out on seven control subjects. The fecal and urinary excretion of radioactivity was determined before treatment with vita-

Table 24. Urinary Radioactivity after a Single "Flushing" Injection of 1 mg. "Cold" B_{12} Given 2 Hours after Oral Dose

Patient	Dose of $Co^{60}B_{12}$		IFC Unit	Urinary Radioactivity, % of Oral Dose		
	μg	μc		1st Day	2nd Day	3rd Day
Control Subjects (6)						
G.W. 0.56		5.0*	0	38.2	0.2	0.1
R.R. 1.12		2.63*	0	17.3	0.6	0.0
E.K. 0.5		0.05	0	18.6	0.0	...
H.B. 0.5		0.05	0	39.4	0.0	...
E.Y. 0.5		0.05	0	26.0	0.0	...
J.H. 0.5		0.07	0	28.3	1.8	...
Uremic Subjects (4)						
D.H. 0.56		5.0*	0	15.2	10.2	3.6
C.S. 0.56		5.0*	0	8.1	1.5	0.0
P.P. 0.5		0.04	0	13.1	3.6	3.7
J.I. 0.5		0.07	0	5.1	2.7	...
Patients with Addison's Anemia and Uremia (2)						
C.S. 0.5		0.07	0	0.9	0.6	0.0
C.S. 0.5		0.05	1	6.9	2.3	0.9
T.L. 0.5		0.07	0	2.7	0.0	0.0
T.L. 0.5		0.07	0.50	9.1	7.0	...
T.L. 0.5		0.07	0.75	13.4	7.6	2.6
T.L. 0.5		0.07	...†	11.9	8.3	0.6
T.L. 0.5		0.07	...†	5.8	5.4	0.0
T.L. 0.5		0.07	...†	6.7	3.8	0.0
T.L. 0.5		0.07	...†	4.1	2.6	0.0
T.L. 0.5		0.07	...†	7.5	4.0	0.0

* $Co^{57}B_{12}$.
† Intrinsic factor concentrates of unknown potency.

min B_{12}, at the end of a treatment course, and again one or three weeks after cessation of the parenteral injections. The treatment course consisted of daily injections of 1,000 micrograms vitamin B_{12} for one week. The results (Table 25) show that the average urinary excretion value during treatment was far below the pretreatment level, and even 1 or 3 weeks after the discontinuation of the injections the average value was still below the control value, although great improvement had taken place by this time.

During treatment the individual urinary excretion values were all below their control levels, four declined below 10 per cent and one even down to zero. One week after cessation of treatment two patients still showed values below 10 per cent, three weeks after two of three subjects had regained their pretreatment levels, while the third was still below his control value.

The individual fecal excretion values were always higher on treat-

Table 25. Fecal and 24-Hour Urinary Radioactivity in Control Subjects before and after Parenteral "Loading" with Large Doses of Non-Labeled B$_{12}$ (1 mg. B$_{12}$ daily for 1 week); 1 mg. "Cold" B$_{12}$ Was Given Intramuscularly 2 Hours after Oral Dose of 0.5 µg Co^{60}B$_{12}$ (0.02 µc)

| | Radioactivity, % of Oral Dose | | | | | |
| | No Premedication | | Preloading with B$_{12}$, 1 mg. I.M. q.d. × 7 | | Off B$_{12}$ 1 or 3 Weeks | |
Patient	Feces	Urine	Feces	Urine	Feces	Urine
J.E.	49.3	28.1	78.5	13.2	66.6	29.5*
D.O.	35.5	32.5	84.8	9.6	79.7	15.4*
M.P.	44.7	14.6	96.7	0	84.7	8.7*
F.S.	34.1	29.4	76.1	6.5	74.8	4.6*
G.H.	44.8	28.9	49.3	21.0	56.6	17.6†
A.M.	63.4	24.0	72.3	10.8	28.1	31.8†
N.R.	67.6	14.2	79.0	9.5	65.0	13.7†
Average ...	48.5	24.5	76.7	10.1	65.1	17.3

* Test performed 1 week after last B$_{12}$ injection.
† Test performed 3 weeks after last B$_{12}$ injection.

ment than their corresponding control values. One to three weeks after cessation of therapy five of the seven patients still showed much elevated fecal excretion values, one subject revealed a value equal to the pretreatment figure, and only one showed a definitely lower value. Apparently the fecal excretion values returned to their pretreatment levels more slowly than the urinary excretion values.

Because of the suppression of the vitamin B$_{12}$ absorption from the gastrointestinal tract seen here during and shortly after pretreatment with large doses of parenteral vitamin B$_{12}$, it is suggested that the absorption test not be performed while this treatment is being given. After cessation of therapy, several weeks should elapse before the Schilling test is attempted. If the test is performed too soon after cessation of therapy and the result is found to be low or borderline, this result may be difficult to interpret.

If the urinary excretion test reveals a normal amount of radioactivity, it indicates that vitamin B$_{12}$ has been absorbed and the test is said to be negative. This is true only if radioactivity from all other sources has been excluded. If the patient has been subjected to treatment or diagnostic procedures involving other radioactive isotopes shortly before the Schilling test is performed, a false negative result may be obtained in patients with malabsorption of cyanocobalamin. Since I^{131} is the most commonly used radioactive isotope in clinical medicine, interference is most often from this source. In order to exclude false negative test results, a sample of urine may be obtained for counting purposes immediately before the Schilling test is started. Such a urine sample will reveal whether the patient is excreting radioactive material which might interfere with the test result.

Results with Varying Time Intervals between the Oral Dose and the Parenteral "Flushing" Injection

The time interval between the oral dose and the parenteral "flushing" injection has been given some attention (73, 415), but no systematic study of this subject exists. Besides, very little is known of the excretion pattern beyond the first day or two after the test material has been given. In order to establish the optimum time for the "flushing" injection and to learn the 24-hour excretion pattern in detail, absorption studies were carried out on 206 control subjects. An oral test dose of 0.56 μg vitamin B_{12} containing 0.39 or 0.50 μc Co^{60} and a single "flushing" intramuscular injection of 1 mg. non-labeled vitamin B_{12} were administered to each of them. Twenty-four-hour urine collections for radioactivity measurements were obtained from the time of the parenteral injections. The subjects were divided into fifteen groups consisting of 10–42 individuals. The injections were given at the time of the oral test dose in the first group. In subsequent groups the injections were administered 2, 4, 6, 8, 10, 12, 24, 48, 72, 96, 120, 144, 168, and 336 hours after the oral dose. The results are shown in Table 26, where the lowest, highest, and average figures are found for each group, together

Table 26. Results of the 24-Hour Urinary Radioactivities in Control Subjects, with Varying Time Intervals between Oral Dose of 0.56 μg B_{12} Containing 0.39 or 0.5 μc Co^{60} and Single "Flushing" Injection of 1 mg. "Cold" B_{12}

No. of Urinary Tests	Time between Oral Dose and I.M. Inj. (hr.)	8-Hr. Plasma Absorption $\mu\mu$g/ml. Plasma			Urinary Radioactivity, % of Oral Dose		
		No. of Tests	Average	Range	Average	S.D.	Range
10	0	0			17.3	± 7.1	10.6–31.0
28	2	0			22.4	± 8.0	6.5–44.7
11	4	3	6.8	5.6–8.6	23.5	± 6.2	11.2–33.1
42	6	42	8.0	3.2–15.1	28.9	± 8.5	13.2–48.2
10	8	10	4.6	3.1–6.0	26.6	± 7.4	16.8–39.7
10	10	10	4.8	2.5–9.9	23.6	± 5.1	16.5–31.7
10	12	10	4.2	3.1–6.4	21.4	± 6.5	12.3–30.8
10	24	10	3.9	2.1–7.3	12.8	± 4.8	5.6–21.6
10	48	5	5.5	3.3–7.0	7.8	± 3.0	3.6–11.4
12	72	7	3.8	2.8–5.6	3.6	± 1.8	0.6–6.8
12	96	8	5.6	2.9–11.4	2.9	± 1.5	0.7–6.2
10	120	7	4.3	3.7–5.3	1.6	± 0.6	0.9–3.1
10	144	10	5.2	3.3–7.5	1.5	± 0.7	0.7–2.8
10	168	10	5.2	3.1–8.1	1.3	± 0.4	0.8–2.0
11	336	11	5.7	2.9–10.3	0.5	± 0.2	0.2–0.7

with the standard deviation of the mean. The maximum average 24-hour urinary radioactivity of 28.9 per cent was found when the "flushing" injections were administered 6 hours after the oral dose. The corresponding figure for the group that received the 2-hour injection was 22.4 per cent. The difference between these two mean values is statistically significant ($p < 0.01$). The mean urinary excretion value was even lower in the group that received the parenteral and oral doses simultaneously, namely 17.3 per cent. From the peak value there was a slow decline during the next 6 hours so that the 12-hour and the 2-hour injections resulted in about the same average urinary excretion values. The greatest decline in the average 24-hour urinary radioactivity occurred between the 6- and the 24-hour injections. From the second day on a slower decline became evident. The average excretion had declined to 2.9 per cent of the oral dose, or 10 per cent of the average maximum excretion value, in the group that received the injection four days after the oral dose. By the end of one and two weeks, the average values had declined to 1.3 and 0.5 per cent respectively.

To be certain to exclude patients with vitamin B$_{12}$ malabsorption in the groups with the low urinary excretion values, another parameter for the absorption of cyanocobalamin had to be employed simultaneously. For this purpose the 8-hour plasma absorption of radiocyanocobalamin was recorded in 143 of the subjects. The values were expressed in $\mu\mu$g/ml. of plasma (Table 26). Because plasma absorption always was normal, the low urinary excretion of radioactivity in the last few groups reflects the true urinary excretion pattern in control subjects.

The study shows that there is a limited time during which vitamin B$_{12}$ is available for excretion into the urine by the procedure of parenteral "flushing." For removing as much of the radioactivity from the body as possible with a single injection the 6-hour injection is our choice. However, the difference between the 6- and the 2-hour values is not so large that a change in the routine performance of the Schilling test seems warranted. In fact, it appears that for diagnostic purposes the injection may be given at any time during the first day. Since so much clinical experience has been accumulated with the 2-hour injection, and since we use a very small dose of radioactivity (0.07 μc Co^{60}) in the routine performance of the Schilling test, the timing of the parenteral injection has not yet been changed in our clinical laboratory due to this observation.

It is understandable that the 24-hour urinary excretion of radioactivity will be higher with the 6- than the 2-hour injections if one keeps in mind the normal plasma absorption curve of cyanocobalamin (60, 158, 162, 163, 234) and the excretion pattern of radioactivity in fractionated urine collections (39, 60, 557). The 6-hour injection is given at the steepest part of the plasma absorption curve and it seems logical that it should be more effective than the 2-hour injection which is administered a couple of hours before the absorption from the intestine really begins (60, 557).

Results with Daily "Flushing" Injections for One Week

It has been reported that additional "flushing" injections given one and two days after the oral test dose of labeled cyanocobalamin will result in the recovery of additional amounts of radioactivity in subsequent urine collections (177, 415, 509, 657). This phenomenon was studied closer in five control subjects. Following the oral test dose of labeled cyanocobalamin, each was given 1 mg. of "cold" vitamin B_{12} intramuscularly at 10 A.M. daily for one week. Urine was collected for 24-hour periods after each injection. The results (Table 27) show that more radioactivity could indeed be recovered in the urine by the procedure of daily "flushing." The average amount of radioactivity regained in the urine decreased rapidly after the second day and was below 1 per cent of the oral dose after the fourth collection period. The average radioactivity in the urine for the first 24-hour collection was 24.0 per cent, for the first four days 36.3 per cent, and for the entire week 38.2 per cent of the oral test dose.

Table 27. 24-Hour Urinary Radioactivity in Control Subjects after Oral Dose of 0.56 μg $Co^{60}B_{12}$ (0.5 μc), with 1 mg. "Cold" B_{12} Given Intramuscularly Daily at 10 A.M. for 1 Week Beginning on the Day of Oral Dose

Patient	Radioactivity, % of Oral Dose in Seven 24-Hour Periods						
	1	2	3	4	5	6	7
L.D.	24.2	10.5	2.6	1.3	0.9	0.7	0.7
M.S.	24.5	7.7	0.9	0.6	0.3	0.3	0.3
K.R.	22.6	8.0	2.4	1.1	0.9	0.7	0.6
A.L.	26.0	9.8	2.7	1.1	0.8	0.6	0.6
T.M.	22.8	9.2	2.5	1.4	0.8	0.7	0.7
Average	24.0	9.0	2.2	1.1	0.7	0.6	0.6
Range	22.6–26.0	7.7–10.5	0.9–2.7	0.6–1.4	0.3–0.9	0.3–0.7	0.3–0.7

Results with "Flushing" Doses of Varying Magnitude

Because a limited amount of the absorbed radioactivity is excreted in the 24-hour urine in the Schilling test (Table 9) (73, 82, 380) and since additional activity can be regained on subsequent days with renewed "flushing" injections (Table 27) (177, 415, 509, 657), it was decided to investigate the possibility of increasing the urinary recovery of radioactivity during the first 24-hour collection period. One possible reason for the fact that only a limited amount of the absorbed radioactivity is excreted in the first 24-hour urine is the use of a suboptimal "flushing" dose. To determine the effect of parenteral doses of varying size, three groups of control subjects were studied with injections of 100, 1,000, and 5,000 μg "cold" vitamin B_{12}, respectively. The three groups consisted of 10, 42, and 10 subjects respectively, and the parenteral injections were administered 6 hours after the oral test dose. The results (Table 28) show that by increasing the "flushing" dose from 0.1 to 1.0 mg. the average urinary excretion value rose from 5.6 to 28.9 per cent ($p < 0.001$). A further five-fold increase in the size of the 1 mg. "flushing" dose led only to a minor increase in the average excretion value from 28.9 to 35.1 per cent. This difference is also statistically significant ($0.02 < p < 0.05$) for the number of tests performed.

Table 28. Comparison of the 24-Hour Urinary Radioactivity with Differing "Flushing" Doses of Non-Labeled B_{12}, Intramuscular Injections Given 6 Hours after Oral Dose of 0.56 μg B_{12} Containing 0.39 or 0.5 μc Co^{60}

| No. of Tests | B_{12} I.M. μg | Radioactivity, % of Oral Dose | | |
		Average	S.D.	Range
10.......	100	5.6	± 4.1	1.8–16.5
42.......	1,000	28.9	± 8.5	13.2–48.2
10.......	5,000	35.1	± 6.9	21.2–42.9

It is apparent that the smallest dose used in this study did not result in maximal "flushing" effect. On the other hand, only minor improvement in the excretion values was observed with increase in the parenteral dose above 1 mg. Thus there seems to be no compelling reason for giving larger than 1 mg. "flushing" doses in the performance of the Schilling test. Lack of "flushing" effect doesn't appear to be the reason why only a minor part of the absorbed radioactivity is excreted in the urine when the Schilling test is performed.

Results with Multiple "Flushing" Injections

Next, it was decided to investigate whether multiple "flushing" injections would increase the radioactivity in the first 24-hour collection period. For this purpose the fecal and urinary excretion tests were performed simultaneously in five control subjects. First, a control test was performed whereby they all were given 0.50 μg B_{12} containing 0.05–0.10 μc Co^{60} orally followed by 1 mg. "cold" cyanocobalamin 2 hours later. The average urinary excretion value in the first 24-hour urine collection period was 22.5 per cent, while no or negligible activity was found in the second 24-hour collection period (Table 29, Column A).

At a different time, the second part of the study was done with a similar oral test dose of radiocyanocobalamin, but now multiple "flushing" injections were given as follows: three during the first and three during the second day, and one on the third day. The first parenteral injection contained 2 mg. vitamin B_{12}, all the others only 1 mg. Urine was collected in 24-hour periods starting immediately after the first injection. The average urinary excretion value during the first collection period was 26.4 per cent (Table 29, Column B). The difference between this figure and the corresponding control value of 22.5 per cent is not statistically significant $(0.3 < p < 0.4)$. It is therefore evident that multiple "flushing" injections do not materially increase the urinary excretion values on the first day over and above what is found after a single injection. The same is also true for the result obtained on the second day. In the present series the average figure was 7.6 per cent, which should be compared with the average 9.0 per cent excretion value observed after a single injection (Table 27). The total average three-day urinary radioactivity after multiple "flushing" injections of 8 mg. "cold" B_{12} in this study was 37.5 per cent (Table 29) compared with 35.2 per cent following a single daily injection of 1 mg. (Table 27). This smaller difference in the total three-day excretion is not statistically

Table 29. Single and Multiple "Flushing" Injections Compared: Results of Urinary and Fecal Radioactivity in Control Subjects after Oral Dose of 0.5 μg B_{12} Containing 0.05–0.1 μc Co^{60}

		Radioactivity, % of Oral Dose					
		A*			B†		
			Urine			Urine	
Patient	Date of Examination	Feces	Day 1	Day 2	Feces	Day 1	Day 2	Day 3
G.P. 11-14-55		32.3	31.6	0				
G.P. 11-29-55					44.2	28.0	8.8	1.8
F.K. 1-9-56		44.8	12.4	0				
F.K. 12-5-55					31.9	27.8	9.1	2.6
W.B. 11-14-55		28.7	23.0	0				
W.B. 12-19-55					50.8	24.5	7.6	5.2
R.N. 12-5-55		46.5	30.2	1.6				
R.N. 12-12-55					45.4	29.4	8.3	3.4
J.M. 12-5-55		71.1	15.4	0				
J.M. 12-12-55					46.3	22.1	4.1	4.5
Average		44.7	22.5	0.3	43.7	26.4	7.6	3.5

* Single "flushing" injections, 1 mg. "cold" B_{12} administered after 2 hours.

† Multiple "flushing" injections, 2 mg. "cold" B_{12} at 2 hours, 1 mg. each at 8, 14, 26, 32, 38, and 50 hours after the oral dose.

significant $(0.3 < p < 0.4)$. Previously it has also been reported that no significant improvement occurred in the 24-hour urinary recovery of radioactivity with multiple "flushing" injections (415).

The average fecal excretion of radioactivity was about the same in the 2 parts of this study. It is, therefore, believed that the multiple injections did not reduce the absorption of cyanocobalamin to any greater extent than the single injection.

Results with Parenteral "Loading" Administered Simultaneously with the Oral Dose

A study was carried out in order to learn whether a small parenteral saturation dose of "cold" vitamin B$_{12}$ given at the time of the oral test dose would result in increased urinary radioactivity in the Schilling test. For this purpose the fecal and urinary radioactivities were determined in 5 control subjects who were given an oral test dose of 0.5 µg Co^{60}B$_{12}$ followed by 1 mg. non-labeled vitamin B$_{12}$ intramuscularly 2 hours later. The average urinary excretion of radioactivity in these control studies was 23.7 per cent (Table 30, Column A). At another time, absorption tests were repeated with the same oral test dose, but this time 50 µg of "cold" vitamin B$_{12}$ was administered intramuscularly simultaneously with the oral test dose. A multiple "flushing" procedure was used in this part of the experiment similar to the one described in

Table 30. Results of Parenteral "Loading" Given at the Time of Oral Dose: Comparison of Urinary and Fecal Radioactivity in Control Subjects after Oral Dose of 0.5 µg Co^{60}B$_{12}$ (0.07 µc)

		Radioactivity, % of Oral Dose						
		A*			B†			
			Urine			Urine		
Patient	Date of Examination	Feces	Day 1	Day 2	Feces	Day 1	Day 2	Day 3
E.Y. 2-20-56		23.0	26.0	0				
E.Y. 1-16-56					29.5	22.3	7.6	1.1
J.B. 1-23-56		65.7	6.8	0				
J.B. 1-30-56					71.3	13.5	2.9	0
U.B. 1-23-56		17.2	27.6	0				
U.B. 1-30-56					37.1	32.0	9.2	5.2
H.B. 1-23-56		31.4	39.4	0				
H.B. 1-30-56					48.1	36.4	5.9	3.4
E.K. 1-23-56		38.3	18.6	0				
E.K. 1-30-56					52.7	19.4	5.5	1.2
Average..............		35.1	23.7	0	47.7	24.7	6.2	2.2

*Single "flushing" injection, 1 mg. "cold" B$_{12}$ given 2 hours after oral dose.

†50 µg "cold" B$_{12}$ given at time of oral dose. Multiple "flushing" injections, 2 mg. "cold" B$_{12}$ after 2 hours, 1 mg. each at 8, 14, 26, 32, 38, and 50 hours after oral dose.

the preceding section (pp. 92–94). The average urinary radioactivity in the first 24-hour collection period was 24.7 per cent (Table 30, Column B). This value is not materially different from the 23.7 per cent control value obtained in the same subjects (Table 30, Column A), and the 26.4 per cent obtained without "loading" at time zero in the group described in the previous section (Table 29, Column B). In other words, the procedure of "loading" at the time of the oral test did not enhance the urinary excretion of radioactivity. Comparison of Tables 29 and 30, Columns B, shows that this is true not only for the values obtained on the first day but also on the two succeeding days. The total average three-day urinary activity with parenteral "loading" at time zero amounted to 33.1 per cent as compared with 37.5 per cent without such treatment.

The average fecal excretion of radioactivity with "loading" at time zero was 47.7 per cent as compared with 35.1 per cent in the control tests in the same individuals. This increment in the fecal excretion of radioactivity together with slightly lowered three-day urinary activity with, rather than without parenteral "loading" at zero time, may even suggest that this procedure reduced the total amount of radiocyanocobalamin absorbed from the intestine.

Results with Parenteral "Preloading" Administered 24 Hours Prior to the Oral Test

A study was made to learn whether a small parenteral saturation dose of "cold" vitamin B_{12} given 24 hours before the oral test dose would result in increased recovery of radioactivity in the Schilling test. For this purpose vitamin B_{12} absorption tests were carried out in seven control subjects in a manner similar to that in the previous section with the only difference that in the second part of the test the "preloading" dose of 50 μg "cold" vitamin B_{12} was administered intramuscularly 24 hours before instead of simultaneously with the oral test dose. In two of the subjects the multiple "flushing" procedure was carried out only on the day of the oral test. The results (Table 31) show that the average urinary radioactivity in the first 24-hour collection period was 38.5 per cent with 24-hour "preloading" and multiple flushing injections as compared with 24.7 per cent without "preloading" and a single "flushing" injection. The difference is statistically significant $(0.01 < p < 0.02)$. The figure of 38.5 per cent is also significantly higher than the corresponding values of 26.4 and 24.7 per cent in the series treated with similar "flushing" procedures without and with "loading" at the time of the oral test (Tables 29 and 30, Columns B). The average

Table 31. Results of "Preloading" Given 24 Hours before Oral Dose: Comparison of the Urinary and Fecal Excretion Methods in Control Subjects after Oral Dose of 0.5 µg $Co^{60}B_{12}$ (0.07 µc)

		Radioactivity, % of Oral Dose						
		A*			B†			
			Urine				Urine	
Patient	Date of Examination	Feces	Day 1	Day 2	Feces	Day 1	Day 2	Day 3
E.C. 10-17-55		17.7	19.8	1.3				
E.C. 10-23-55					35.5	35.1	10.9	3.7
J.H. 10-17-55		21.3	28.3	1.8				
J.H. 10-23-55					21.7	46.7	4.9	1.7
R.N. 10-24-55		18.1	21.9	0				
R.N. 10-30-55					25.8	25.4	6.3	0.8
E.H. 10-31-55		34.2	30.5	1.8				
E.H. 11-27-55					51.3	34.9	5.7	2.5
A.T. 10-31-55		22.6	33.3	0				
A.T. 11-6-55					14.2	50.5	10.1	2.0
W.B. 10-3-55		28.2	9.5	0				
W.B. 10-10-55					30.5	43.9	...	...
C.G. 10-3-55		15.2	29.5	0				
C.G. 10-10-55					34.3	32.9	...	...
Average		22.5	24.7	0.7	30.5	38.5	7.6	2.1

*Single "flushing" injection, 1 mg. "cold" B_{12} given 2 hours after oral dose.

† 50 µg "cold" B_{12} intramuscularly 24 hours before oral dose. Multiple "flushing" injections, 2 mg. "cold" B_{12} at 2 hours, 1 mg. each at 8, 14, 26, 32, 38, and 50 hours after oral dose.

amounts of radioactivity excreted on the second and third day were not materially different from those observed on the corresponding days in the previous experiment (Table 30, Column B). The total three-day urinary radioactivity regained when "preloading" was given 24 hours before the oral test was 48.2 per cent of the ingested dose. This figure is almost twice the 24-hour control value in the same individuals (Table 31, Column A), and 10.7 and 15.1 per cent above the three-day values obtained in the preceding two series subjected to a similar "flushing" procedure without and with "loading" at zero time. A comparison of Columns B, Tables 29–31, shows that the entire increment in the urinary radioactivity with 24-hour "preloading" occurred in the first 24-hour collection period. Even though the 24-hour "preloading" procedure resulted in a great increase in the radioactivity excreted in the first day of collection, there was no decrease in the activity excreted on the second or the third day.

When daily parenteral injections of vitamin B_{12} are given, the urinary excretion of the vitamin is lower in the first 24-hour period than on subsequent days (630). This observation is best classified as a saturation phenomenon. The fact that the first 24-hour urinary radioactivity is higher with than without 24-hour "preloading" is probably related to this saturation phenomenon.

The average fecal excretion of radioactivity with the 24-hour "preloading" technique was 30.5 per cent. This value is only slightly above the control value of 22.5 per cent. It is therefore believed that there cannot be much, if any, impairment of the absorption of vitamin B_{12} by a single 50 μg injection of vitamin B_{12} 24 hours before the oral test.

Because both fecal and urinary radioactivities were measured in all patients included in the last three series (Tables 29–31), it was also possible to express the urinary excretion of radioactivity as a percentage of the absorbed vitamin (Fig. 1). The results show that with a single "flushing" injection at two hours the average first-day urinary radioactivity ranged between 34.8 and 42.1 per cent of the absorbed dose in the three series. With multiple injections without and with zero-hour "loading," the corresponding figures were 47.2 and 46.9 per cent, while an increase to 55.7 per cent was noted with the 24-hour "preloading" technique.

These findings show that there is an upper maximal limit to the amount of vitamin B_{12} that can be regained in the first-day urine even with the 24-hour "preloading" technique. Furthermore, it can be seen that the maximum average radioactivity regained in the three-day urine collections was 70.0 per cent of the absorbed amount. This is almost twice the average amount recovered in the 24-hour urine when

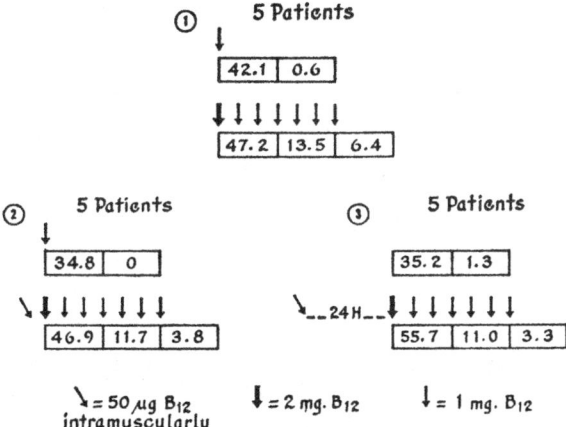

Figure 1. Average urinary radioactivity on the 1st, 2nd, and 3rd day, expressed as a percentage of absorbed activity, with single or multiple parenteral injections; in the 2nd part of the experiments the subjects in groups 2 and 3 received parenteral loading injections at zero time or 24 hours before oral dose.

the Schilling test is performed in the routine manner (82, 380) (Table 9). It can be seen from Tables 29–31 that multiple "flushing" injections given over a three-day period with or without "preloading" lead to a retention in the body of approximately 20 per cent of the oral test dose of radioactivity as compared with 33–52 per cent with only a single injection as given in the routine performance of the Schilling test. Since one single daily injection was almost as effective in removing radioactivity from the body as multiple injections, it should be kept in mind that the total body burden of radioactivity after a Schilling test can readily be halved by a few injections of vitamin B$_{12}$ if use is made of the knowledge presented here. It is also worth remembering that the "flushing" procedure becomes less and less effective in removing radioactivity from the body as time goes on (Table 26). A few injections given during the first three days after the test might remove from the body as much radioactivity as a hundred injections given later (165).

3 | THE PLASMA ABSORPTION TEST

Results in Control Subjects and Patients with Pernicious Anemia
after Test Doses of 0.46 µg Vitamin B_{12} Containing
0.5 µc Co^{60} or 0.92 µg B_{12} with 1.0 µc Co^{60} *

It has been said that radioactivity was not present in measurable
quantities in the plasma after the ingestion of labeled cyanocobalamin
(557). In order for the orally administered radioactivity to appear in
the urine in the Schilling test it has, however, to pass through the blood
stream. It was therefore reasoned that if a sensitive method was used it
should be possible to detect the activity in the blood or plasma. This
reasoning soon proved to be correct. Three factors more than anything
else were responsible for the successful measurement of the radioactivity in the plasma: (a) the use of radiocyanocobalamin with a relatively
high specific activity (around 1 mc/mg.), (b) the use of a large volume
of plasma for counting purposes (20 ml.), and (c) the use of a prolonged
counting time. The earliest batches of $Co^{60}B_{12}$ available probably did
not have high enough specific activity to allow measurement of plasma
radioactivity following the ingestion of small test doses. The subsequent availability of material with higher specific activity was in this
respect fortunate. A specially made scintillation detector capable of
accommodating 20 ml. vials made it possible to measure the radioactivities of larger volumes of plasma, and by employing a preset count of
12,800 the background counts became very stable so that even small
amounts of radioactivity became very significant. By using this technique it was possible to define the normal absorption of cyanocobala-

* This section appeared in slightly different form in Doscherholmen and Hagen,
Blood, 12:336, 1957, Grune & Stratton, New York (162); and Proc. 6th Congr.
Internat. Soc. Hemat., Boston 1956, Grune & Stratton, New York, 347, 1958 (163).
An abstract of this material appeared in J. Clin. Invest., 35:699, 1956, American So-
ciety for Clinical Investigation (164).

Table 32. Radioactivity in 20 ml. of Blood or Plasma after Oral Dose of 0.46 μg $Co^{60}B_{12}$ (0.5 μc) (all patients male)

Columns 1–216 give "Net cpm at Different Hours after the Oral Dose."

Patient	Age	Diagnosis	Substance Tested	1	2	3	4	5	6	8	10	12	16	20	24	28	32	36	48	52	72	96	120	144	168	192	216
M.R.J.	59	pneumonia	blood	1	5	4	2		15	18																	
H.L.O.	82	rheumatoid arthritis	blood	8	4	7	8		25	34																	
C.F.C.	48	coronary disease	blood	6			18	33	33																		
R.V.	22	bronchiectasis	blood	5	7	8	10		18	21		17			17						16	15				14	
			plasma	0	1	4	10		33	47		36			27						22	19				18	
S.P.	26	peptic ulcer	blood	4	7	11	12		20	22		22			16						14	18				12	
			plasma	5	0	7	9		36	44		37			32						23	19				18	
W.W.C.	64	psychoneurosis	plasma	6	10	5	6		36	38		31			18				17		10	11					
G.W.S.	67	asthma	plasma	7	6	4	6		15	30		31			29				21		24	24		20	17		
R.W.D.	66	osteoarthritis	plasma	1	9	5	7		35	47		39			36				22		19	21				17	18
L.C.	25	healthy	plasma												26				18		16	11	8		8		
E.A.P.	25	psychoneurosis	plasma							40	43				24				17		15	13	9	9	8		
B.B.	23	healthy	blood				7			17					7				11		5	13	8	6	0		
			plasma				5			19		21			15				10		12	9	4	11	7		
D.M.	24	healthy	blood								41				19				13		11	8					
			plasma								54				28				22		16	15					
D.B.	24	pulmonary infiltr.	blood				16			22		24	12	15	19	10	18	17		14							
			plasma								41†																
L.S.	28	nephrolithiasis	blood				18			24		24	17	18	17	17	12	19									
			plasma								85†																
G.H.D.	46	hypertension	plasma				5	9	24																		
J.E.B.	42	pulmonary fibrosis	plasma				6	16	28																		
H.R.S.	32	bronchiectasis	plasma			8	11		18																		
J.A.L.	36	bronchial asthma	plasma				13	19	30	54					89												
H.E.M.	56	Parkinsonism	plasma				12	17	36	48					40												
E.L.	50	pernicious anemia	blood		1		2		2	2	3																
			plasma																								
E.L.*	59	pernicious anemia	blood		4		9		28	24																	
			plasma							42																	

(From Doscherholmen and Hagen: Radioactive vitamin B12 absorption studies: Results of direct measurement of radioactivity in the blood. Blood, 12:336, 1957.)

* With 100 mg. intrinsic factor concentrate.

† Plasma obtained from 8- and 12-hour specimens.

min and to separate control subjects from patients with pernicious anemia (162).

Forty-one tests were carried out on 36 non-pernicious anemia control subjects and seventeen tests on 9 patients with Addison's pernicious anemia. The oral test dose was either 0.46 μg vitamin B_{12} containing 0.5 μc Co^{60} or 0.92 μg B_{12} containing 1.0 μc Co^{60}. Peripheral venous blood was obtained at different time intervals up to one week or more after the dose was administered.

Tables 32 and 33 include the results of measurements of radioactivity in blood and plasma at different time intervals in 28 control subjects and 8 pernicious anemia patients examined with the smaller test dose. In the control subjects it was difficult to detect activity during the first three hours of the test. Out of 28 blood or plasma samples counted from

Table 33. Comparison of the Radioactivity in 20 ml. of Plasma and the 24-Hour Urinary Excretion of Radioactivity after the Administration of 1,000 μg B_{12} Intramuscularly 24 Hours after the Oral Dose of 0.46 μg $Co^{60}B_{12}$ (0.5 μc)

Patient	Age	Diagnosis	Net cpm at Different Times after Oral Dose		Urinary Excretion, % of Oral Dose
			10 Hr.	24 Hr.	
J.A.L.	36	bronchial asthma	54	39	18.2
M.L.*	23	healthy	50	30	17.7
H.E.M.	56	Parkinsonism	48	40	17.4
S.S.	63	arteriosclerosis	39	17	10.9
F.J.O.	39	bronchiectasis	37	26	11.8
H.A.G.	63	coronary disease	31	20	10.4
E.A.	67	lung tumor	27		8.2
D.C.	57	optic atrophy	25	23	7.0
D.M.*	27	healthy	21	15	4.9
I.W.B.	59	psychoneurosis	20		9.3
S.F.P.	33	cholelithiasis	19		12.7
P.L.	67	pernicious anemia	2	0	0
P.L.†	67	pernicious anemia	22	10	5.3
F.B.	64	pernicious anemia	6		1.3
F.B.†	64	pernicious anemia	27		8.6
H.A.G.	62	pernicious anemia	8		0.6
H.A.G.†	62	pernicious anemia	32		12.4
F.C.	59	pernicious anemia	8		0.6
F.C.†	59	pernicious anemia	42		11.0
O.F.K.	56	pernicious anemia	7		0.8
O.F.K.†	56	pernicious anemia	40		14.1
L.E.	81	pernicious anemia	8		1.6
L.E.†	81	pernicious anemia	44		12.5
A.M.	85	pernicious anemia	5		0.9

(From Doscherholmen and Hagen: Radioactive vitamin B_{12} absorption studies: Results of direct measurement of radioactivity in the blood. Blood, 12:336, 1957.)

* Female patient.

† 100 mg. intrinsic factor concentrate administered.

this interval, only 4 contained more than 7 cpm. After 4 hours, measurable activity appeared in 11 out of 19 blood and plasma samples. After 5 hours, activity was present in all 5 cases examined at that time. From then on there was an increase in radioactivity until a peak was reached in the 8- to the 12-hour period. The average peak plasma value, 38 cpm, was found at 8 hours, but in some individual tests the 12-hour value was just as high as the 8-hour value. Following the peak there was a slow decline in radioactivity over the ensuing days. Even after a week significant activity was still present in the plasma in 3 out of 5 instances. One patient with pernicious anemia (E.L.) was followed with blood measurement every two hours for ten hours after the ingestion of the oral test dose without showing any definite radioactivity. When the same procedure was repeated one month later with the addition of 100 mg. IFC, blood and plasma counts were within the range found in control subjects. Seven more patients with pernicious anemia were examined with similar test doses and no definite radioactivity or only traces were found at ten hours unless IFC was added to the test dose.

A comparison between the results of the direct blood measurement technique and those obtained with a modified Schilling test is found in Table 33. To avoid possible alteration of the plasma absorption curve the "flushing" parenteral dose of ordinary crystalline vitamin B_{12} was given 24 hours after the oral dose instead of 2 hours as called for in Schilling's original method (557). The study was carried out in 11 control subjects and 7 patients with pernicious anemia with the smaller tracer dose. In 6 of the latter patients, the same procedure was repeated after the addition of IFC to the test dose. The blood sampling was done after 10 hours in all cases and in 11 cases also after 24 hours. A good correlation was found between the radioactivity in urine and the 10-hour ($r = 0.94$) and the 24-hour ($r = 0.93$) plasma samples; i.e., with increased plasma values there was increased urinary excretion of radioactivity and vice versa. This was especially well demonstrated in the 6 patients with pernicious anemia tested with and without IFC. Positive correlation between the plasma absorption test and the urinary excretion test was also found in a different study (159).

The larger dose of 0.92 μg vitamin B_{12} containing 1.0 μc of Co^{60} was given to three control subjects and one patient with pernicious anemia. The results (Table 34) revealed the same general findings, except that higher counts were obtained. The patient with pernicious anemia showed traces of radioactivity in blood and plasma at 4 and 8 hours, but when IFC was added to the test dose of labeled vitamin B_{12}, there was a five-fold increase in his maximum plasma counts.

Although whole blood or plasma could be used for counting purposes,

Table 34. Radioactivity in Blood or Plasma after the Administration of 0.92 μg $Co^{60}B_{12}$ (1.0 μc) Orally to 3 Control Subjects and 1 Pernicious Anemia Patient (all male)

Patient	Age	Diagnosis	Substance Tested	Net cpm at Specified Number of Hours after Oral Dose													Modified Schilling Test‡
				0	4	8	10	12	24	36	48	72	96	120	144	168	
M.R.K.	61	bronchial asthma	blood		3	54		55	47		33	32	22	13	14	21	
			plasma				108†										
F.H.	24	psychoneurosis	blood		22	33		31	29	31							
			plasma				56†										
C.C.	62	emphysema	blood			38	38		28								15.6
			plasma				60		53								
F.McA.	75	pernicious anemia	blood		9	10		6	0								0.8
			plasma		11	10		5	2								
F.McA.*	75	pernicious anemia	blood	7	0	29		30	26								8.4
			plasma	4	9	53		44	32								

(From Doscherholmen and Hagen: Radioactive vitamin B_{12} absorption studies: Results of direct measurement of radioactivity in the blood. Blood, 12:336, 1957.)

* 200 mg. intrinsic factor concentrate administered.

† Plasma obtained from pooled 8- and 12-hour blood specimens.

‡ Urinary excretion of radioactivity as a percentage of oral tracer dose, with 1,000 μg B_{12} given intramuscularly 24 hours after oral dose.

103

it was found early that plasma gave higher counts. Except for a few instances where the radioactivity was so close to the background that it was difficult to evaluate, plasma counts were consistently higher than whole blood counts. This was well borne out by the experiments cited in Table 35. Unwashed red blood cells contained some radioactivity, but always less than whole blood. This could have been due to the trapping of plasma. When red blood cells were washed twice with normal saline, they contained no definite radioactivity.

Table 35. Radioactivity of 20 ml. of Whole Blood, Plasma, and Unwashed and Washed Red Blood Cells

Patient	Plasma	Whole Blood	RBC Unwashed	RBC Washed
E.L.	42	28	17	
F.H.	56	32	22	
M.R.K.	108	55	20	
C.C.	60	38		6
E.L.	33			0

(From Doscherholmen and Hagen: Radioactive vitamin B_{12} absorption studies: Results of direct measurement of radioactivity in the blood. Blood, 12:336, 1957; and from Doscherholmen and Hagen: Radioactive vitamin B_{12} absorption studies: Results of direct measurement of radioactivity in the blood. Proc. 6th Congr. Internat. Soc. Hemat., Grune & Stratton, New York, 347, 1958.)

The question arose whether smaller scintillation counters could be used. To explore this possibility the same sample of whole blood was counted in three different-sized well-type scintillation counters using volumes of 20, 8, and 4 ml., respectively. Table 36 shows that in the case of whole blood definite radioactivity was detected in volumes of 20 and 8 ml., but not in 4 ml. However, when plasma was counted, significant activity could be found even with the 4 ml. well counter.

The reproducibility of the plasma counting technique was compared with that of the urinary excretion method by duplicate tests on five control subjects. The second study was made in each instance after the radioactivity had disappeared from the plasma. The 0.46 μg (0.5 μc) oral dose was given and blood samples were drawn ten hours later. Thereupon, 1,000 μg of non-radioactive vitamin B_{12} were injected parenterally and the urine collected for the ensuing 24 hours for radioactivity measurements. The results are summarized in Table 37. In general there was good reproducibility but with some variations. However, in this small series the repeated plasma values correlated a little better than the duplicate urinary excretion percentages.

After physiologic amounts of labeled vitamin B_{12} were administered

Table 36. Radioactivity of the Same Sample of Blood or Plasma in Three Different-Sized Well-Type Scintillation Counters, 20, 8, and 4 ml.

Patient	Efficiency of Counter (%)	Volume Counter (ml.)	Net cpm
Blood			
F.H. 24		20	29
F.H. 30		8	10
F.H. 30		8	8
F.H. 42		4	5
F.H. 42		4	0
Plasma			
S.P. 24		20	19
S.P. 30		8	10
S.P. 42		4	9
D.M. 24		20	54
D.M. 30		8	25
D.M. 42		4	19

(From Doscherholmen and Hagen: Radioactive vitamin B_{12} absorption studies: Results of direct measurement of radioactivity in the blood. Blood, 12:336, 1957.)

Table 37. Comparison between the Reproducibility of the Plasma Radioactivity and the 24-Hour Urinary Excretion Test: 1,000 µg B_{12} Was Given Intramuscularly 10 Hours after Oral Dose of 0.46 µg $Co^{60}B_{12}$ (0.5 µc)

Patient	cpm in 20 ml. of Plasma at 10 Hr.		Urinary Radioactivity, % of Oral Dose	
	Test A	Test B	Test A	Test B
E.B. 31		23	25.8	14.4
P.B. 34		39	28.5	27.4
E.H. 33		38	18.2	20.6
W.P. 51		49	34.9	26.8
L.K. 17		28	9.9	20.7

(From Doscherholmen and Hagen: Radioactive vitamin B_{12} absorption studies: Results of direct measurement of radioactivity in the blood. Blood, 12:336, 1957.)

orally, the peak of the radioactivity in the blood and plasma was found 8 to 12 hours later. Insignificant activity was present during the first three hours. This trend was found consistently not only in control subjects but also in patients with pernicious anemia when IFC was given simultaneously with the test dose. Therefore, the delay in appearance of blood radioactivity could not be attributed to lack of readily available intrinsic factor for interaction with vitamin B_{12}. Although significant activity in the plasma started to appear at 3–4 hours, it was not consistently found until 5 hours after the test material was given. This finding was in line with Schilling's original observation that significant excretion in the urine usually began 4–6 hours after the parenteral "flushing" dose of vitamin B_{12} (557).

Our absorption curves after physiologic doses of labeled vitamin B$_{12}$ were strikingly different from those observed by Ross *et al.* (551), who determined serum levels of vitamin B$_{12}$ with bioassay after massive oral doses. They found peak serum concentrations between 1 and 2 hours after the ingestion of the test dose, absorption closely resembling that of glucose. These differences indicate that physiologic amounts of vitamin B$_{12}$ were absorbed in a different manner from massive doses.

In our studies, after the peak values of gamma radiation were attained there was a comparatively slow and gradual decline of the blood radioactivity. This rather slow disappearance was in marked contrast to the rapid clearance after parenteral administration previously reported. Conley and associates (122), using a microbiological method, were unable to demonstrate increased serum vitamin B$_{12}$ concentrations six hours after the intravenous administration of 1,000 μg of vitamin B$_{12}$. Mollin *et al.* (437) injected intravenously 1.5 μg doses of Co^{58}-labeled vitamin B$_{12}$ and found a rapid clearance of plasma radioactivity. Indeed, 50 per cent had disappeared in 0.3 to 0.9 hours. After 10 hours only 5 to 29 per cent of the peak activity remained, with an average of approximately 17.5 per cent. Our plasma clearance curves after oral administration of physiologic doses were strikingly different. If we accept the 10-hour value as close to the highest concentration, 14 hours later from 43.6 to 92.0 per cent with an average of 68.1 per cent of the peak radioactivity persisted in the plasma in 13 control subjects (Tables 32 and 33). Similar figures were found with the larger test dose (Table 34) when whole blood samples were counted, and in 2 patients with pernicious anemia when IFC was added to the oral test dose of vitamin B$_{12}$ (patient P.L., Table 33, and patient F.McA., Table 34).

The 8-hour plasma radioactivity ranged from 19 to 47 cpm with an average of 38 cpm. Assuming that the Co^{60} remained with the vitamin, this corresponded to from 1.9 to 4.7 $\mu\mu$g vitamin B$_{12}$ per ml. of plasma with an average of 3.8 $\mu\mu$g. This was equal to approximately 1.0 per cent of the total concentration of vitamin B$_{12}$ present in serum which averaged 337 $\mu\mu$g per ml. in 48 tests in our laboratory.

Assuming an average plasma volume of approximately 2,800 ml. (444), it can be determined from Tables 32 and 33 that the plasma radioactivity at its peak was only 2 per cent of the amount given (230,000 cpm). This figure was in contrast to the average of 11.7 per cent we were able to flush out in the urine on the second day of the studies. It is also of interest that we were able to detect definite radioactivity in the plasma 24 hours after such a flushing procedure. It is apparent, then, that only a fraction of the absorbed vitamin was present in the circulating blood at a given moment.

The relatively late accumulation of radioactivity in the plasma, the slow clearance from the plasma, the fact that five to six times more radioactivity was excreted in the urine on the second day of the experiments than was circulating at the peak of the radioactivity, and the finding of definite radioactivity in the plasma even after such a flushing procedure may all be taken as evidence of a prolonged influx of radioactivity into the blood stream after oral administration of physiologic amounts of vitamin B_{12}. A slow transport of the vitamin through the intestinal wall with gradual release into the blood could explain all of these phenomena, although alternative explanations are possible.

Nine patients with pernicious anemia were examined and in all instances we were able to separate them from the control subjects. The plasma counts obtained in 7 given the smaller test dose ranged from 2 to 8 cpm, while the normals given a similar test dose had activity ranging from 19 to 54 cpm. When IFC was added to the test dose the patients with pernicious anemia had plasma radioactivity ranging from 22 to 44 cpm. In the eighth case whole blood was examined, and here also a good differentiation from normals was obtained. The ninth case was tested with the larger test dose and revealed a maximum plasma radioactivity of 11 cpm. With the addition of IFC the radioactivity increased to 53 cpm. The three control subjects given a similar test dose had peak plasma activity ranging from 56 to 108 cpm.

Although we had no difficulty in separating control subjects from patients with pernicious anemia, 4 of the 9 latter nevertheless had activity in the plasma slightly above three times the standard deviation of the background, while the rest had less activity. We interpret this finding as evidence for slight absorption of vitamin B_{12}. An additional confirmation of this opinion is the fact that in all but 1 case we were able to detect a definite but subnormal amount of radioactivity in the urine after a "flushing" parenteral dose of 1,000 μg non-radioactive vitamin B_{12} given 24 hours after the start of the test. Over the past few years it has become increasingly evident that patients with pernicious anemia can absorb small but insufficient amounts of vitamin B_{12} (435). Our findings are in agreement with this opinion.

Smaller scintillation counters have a higher absolute efficiency and it was therefore expected that they also could be used for counting purposes. Our failure to detect radioactivity in the 4 ml. counter when whole blood was used (Table 36) must be ascribed to the diluent effect of the red blood cells and the fact that their presence makes it difficult to ensure a homogeneous mixture of whole blood. The activity obtained with the smaller counters is of a lower magnitude, thus reducing the margin of accuracy when work is done with such small quantities of radioactivity. The availability of Co^{58} and Co^{56} with half-lives of 72 days in contrast to 5.3 years for Co^{60} will permit the use of larger test doses. Indeed, we have been able to obtain the same average activity in 4 ml. of plasma after an oral test dose of 2 μc Co^{58} (2.5 μg B_{12}) as with 20 ml. plasma after 0.5 μc Co^{60}-labeled vitamin B_{12}.

Since the direct measurement of radioactivity in the plasma has differentiated between normal subjects and patients with pernicious anemia, it appears to have certain advantages in the diagnosis of this disease. The test is easy to perform, requires less cooperation from the patient in comparison with the Heinle and the Schilling methods, and the result can be obtained within 12 hours. There is no interference with the bone-marrow morphology, since no parenteral vitamin B_{12} is given and the test dose is less than the daily intake of vitamin B_{12} on a normal diet.

Comparison of the Plasma Absorption Method and the Schilling Test *

The purpose of this study was to compare the efficacy of the plasma absorption and urinary excretion tests in a number of patients with pernicious anemia and control subjects. At the same time comparisons were made between 6- and 8-hour plasma samples and between 2- and 24-hour urine collections. The oral test doses, 0.56 μg B_{12} containing 0.5 μc Co^{60}, were administered to the fasting subjects at 8 A.M. Blood samples were collected at 6 and 8 hours. The "flushing" parenteral dose of 1 mg. non-labeled vitamin B_{12} was given immediately after the 6-hour blood sample was taken. Urine was collected quantitatively for 24 hours from the time the parenteral dose was administered. The radioactivity was determined on the 2-hour urine sample obtained between 6 and 8 hours and on the subsequent 22-hour collection. The 24-hour urinary excretion of radioactivity in each case is the sum of these two individual determinations.

The results obtained in 42 control subjects and 14 patients with Addison's pernicious anemia are shown in Table 38. The averages with their standard deviations and ranges for all four measurements are tabulated. The differences between the mean values for each of the four measurements in the two groups are statistically significant (p < 0.01). The 8-hour plasma absorption and the 24-hour urinary radioactivity values furthermore revealed no overlap between the two groups. The 6-hour plasma and the 2-hour urine tests, however, showed overlap in 4 and 6 subjects respectively. Under the experimental conditions

* An abstract of this section, by Doscherholmen and Hagen, appeared in J. Lab. Clin. Med., 52:809, 1958, published by the C. V. Mosby Company, St. Louis (159).

Table 38. Results of the Plasma-Absorption and Urinary Excretion Tests after Oral Dose of 0.56 μg $Co^{60}B_{12}$ (0.5 μc), with 1 mg. "Cold" B_{12} Given Intramuscularly 6 Hours after Oral Dose

| Test Subjects | No. | Plasma Absorption, μμg $Co^{60}B_{12}$/ml. | | | | Urinary Radioactivity, % of Oral Dose | | | |
| | | 6 Hr. | | 8 Hr. | | 2-Hr. Test | | 24-Hr. Test | |
		Range	Mean S.D.	Range	Mean S.D.	Range	Mean S.D.	Range	Mean S.D.
Control subjects	42	0.9–10.4	3.6 ± 1.9	3.2–15.1	8.0 ± 2.8	0.3–10.9	3.2 ± 2.0	13.2–48.2	28.9 ± 8.5
Pernicious anemia without IFC....	14	0–1.5	0.4 ± 0.4	0–2.3	0.7 ± 0.6	0–0.6	0.2 ± 0.2	0.2–7.2	2.2 ± 2.0
Pernicious anemia with IFC	14	0.4–3.9	2.0 ± 1.0	0.7–7.3	5.0 ± 1.9	0.4–5.0	2.1 ± 1.3	4.1–35.3	23.2 ± 10.4

109

of this study the 8-hour plasma absorption was just as valuable as the 24-hour urine test in the diagnosis of malabsorption of cyanocobalamin. The 6-hour plasma absorption was just as valuable as the 2-hour urine test, but both were inferior to the 8-hour plasma and the 24-hour urine tests in the diagnosis of vitamin B$_{12}$ malabsorption states.

The 14 patients with malabsorption of vitamin B$_{12}$ had the tests repeated with the addition of 1 USP unit of IFC. The averages of these tests with their standard deviations and ranges are also given in Table 38 and the individual results with and without IFC are found in Fig. 2. Great improvement was observed in the average values of all four measurements after the addition of IFC (Table 38), although the individual response varied greatly (Fig. 2). If one studies closer the results of the two most discriminating measurements, namely the 8-hour plasma and the 24-hour urine tests, it becomes apparent that IFC increased the 8-hour plasma values in all instances. In two of them, however (Nos. 8 and 13, Fig. 2), it failed to raise the level above 3.2 $\mu\mu$g per ml. plasma which was the lower normal limit found in the control subjects, while in three of them (Nos. 8, 10, and 13) it failed to raise the 24-hour urine value above 13.2 per cent, the lower normal limit in the control group. There was no clinical evidence of sprue or steatorrhea in these three patients and no known premedication with heterologous intrinsic factor

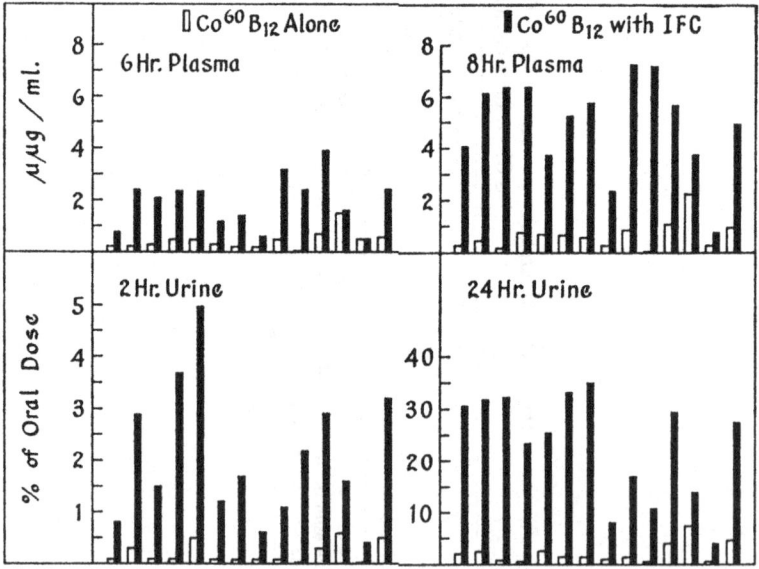

Figure 2. Radioactive B$_{12}$ of plasma and urine in patients with Addison's pernicious anemia with and without intrinsic factor concentrate; oral dose 0.56 μg B$_{12}$ (0.5 μc Co^{60}); 1 mg. "cold" B$_{12}$ given 6 hours after oral dose.

concentrate to explain the below-average response to the intrinsic factor. Their subnormal response to IF may indicate a latent intestinal absorption defect that was unrecognized or it may represent a more extreme variation in the normal response to heterologous intrinsic factor. The findings bring to mind the unexplained variation in the absorption gradient in patients with Addison's pernicious anemia described by Baker and Mollin (20), and by Callender and Evans (81).

From Table 38 it is evident that approximately two thirds of control subjects will show 2-hour urinary radioactivities between 1.2 and 5.2 per cent of the ingested dose. Half of the remainder would be expected to show 2-hour urinary radioactivities below 1.2 per cent. In fact, in the present control series four subjects had values below this figure. Because carbamylcholine chloride has been found to stimulate the secretion of intrinsic factor in control subjects with low absorption of vitamin B_{12} but not in patients with Addison's pernicious anemia (436), it was decided to test the effect of this stimulant in the subjects with low 2-hour urinary excretion values. Consequently, the absorption tests were repeated with 0.25 mg. of this substance given intramuscularly immediately before the oral test dose was administered to three of the above-mentioned subjects (W.P., L.D., and P.I., Fig. 3). The fourth subject (C.D.) suffered from emphysema and since it was

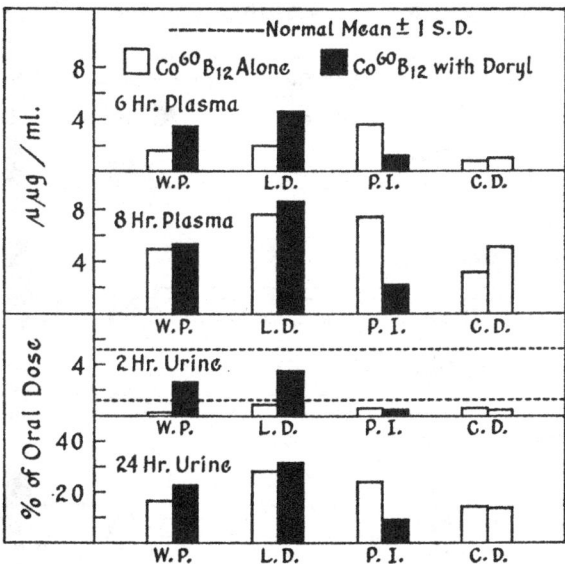

Figure 3. Radioactive B_{12} of plasma and urine in control subjects with and without carbamylcholine chloride (Doryl[R]); oral dose 0.56 μg B_{12} (0.5 μc Co⁶⁰); 1 mg. "cold" B_{12} given intramuscularly 6 hours after oral dose.

found unadvisable to administer a parasympathetic stimulant to such a patient, he had the absorption test repeated without the addition of this drug. The results show that in subjects W.P. and L.D. there was improvement in all four measurements of the B$_{12}$ absorption, although the greatest increase was in the 6-hour plasma and the 2-hour urine values. In the third subject, P.I., there was, if anything, a decrease in the absorption of vitamin B$_{12}$ with carbamylcholine chloride. In the fourth subject, C.D., no essential change took place when the test was repeated. In certain control subjects it seems therefore that carbamylcholine chloride stimulates the absorption of cyanocobalamin.

Vitamin B$_{12}$ absorption was also tested in five of the patients with Addison's pernicious anemia after stimulation with carbamylcholine chloride. The results obtained with and without this stimulation are shown in Fig. 4. In three of the patients, J.M., H.P. and A.M., the addition of this drug effected no change in any of the measurements of absorption. When the labeled vitamin B$_{12}$ only was given to patient J.S. all four measurements of absorption were abnormally low. However, with the addition of carbamylcholine chloride they were all raised to the border zone between definite normal and abnormal values. Borderline values in this respect are those below two S.D. of the mean in the control group and above two S.D. of the mean in the pernicious anemia group. The border zone for the 8-hour plasma and the 24-hour urine values lies between the interrupted and the continuous horizon-

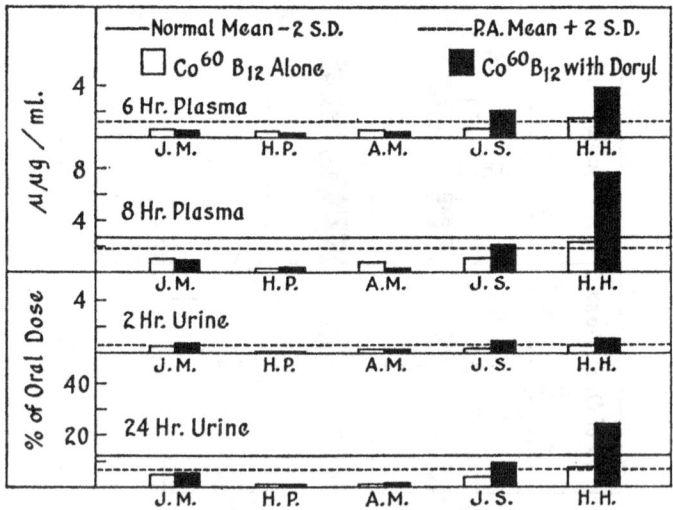

Figure 4. Radioactive B$_{12}$ of plasma and urine in patients with Addison's pernicious anemia with and without carbamylcholine chloride (Doryl^R); oral dose 0.56 µg B$_{12}$ (0.5 µc Co^{60}); 1 mg. "cold" B$_{12}$ given intramuscularly 6 hours after oral dose.

tal lines in Fig. 4. One subject, H.H., showed borderline absorption when the labeled vitamin was administered alone, while all four measurements of absorption became normal with the addition of carbamylcholine chloride. Both of these subjects (J.S. and H.H.) had histamine-fast achlorhydria, macrocytic anemia with megaloblastic bone marrow, and low serum vitamin B_{12} concentrations of 70 and 58 $\mu\mu g$ per ml.; both responded to parenteral vitamin B_{12} treatment.

It is believed that both J.S. and H.H. suffered from vitamin B_{12} deficiency. The nutritional history did not indicate a pure dietary type of B_{12} avitaminosis. Since the absorption of cyanocobalamin was impaired and could be corrected with intrinsic factor these patients were believed to suffer from Addison's pernicious anemia. If the secretion of intrinsic factor under conditions of normal food intake was as low as observed when vitamin B_{12} was given alone, it is quite understandable that the absorption of cyanocobalamin was inadequate and gradually led to a depletion of the body's stores of the vitamin. Their ability to secrete IF was not totally lost, however, as shown by the results after stimulation with carbamylcholine chloride.

Apparently there are varying degrees of secretion of intrinsic factor. On the one hand is the completely normal individual with abundant secretion of this factor; on the other is the patient who secretes none. Between these extremes all degrees of secretion exist. An analogy may be made between the secretion of IF and hydrochloric acid in this respect. It has been known for many years that patients with Addison's pernicious anemia do not completely lack intrinsic factor (236, 237). The present study clearly shows the great variation in the ability to absorb cyanocobalamin among patients with Addison's pernicious anemia. Indirectly this means a great variation in the secretion of intrinsic factor. Furthermore, the study also shows that by proper stimulation, the intrinsic factor production can be increased considerably in certain instances of pernicious anemia.

If carbamylcholine chloride stimulation of the IF production had been accepted as a routine procedure in the plasma absorption test or the Schilling test, the diagnosis of Addison's pernicious anemia would have been missed in subject H.H. and the result would have been difficult to interpret in patient J.S. It is therefore believed that routine use of this drug in the plasma absorption test or the urinary excretion method is not advisable.

The correlations of the four measurements of absorption were also studied. In Table 39 the correlation coefficient has been given for the observations in the control group. The standard error for these r-values is 0.15. Positive correlations existed among all four measurements of

Table 39. Correlations among 4 Measurements of the Absorption of B_{12} in 42 Control Subjects: Oral Dose 0.56 µg $Co^{60}B_{12}$ (0.5 µc), with 1 mg. "Cold" B_{12} Given Intramuscularly 6 Hours after Oral Dose

Measurements	Correlation Coefficient, r-Value
6-hour plasma versus 8-hour plasma	+0.81
6-hour plasma versus 24-hour urine	+0.66
2-hour urine versus 24-hour urine	+0.63
8-hour plasma versus 24-hour urine	+0.53
6-hour plasma versus 2-hour urine	+0.48
8-hour plasma versus 2-hour urine	+0.34

absorption since all r-values exceeded 2 standard errors. Best correlation was found between the 6- and 8-hour plasma values and the poorest between the 8-hour plasma and the 2-hour urine values.

The 8-hour plasma absorption value obtained 2 hours after a parenteral dose of 1 mg. non-labeled vitamin B_{12} averaged 8.0 µµg/ml. (S.D. 2.8 µµg/ml.) in the 42 control subjects in this series. This figure was significantly higher than the average value of 4.7 µµg/ml. (S.D. = 1.5 µµg/ml.) plasma observed in 100 different control subjects who did not receive any parenteral injection before the 8-hour plasma sample was obtained (p < 0.01). In 9 patients with pernicious anemia who received similar oral doses but no parenteral injections, the average 8-hour plasma absorption figures were 0.5 and 3.8 µµg/ml. without and with IFC. Thus it appears that the "flushing" dose resulted in increased plasma radioactivity. This subject is dealt with in more detail later.

Results of the Plasma Absorption Test Using 0.56 µg Cyanocobalamin Containing 0.25 µc Co^{60}

When radioactive isotopes are used for diagnostic purposes, it is imperative to use as small a dose as possible in order to keep the body's burden of radioactivity at a minimum. This is especially important when one is dealing with an isotope with a long physiologic half-life, such as Co^{60}. On the other hand, if too small a test dose is used, the accuracy of the test may suffer. The problem then is to find the smallest dose that will still give reliable results with the equipment at hand. With this principle in mind, it was decided to test the plasma absorption with half the amount of radioactivity used in the study just described. The amount of vitamin B_{12} in the test dose was not altered.

The present study includes 37 control subjects and 10 patients with Addison's pernicious anemia, all of whom received the oral dose of 0.56 µg B_{12} containing 0.25 µc Co^{60} after an overnight fast followed by an intramuscular injection of 1 mg. non-labeled cyanocobalamin 6 hours

Table 40. Results of the 8-Hour Plasma-Absorption Test after Oral Dose of 0.56 µg $Co^{60}B_{12}$ (0.25 µc), with 1 mg. "Cold" B_{12} Given Intramuscularly 6 Hours after Oral Dose to Subjects in Group A Only

| Test Subject | No. | 8-Hr. Plasma Absorption, µµg $Co^{60}B_{12}$/ml. | | |
		Average	S.D.	Range
		Group A		
Control subjects	37	7.6	2.4	4.5–16.1
Pernicious anemia without IFC	10	0.2	0.3	0–0.7
Pernicious anemia with IFC	10	5.0	2.3	2.0–10.4
		Group B		
Control subjects	20	4.6	1.4	1.9–7.1

later. Peripheral venous blood was taken 8 hours after the oral doses were given. In addition, the 8-hour plasma absorption was also recorded in 20 control subjects, each of whom received a similar oral test dose but no parenteral injection.

Table 40 shows the averages, standard deviations, and ranges for the 8-hour plasma absorption values in the subjects who received the parenteral injections. The results are essentially the same as found in the previous study (Table 38). Thus the average control value was 7.6 µµg/ml. in the present group as compared with 8.0 µµg/ml. in the group that received twice as much radioactivity. Patients with Addison's pernicious anemia in the present study showed average values of 0.2 and 5.0 µµg/ml. without and with IFC while the corresponding figures were 0.7 and 5.0 when twice as much radioactivity was administered.

Since there was no overlap between the control group and patients with pernicious anemia in the present study, it is evident that the plasma absorption technique can be used even with as little radioactivity as 0.25 µc Co^{60} in the oral test dose.

The average 8-hour plasma absorption value in the 20 control subjects who did not receive parenteral injections in this study was 4.6 µµg/ml., range 1.9 to 7.1 µµg/ml. (Table 40, Group B). In other words, the difference in the 8-hour plasma values with and without parenteral injections mentioned in the previous section (p. 114) was also reproduced in this study.

From this study it was concluded that the plasma absorption test can be used successfully in the diagnosis of pernicious anemia with as little as 0.25 µc Co^{60} in the 0.56 µg B_{12} oral test dose. The parenteral dose given 6 hours after the oral ingestion of the labeled cyanocobalamin is not needed for a successful separation of control subjects from patients with pernicious anemia, but it had the advantage of increasing the circulating radiocyanocobalamin in control subjects by an average of 65 per cent in the present series and by 70 per cent in that of the preceding section. It remains for future studies to determine whether even smaller doses of radioactivity can be used successfully in the plasma absorption test.

Scintillation Spectrometry of $Co^{57}B_{12}$ in the Diagnosis of Pernicious Anemia *

In the preceding three sections the values for the absorption were obtained by measuring the radioactivity in 20 ml. volumes of plasma. Because many laboratories are equipped only with smaller scintillation detectors and since the volume of blood needed to obtain 20 ml. of plasma may seem large and objectionable, the decision was made to work out a satisfactory method using only 4 ml. of plasma. For this purpose scintillation spectrometry of Co^{57}-labeled cyanocobalamin was chosen. The unique energy spectrum of Co^{57} with a single photo peak makes it extremely well suited for differential counting (170, 538). By excluding all impulses coming from the spectrum outside the area where the Co^{57}-peak was located, it was possible to reduce the background count from approximately 190 cpm to 10 cpm with a simultaneous loss of 46.2 per cent of the experimental counts. Since the background count was reduced by 95 per cent the small experimental counts should become more significant.

For the scintillation spectrometry we used a previously described 4 ml. well scintillation detector (24) with a model 172 Nuclear Chicago scaler without internal amplifier. The pulse height analyzer (Model 115, Radiation Instrument and Development Laboratory) with an internal amplifier with a gain of 125 was set at a channel width (window) of 7 volts and channel level (threshold) of 12 volts. Each vial was counted twice with a preset count of 640 and the average cpm used. Four unknown samples were preceded and followed by a background count. The average of these was used as the true background count for the 4 experimental counts. Integral counting was also performed on 4 ml. plasma with the same equipment with no window and with a channel level of 7 volts. Integral counting was furthermore carried out on 4 ml. samples of plasma in the 20 ml. well counter for comparison. For the integral counting the counting time was 1 hour for the smaller detector and 10,000 preset counts for the 20 ml. counter.

* This section is adapted from Doscherholmen, Vitamin B_{12} und Intrinsic Factor, 2. Europäisches Symposion, Hamburg, 1961, Ferdinand Enke Verlag, Stuttgart, 345, 1962 (154).

Ten control subjects and four patients with malabsorption of cyan-ocobalamin are included in this series. Three of the latter suffered from Addison's pernicious anemia in remission and one had undergone a total gastrectomy for carcinoma of the stomach. An oral test dose of 0.56 μg vitamin B_{12} containing 0.5 μc Co^{57} was given to each subject at 8 A.M. after an overnight fast and breakfast was served 2 hours later. A 4 P.M. plasma sample was obtained from an antecubital vein. One mg. "cold" cyanocobalamin was injected intravenously through the same needle immediately after the 8-hour blood sample was obtained. At 5 P.M. a second venous blood sample was taken from the other arm. A preliminary study on two control subjects given 0.56 μg vitamin B_{12} containing 3.42 μc Co^{57} had shown that the absorption values reached their peaks 1 and 2 hours after the 4 P.M. injections (Table 41). It was decided to draw the second blood sample in the experimental subjects in the present series at 5 P.M. because the post-injection values should then be at or near their maximum. The values of the second plasma sample in these subjects represent an augmented plasma absorption test.

The results are shown in Tables 42 and 43. With differential counting the background counts ranged from 9 to 11 cpm and the experimental counts in the 8-hour plasma samples from the 10 control subjects ranged from 6 to 20 cpm with an average of 13 cpm. In the augmented plasma absorption test the corresponding figures ranged from 11 to 41 with an average of 23 cpm. With integral counting in the 4 ml. detector the background count ranged from 185 to 193 cpm and the radioactivity in the 8-hour plasma samples in the control subjects varied from 12 to 37 with an average of 24 cpm. In the augmented plasma absorption test the corresponding figures were 21 and 70 with an average of 43 cpm. The integral counting in the 20 ml. detector showed from 10 to 37, average 23 cpm, in the 8-hour plasma samples in the control subjects while the corresponding figures in the augmented plasma absorption test ranged from 25 to 72 cpm with an average of 44 cpm. Thus the augmented plasma absorption test showed an almost 100 per cent increase

Table 41. Plasma-Absorption Values in 2 Control Subjects after Oral Dose of 0.56 μg $Co^{57}B_{12}$ (3.42 μc), with 1 mg. "Cold" B_{12} Given Intravenously Immediately after the 8-Hour Blood Sampling

	Radioactivity, cpm/20 ml. Plasma at Different Numbers of Hours after Oral Dose						
Subject	8	8.25	8.5	8.75	9	10	12
1	337	494	552	582	583	571	460
2	249	402	424	464	475	530	437

Table 42. Plasma Absorption 8 and 9 Hours after Ingestion of 0.56 µg $Co^{57}B_{12}$ (0.5 µc), with 1 mg. "Cold" B_{12} Given Intravenously Immediately after the 8-Hour Blood Sampling

Patient	Radioactivity, cpm/4 ml. Plasma					
	4 ml. Well Counter				20 ml. Well Counter	
	8-Hr. Plasma		9-Hr. Plasma		8-Hr. Plasma	9-Hr. Plasma
	Integral	Diff.	Integral	Diff.	Integral	Integral
Control Subjects						
J.A.	37	20	70	41	37	72
F.W.	12	10	29	15	13	28
A.F.	22	14	37	22	23	34
J.M.	15	9	21	16	10	25
G.O.	22	8	43	18	20	42
G.S.	31	14	52	23	29	54
A.H.	13	6	26	11	14	28
D.A.	26	17	51	30	31	57
H.B.	23	10	45	23	21	43
J.C.	34	17	56	33	36	60
Average	24	13	43	23	23	44
Pernicious Anemia						
B.S.	0	0	0	0	0	0
B.S.*	20	11	40	18	25	47
L.M.	0	0	0	0	2	0
L.M.*	14	6	26	12	17	26
W.H.	0	1	0	2	2	4
W.H.*	16	7	30	14	13	26
Total Gastrectomy						
C.C.	2	1	1	0	0	0
C.C.*	18	10	28	15	17	31

(From Doscherholmen: Scintillation spectrometry of Co^{57}-vitamin B_{12} in the diagnosis of pernicious anemia. Vitamin B_{12} und Intrinsic Factor, 2. Europäisches Symposion, Hamburg, 1961, Ferdinand Enke Verlag, Stuttgart, 345, 1962.)
* 1 USP unit intrinsic factor concentrate administered.

Table 43. Plasma Absorption of $Co^{57}B_{12}$ in 10 Control Subjects, Comparison between the Results Obtained by Integral and Differential Counting Techniques

	Type of Counting	$Co^{57}B_{12}$, µµg/ml. Plasma			
		8-Hr. Plasma		9-Hr. Plasma	
		Average	Range	Average	Range
4 ml. detector.......	integral	3.6	1.8–5.6	6.6	3.2–10.7
4 ml. detector.......	differential	3.5	1.7–5.6	6.5	3.1–11.5
20 ml. detector.......	integral	3.7	1.6–5.8	7.0	3.9–11.3

(From Doscherholmen: Scintillation spectrometry of Co^{57}-vitamin B_{12} in the diagnosis of pernicious anemia. Vitamin B_{12} und Intrinsic Factor, 2. Europäisches Symposion, Hamburg, 1961, Ferdinand Enke Verlag, Stuttgart, 345, 1962.)

in the average radioactivity over and above the average 8-hour plasma absorption values.

In the three patients with pernicious anemia and the one with total gastrectomy no amount or negligible amounts of radioactivity were present in the plasma samples and no overlap occurred in the counting between them and the control group. Differential counting was just as discriminatory as integral counting in this regard. When the tests were repeated in these four patients with the addition of one unit IFC, the plasma values were all within the range found in the control subjects.

Table 43 shows the averages and ranges for the absorption values expressed in $\mu\mu g$ per ml. of plasma. Generally speaking, there was good agreement regarding the plasma content of $Co^{57}B_{12}$ whether the counting was performed by integral or differential counting.

This study shows that the plasma absorption test can be used successfully in the diagnosis of vitamin B_{12} malabsorption states with the use of as little as 0.5 μc Co^{57} and 4 ml. of plasma. With the augmented plasma absorption test it should be possible to make the diagnosis with half this amount of radioactivity or plasma. Integral or differential counting can be used with equal success. Scintillation spectrometry may be preferred because it results in such stable and low background counts.

The purpose of this study was to show that the plasma absorption test could be performed successfully with the average equipment in an isotope laboratory and on a reasonable amount of plasma. The oldest equipment available was used, in order to rule out the need for additional investment in new and expensive equipment. Initially no great effort was made to find a setting that would give the greatest reduction in the background count with the smallest loss of experimental counts. Subsequent investigations showed that a window width of 9 volts would have been slightly more ideal than the 7 volts originally chosen (Table 44). With the use of newer equipment and a window width of 9 volts, better results than those obtained might have been possible. Although

Table 44. Counting Efficiency as a Function of Window Width

Window Width (volts)	$Co^{57}B_{12}$ (net cpm)	Background (cpm)	Efficiency (%)	Figure of Merit $\times 10^6$
1	4,216	3	8	5.9
3	11,891	6	23	23.6
5	19,471	10	38	37.9
7	27,136	13	53	56.6
9	34,362	17	67	69.5
∞	51,491	200	100	13.3

the results of the differential counting may not have been the best obtainable, it was gratifying to find such a good separation of the two groups of patients.

Results in Patients with Partial and Total Gastrectomy

A number of patients with gastric resection or gastrectomy had impaired vitamin B_{12} absorption as judged by the Schilling test (44, 68, 349, 372A, 372, 379, 507, 558–560), the Heinle test (17, 86, 182, 270, 272, 278, 366, 378, 611, 629), and the Glass test (214, 219, 231). This impaired absorption of cyanocobalamin may lead to vitamin B_{12} deficiency both in total (497) and partial (393) gastrectomy in the same way as the impaired absorption of cyanocobalamin leads to vitamin B_{12} deficiency in pernicious anemia (598). Consequently it was decided to evaluate the absorption of cyanocobalamin with the plasma absorption method in a group of such patients. Ten subjects who had undergone various types of gastrectomy prior to the test were given oral test doses of 0.56 μg vitamin B_{12} containing 0.5 μc Co^{60}. In each instance an 8-hour blood sample was obtained for radioactivity measurements. Immediately after the blood was drawn, 1 mg. "cold" vitamin B_{12} was administered intramuscularly and the urine was collected for 24 hours thereafter. Thus the plasma absorption as well as the urinary excretion tests were performed in this series. A week later the test was repeated in a similar manner in eight of the patients but with the addition of one USP unit of hog stomach intrinsic factor concentrate to the oral test dose of the labeled vitamin. The results of the radioactivity measurement of the plasma and urine samples (Table 45) show a very good correlation between the two parameters of absorption (r = 0.91). And, as the table also shows, low urinary excretion figures correlated well with low plasma values.

Of the first seven patients, who had partial gastrectomy, five showed normal absorption of cyanocobalamin without the addition of IFC. In one of these (H.C.) IFC improved the absorption figures, in two (S.D. and L.T.) the addition of this factor resulted in somewhat lowered absorption values. Patient S.K. showed low absorption figures shortly after being admitted for psychogenic diarrhea. When the test was repeated a week later, borderline plasma and urinary excretion values were observed. With IFC the urine and plasma tests both were within the normal range. Subject B.M. had undergone partial gastrectomy and also suffered from a transverse myelitis. This latter occurred suddenly the year prior to admission when he had an operation for an abscess of the spine at the level of the 7th–8th thoracic vertebrae. Both measurements indicated no or negligible absorption of vitamin B_{12} without, but

Table 45. Plasma Absorption and 24-hour Urinary Excretion Values in Patients with Various Types of Gastrectomy: Oral Dose 0.56 µg Co⁶⁰B₁₂ (0.5 µc), with 1 mg. "Cold" B₁₂ Given Intramuscularly 8 Hours after Oral Dose

| | | | Radioactivity | | | |
| | | | Plasma, cpm/20 ml. | | 24-Hour Urine, % of Oral Dose | |
Patient	Age	Type of Operation	Without IFC	With IFC*	Without IFC	With IFC*
J.M.	64	Billroth II, 75% gastric resection	60		22.6	
S.D.	62	Billroth II, subtotal gastric resection	53	44	28.9	25.6
R.F.	36	segmental gastric resection	49		24.6	
H.C.	68	Billroth II, 75% gastric resection	40	61	17.8	32.5
L.T.	67	gastric resection	29	18	13.8	7.9
S.K.	27	Billroth II, 75% gastric resection	1		2.5	
S.K.	27	Billroth II, 75% gastric resection	12	32	10.9	21.8
B.M.	60	subtotal gastrectomy	9	49	1.2	17.3
F.C.	70	esophagectomy, gastrectomy, duodenectomy, feeding antrostomy	11	33	2.8	9.6
P.T.	63	total gastrectomy	8	17	0.1	5.1
C.J.	62	total gastrectomy	7	50	0.1	15.4

*One USP unit of hog-stomach intrinsic factor concentrate.

121

normal absorption with, intrinsic factor. Vitamin B$_{12}$ therapy given parenterally did not influence his transverse myelitis.

One patient (F.C.) had undergone esophagectomy, duodenectomy, and almost complete gastrectomy. Only a small part of antrum was left behind and used as a feeding antrostomy. This patient had practically no absorption of cyanocobalamin unless intrinsic factor was added. The last two patients (P.T. and C.J.) had both had total gastrectomy. They showed negligible absorption of labeled vitamin B$_{12}$ when the vitamin was administered alone. Both tests showed, however, considerable improvement in the absorption when IFC was supplied.

The conclusion drawn from these tests is that the plasma test gives just as valuable information about the ability to absorb cyanocobalamin as does the urinary excretion test in subjects with various types of gastrectomy.

Results in Patients with Leukemia

Patients with acute and chronic myelogenous leukemia have been found to have increased vitamin B$_{12}$ serum concentrations (26, 27, 178, 342, 443A, 510, 512) and an increased in-vitro (26, 405, 414, 437, 443A, 510) and in-vivo (69, 131, 179, 180, 264, 265, 295, 296, 404, 437, 536, 600) binding capacity for cyanocobalamin. These findings might be attributed to the presence in the blood stream of an increased amount of the normal B$_{12}$-binding protein or to an abnormal protein circulating in the blood of these patients. Most observations are in favor of a quantitative alteration in the B$_{12}$-binding protein in the blood from patients with chronic myeloid leukemia (394, 418, 419), although qualitative differences are not yet completely ruled out (265).

The plasma absorption of vitamin B$_{12}$ following the oral administration of radiocyanocobalamin to patients with leukemia has not been given proper attention as yet. Mollin and Ross (443B) measured the plasma radioactivity in one patient with chronic myeloid leukemia after the oral administration of 1 μg vitamin B$_{12}$ containing 5 μc Co^{56} and found the peak value 24 hours after the oral dose was given as compared with 8–12 hours in control subjects. Since only one subject with leukemia was included in this report, it was thought worthwhile to investigate the plasma absorption of cyanocobalamin from the gut in a group of patients with myeloid leukemia as well as other types of leukemia and make comparison with the absorption pattern in normal subjects and patients with non-leukemic neutrophilic leukocytosis. This study includes six patients with chronic myeloid, fourteen with chronic lymphatic and nine with acute or subacute myeloid leukemia, and fourteen control subjects. Three of the latter had non-leukemic neutrophilic

Table 46. Laboratory Data on 29 Male Patients with Leukemia and 3 Male Patients with Non-Leukemic Leukocytosis

Patient	Age	Diag.*	Hgb.	WBC	N	L	M	E	B	Platelet	Retic. (%)	Serum B$_{12}$, $\mu\mu g$/ml. Free	Serum B$_{12}$, $\mu\mu g$/ml. Total	Maximum Co^{60}B$_{12}$, $\mu\mu g$/ml.	Therapy At time of Co^{60}B$_{12}$ Test	Therapy Previously
										Chronic Myeloid Leukemia						
V.O.	66	C	15.5	69,000	80	12		2	6	328,000	...	...	...	7.5	None for leuk.	X-ray to spleen
V.L.	68	C	10.7	19,200	88	8		4		177,000	6.1	280	800	7.6	6-mercaptopurine; prednisone	X-ray to spleen; 6-mercaptopurine; prednisone; busulfan
E.C.	73	AC	8.9	84,000	85	5		4	6	133,000	1.0	...	...	16.3	X-ray to spleen	X-ray to spleen
H.H.	56	AC	8.0	570,000	85	3	6	6		101,000	3.2	...	...	15.8	Busulfan	Busulfan
V.P.	27	C	11.9	10,000	78	23	1	1		105,000	2.8	20	460	2.8	None for leuk.	Busulfan
J.M.	62	AC	11.2	15,900	93	4	2	1		91,000	3.4	0	528	10.2	None for leuk.	X-ray to spleen
										Chronic Lymphatic Leukemia						
R.A.	62	AC	9.0	83,000	8	97				1,000	5.2	25	145	2.1	Prednisone	X-ray to cervical, inguinal, and aortic nodes and spleen; chlorambucil
A.P.	69	C	11.4	19,000	22	75	8			185,000	5.0	0	90	1.6	None for leuk.	None for leuk.
M.O.	60	C	11.0	348,000	8	96	1			74,000	2.0	0	140	2.6	Chlorambucil	X-ray to rt. and lt. axilla, chest, and neck; spray X-ray; HN$_2$; P^{32}; chlorambucil
H.A.	47	C	10.0	199,000	5	95				56,000	2.2	48	155	4.0	Prednisone	Prednisone
E.F.	69	AC	14.6	11,500	26	73	1			46,000	3.3	80	258	3.5	X-ray to spleen	X-ray to spleen; chlorambucil
E.Y.	60	AC	7.6	735,000	1	99				25,000	3.3	...	...	3.0	Prednisone	X-ray to spleen and neck; prednisone; P^{32}
C.L.	45	AC	13.1	271,000	1	99				40,000	...	...	...	2.2	X-ray to spleen and mediastinum; prednisone	X-ray to neck and spleen; prednisone
H.B.	68	C	10.8	29,700	5	93	1	1		42,000	1.5	0	145	2.0	X-ray to spleen	X-ray to spleen
J.H.	64	AC	9.6	64,000	18	79		2		114,000	2.6	...	...	3.8	X-ray to inguinal regions	X-ray to cervical, inguinal and axillary nodes
E.K.	62	C	13.5	58,600	7	93				118,000	2.8	...	...	4.0	None for leuk.	None for leuk.
A.M.	66	C	11.6	211,000	3	97				120,000	1.0	...	...	2.0	None for leuk.	None for leuk.
C.L.	67	C	14.0	38,000	24	72	2			167,000	2.5	70	215	4.6	None for leuk.	None for leuk.
R.K.	64	C	9.2	42,000	3	97				80,000	8.0	10	110	2.9	X-ray to spleen	X-ray to spleen
I.W.	70	C	9.6	18,500	18	79	1	2		86,000	2.8	5	348	6.3	X-ray to inguinal regions	X-ray to cervical and inguinal areas

Table 46. (Continued)

Patient	Age	Diag.*	Hgb.	WBC	N	L	M	E	B	Platelet	Retic. (%)	Serum B12, μμg/ml		Maximum Co60B12, μμg/ml	Therapy	
												Free	Total		At time of Co60B12 Test	Previously
										Acute/Subacute Myeloid Leukemia						
W.W.	42	AC	6.8	153,000	90	9	7		1	18,000	3.8	43	235	2.7		Prednisone
E.F.	63	C	8.9	5,250	68	25				70,000	1.5	15	200	3.3	Prednisone	Prednisone; 6-mercaptopurine; methotrexate; methyl-prednisolone
O.V.	81	AC	8.0	30,000	67	29	8		1	25,000	0.1	200	348	2.0	Prednisone; 6-mercaptopurine	
J.V.	69	AC	7.7	1,800	13	88	1	1	2	22,000	0.4	155	3080	7.7	Prednisone	Prednisone; 6-mercaptopurine
S.J.	69	AC	7.8	1,250	22	75		3		14,000	0.1	103	240	1.2	Prednisone	Prednisone; 6-mercaptopurine
A.H.	19	AC	8.2	4,000	71	23	6			80,000	0.4	38	205	1.4	None for leuk.	Prednisone; 6-mercaptopurine
J.L.	39	C	9.2	67,000	93	4		3		20,000	1.7	0	370	8.0	None for leuk.	None for leuk.
J.R.	29	AC	11.1	40,600	85	15				9,000	0.4	…	…	5.2	Cortisone	Cortisone
J.B.	74	C	9.5	30,750	23	26		51		7,000	…	10	380	8.7	Prednisone	Prednisone
										Control Group						
M.P.	68	Carcinomatosis	11.6	38,000	96	4				…	…	3	318	1.7	Chlorpromazine hydrochloride	Prednisone; antibiotics; ACTH
P.C.	62	Pyelitis; heart failure	10.5	24,750	90	10				…	…	0	750	5.7	Digitoxin; thyroid extract; nitrofurantoin	Digitalis; thyroid extract
A.F.	38	Lung abscess; glomerulonephritis	9.4	19,000	88	9	1		2	…	…	20	240	2.6	Erythromycin	Several antibiotics
J.A.	78	Cerebral arteriosclerosis	14.0	11,550	69	30		1		…	…	60	375	4.7	None	None

*A = autopsy diagnosis, C = clinical diagnosis.
WBC = white blood count.
N = neutrophils.
L = lymphocytes.
M = monocytes.
E = eosinophils.
B = basophils.

leukocytosis. They all received an oral test dose of 0.56 μg vitamin B_{12} containing 0.5 μc Co^{60}. Blood was obtained at various time intervals up to one week after the oral dose was administered. Clinical data with blood values, serum vitamin B_{12} concentrations, maximum plasma absorption values and therapy are found in Table 46. Blood and serum vitamin B_{12} values are those obtained closest to the dates on which the B_{12} absorption tests were performed. Tables 47 to 52 show the contents of radioactive vitamin B_{12} in the plasma at various time intervals after the oral tests in the various groups.

The six patients with chronic myelogenous leukemia showed abnormal plasma absorption curves. In all of them it took a longer than normal time interval for the plasma radiocyanocobalamin to attain its maximum concentration. Thus the peak concentrations of radioactive vitamin B_{12} in the plasma were found in the 24–72 hour interval after the oral dose was administered (Table 47) instead of in the 8–12 hour period usually seen in control subjects (Table 48). The disappearance

Table 47. Plasma-Absorption Values in 6 Patients with Chronic Myelogenous Leukemia at Various Times after Oral Dose of 0.56 μg $Co^{60}B_{12}$ (0.5 μc)

Patient	$Co^{60}B_{12}$ in μμg/ml. Plasma at Specified Hours after Oral Dose									
	2	4	6	8	12	24	48	72	120	168
V.L.	0.5	0.6	2.3	5.1	5.9	7.6		6.4	5.1	4.4
V.O.		1.1		5.0	5.9	7.3		7.5	5.5	5.7
E.C.		0.2		6.5	10.7	16.3		14.7	13.8	11.6
H.H.		1.6		8.7	12.1	15.3		13.2	10.4	8.8
V.P.				2.0		2.8		2.5	2.4	
J.M.				7.9		10.2	9.7	7.8		
Average		0.9		5.9	8.7	9.9		8.7	7.4	7.6

Table 48. Plasma-Absorption Values of $Co^{60}B_{12}$ in 10 Control Subjects: Oral Dose 0.56 μg $Co^{60}B_{12}$ (0.5 μc)

Control Subject	$Co^{60}B_{12}$, μμg/ml. Plasma at Specified Hours after Ingestion									
	2	4	6	8	10	12	24	72	120	168
1	0.3	2.0	3.2	3.2	3.0	2.3	1.6	1.2	0.8	0.7
2	0.1	3.5	6.7	7.0	6.1	5.4	3.9	2.7	2.4	2.1
3	0.2	1.0	3.8	4.5	4.0	3.5	3.5	2.3	2.1	1.9
4	0.1	0.2	1.8	3.4	4.0	3.6	2.6	0.8	0.5	0.3
5	0.1	3.0	6.8	8.5	9.0	8.2	6.5	3.9	3.2	2.5
6	0	0.6	3.9	5.1	5.2	4.2	2.8	1.4	1.2	0.8
7	0.2	0.7	3.7	4.0	3.7	3.3	2.7	1.8	1.8	1.6
8	0	0.5	3.4	3.9	3.5	3.6	3.1	2.8	2.3	2.1
9	0	0.2	2.7	3.8	3.2	2.9	2.1	1.4	1.0	0.8
10	0.7	0.8	6.6	8.3	8.3	7.4	5.0	2.8	2.1	1.9
Average	0.2	1.3	4.3	5.2	5.0	4.4	3.4	2.1	1.7	1.5

Table 49. Comparison of the Absorption Indices in Patients with Various Types of Leukemia with Those of Control Subjects

Hours after Oral Dose	Control Subjects		Chronic Myeloid Leukemia		Chronic Lymphatic Leukemia		Acute and Subacute Myeloid Leukemia		Non-Leukemic Leukocytosis	
	Average	Range	Average	Range	Average	Range	Average	Range	Average	Range
24	64.8	50.0–79.5	165.1	129.1–250.8	62.6	47.5–85.0	89.0	25.0–176.2	76.5	70.2–82.4
72	41.1	23.5–71.8	146.2	98.7–226.2	31.6	19.0–57.9	54.9	5.0–157.1	43.6	31.6–52.9
120	33.0	14.7–59.0	132.4	100.0–212.3	27.6	13.8–42.3	48.4	18.2–133.3	43.4	21.1–70.6
168	28.6	8.8–53.8	120.0	86.3–178.5	22.0	5.0–42.1	45.5	6.1–128.6	31.2	21.1–41.2

rate of radioactivity from the plasma also seemed to be slower than normal in all instances.

The average 8-hour plasma absorption value in these 6 patients with chronic myeloid leukemia was 5.9 $\mu\mu$g/ml. of plasma which is close to the corresponding figure of 5.2 $\mu\mu$g/ml. found in the 10 control subjects (Table 48). Great differences were found, however, between the control subjects and the patients with chronic myeloid leukemia when all the later average absorption values were compared. Thus the leukemic patients showed average values that were two to five times higher than those obtained in the control subjects (Tables 47 and 48). Comparing the individual absorption figures obtained 24 hours or more after the oral dose only one of the 6 leukemic subjects (V.P.) had values within the normal range (Tables 47 and 48). Except for mild anemia this patient was in hematologic remission when the absorption test was performed. Although all of this patient's absorption values were low, the peak value was still found 24 hours after the oral test dose was given.

To give a numerical expression for the abnormality of the absorption curve a simple absorption index was devised: $A/B \times 100$, with A the plasma value for a specified time and B the 8-hour plasma value. The index values obtained 24, 72, 120, and 168 hours after the test doses were given are shown in Table 49, where they can be compared with the corresponding indices in control subjects and in the other types of leukemia. All cases of chronic myelogenous leukemia had abnormally high indices; no overlap occurred between them and the 10 controls.

The average absorption values for the 14 patients with chronic lymphatic leukemia (Table 50) were considerably lower than those for the 10 control subjects (Table 48) or the 6 patients with chronic myeloid leukemia (Table 47). The individual values in patients with chronic lymphatic leukemia were frequently below normal. Thus, eight of the fourteen values obtained 8 hours after the administration of the labeled vitamin B_{12} were below the lowest corresponding value in the 10 control subjects. The corresponding numbers of below-normal values at 24, 72, 120, and 168 hours were 4 of 14, 4 of 11, 3 of 8, and 1 of 8. Even though the averages and so many of the individual absorption values were abnormally low, the configurations of the absorption curves were normal in chronic lymphatic leukemia. Thus, the maximum absorption values occurred in the 8–12 hour interval in these patients as in the control subjects. The individual as well as the average absorption indices consequently were generally in the same range as those found in the control subjects (Table 49).

The reason for the many low plasma values in patients with chronic lymphatic leukemia is not entirely clear. The lower than normal values

Table 50. Plasma-Absorption Values in 14 Patients with Chronic Lymphatic Leukemia at Various Times after Oral Dose of 0.56 µg Co⁶⁰B_{12} (0.5 µc)

Patient	Co⁶⁰B_{12} in µµg/ml. Plasma at Specified Hours after Oral Dose									
	2	4	6	8	12	24	48	72	120	168
J.H.	0.2	0.1	1.2	3.3	2.9	2.0		1.3	1.0	0.6
E.K.	0.0	0.3	3.0	4.0	3.5	2.0		1.0	0.6	0.2
A.M.	0.5	0.8	0.6	2.0	2.0	1.7	1.2			
H.B.		0.6		1.9	2.0	1.2		1.1	0.8	0.8
C.L.L.		0.5		1.9	2.2	1.4		0.4	0.4	0.8
E.F.		0.6		3.5	3.0	2.2				
E.Y.		0.0		3.0	2.8	1.8				
R.A.				2.1		1.2		0.4	0.4	0.4
M.O.				2.6		1.8		1.1	1.1	0.6
R.K.				2.9		2.0		0.6	0.4	0.4
H.A.				4.0		1.9		0.8		0.5
A.P.				1.6		0.9		0.6	0.6	
I.W.				6.3		4.1	3.0	2.4		
C.A.L.				4.6		2.6		1.2		
Average	0.2	0.4	1.6	3.1	2.6	1.9	2.1	1.0	0.7	0.5

could be due to low absorption from the intestinal tract, rapid clearance from the blood of the absorbed vitamin, or a combination of these two. Since plasma clearance of intravenously injected vitamin B_{12} has been found to be normal in chronic lymphatic leukemia (264, 437, 536), it is possible that some of these patients may have a decreased absorption of cyanocobalamin from the intestinal tract. The two patients with chronic lymphatic leukemia examined with the Schilling test (Table 23) both showed normal excretion values. One of these is also included in this series (C.L.L., Table 50), where he showed rather low absorption values throughout. More investigation is needed to ascertain the reason for the generally low plasma absorption values of cyanocobalamin found in patients with chronic lymphatic leukemia. Because X-ray therapy may reduce the gastric secretory activity (49), the question arose whether the Roentgen therapy these patients had received to the left upper quadrant (spleen) could have reduced the secretion of intrinsic factor. From Tables 46 and 50 it can, however, be seen that low absorption values were observed in the absence of X-ray treatment or any other therapy. If the low plasma absorption values found in patients with chronic lymphatic leukemia should be found to be the result of decreased absorption of vitamin B_{12}, the therapy these patients have received cannot be the cause of the impaired absorption.

The 9 patients with acute or subacute myelogenous leukemia (Table 51) showed average absorption values below those in control subjects (Table 48) and patients with chronic myeloid leukemia (Table 47),

Table 51. Plasma-Absorption Values in 9 Patients with Acute or Subacute Myelogenous Leukemia at Various Times after Oral Dose of 0.56 µg $Co^{60}B_{12}$ (0.5 µc)

Patient	$Co^{60}B_{12}$ in µµg/ml. Plasma at Specified Hours after Oral Dose									
	4	8	12	24	48	72	96	120	144	168
A.H.	0.4	1.4	1.3	1.0		0.9		0.6		0.3
O.V.	0.8	2.0	1.3	0.5		0.1		0.4		
J.R.	2.0	4.2	4.3	4.8	5.2		5.1		3.4	
W.W.		2.7		1.8		0.8		0.7		0.7
E.F.		3.3		2.1		0.6		0.6		0.2
S.J.		1.1		1.2		0.3		0.7		0.5
J.B.		2.1		3.7		3.3		2.8		2.7
J.V.		7.7		5.0		4.3		2.7		
J.L.		7.3		8.0		6.0				3.7
Average	1.1	3.5	2.3	3.1		2.0		1.2		1.4

but higher than those in patients with chronic lymphatic leukemia (Table 50). The individual absorption figures varied greatly and ranged from normal to below normal. Thus, five of the nine 8-hour values, three of the nine 24-hour values, and three of the eight 72-hour values were below the lowest corresponding figures found in the 10 control subjects. The configuration of the absorption curves was normal in 5 subjects; that is, the peak values were observed 8 hours after ingestion of the oral test dose. In 4 patients, however, the maximum absorption values were recorded 24 to 48 hours after the tests were started. Thus this group of patients did not show such uniform behavior in their vitamin B_{12} absorption curves as had been noted in the two previous groups of leukemic subjects. In fact, from the absorption curves one is tempted to believe that two kinds of patient are included in the group of acute and subacute myeloid leukemias. The question may rightfully be raised whether patients with acute or subacute lymphatic leukemia have inadvertently also been included in this group. It should be remembered that the morphological differentiation between acute and subacute leukemia of the myeloid and lymphatic variety is notoriously difficult. Autopsies were performed in 6 of the 9 patients with acute or subacute myeloid leukemia and the findings in all of them were consistent with acute/subacute myeloid leukemia. Although the morphological and autopsy findings indicated myeloid leukemia in each case, the possibility that we are dealing with two variants of leukemia is still not excluded.

One of the subjects (J.B.) suffered from eosinophilic leukemia, which was thought in the beginning to be of a chronic type. His absorption curve showed a pattern similar to those seen in chronic myeloid leukemia. The clinical course of this patient was, however, rapidly downhill; he died within seven months from the time eosinophilia was first noted.

Since the absorption study was performed at a time when the disease was in a subacute stage he was included in this series.

The average absorption indices in patients with acute or subacute myeloid leukemia were slightly higher than the corresponding values in control subjects (Table 49). The individual values showed a great variation with normal as well as definitely abnormal values. This may be taken as suggestive evidence that we are dealing with more than one type of leukemia, but that we are unable to differentiate them because of the inadequacy of the available laboratory criteria.

Table 52. Plasma-Absorption Values in 3 Patients with Non-Leukemic Neutrophilic Leukocytosis at Various Times after Oral Dose of 0.56 μg Co^{60}B$_{12}$ (0.5 μc)

Patient	Co^{60}B$_{12}$ in μμg/ml. Plasma at Specified Hours after Oral Dose				
	8	24	72	120	168
M.P.	1.7	1.4	0.9	1.2	0.7
P.C.	5.7	4.0	1.8	1.2	1.2
A.F.	2.6	2.0	1.2	1.0	
Average	3.3	2.5	1.3	1.1	1.0

The 3 control subjects with non-leukemic neutrophilic leukocytosis (Group 4, Tables 46 and 52) showed absorption values indicating a normal configuration of the absorption curves. Consequently the absorption indices were also within the range found in the 10 control subjects (Table 49). The average absorption values tended to be lower among these patients than in the control subjects. This was caused by definitely decreased absorption figures in 2 of the patients. All 3 patients were seriously ill and died between eight and twenty-seven days after the absorption tests. The low absorption values may be related to their serious illnesses, because both infections (415) and fatal diseases (156) may be associated with reduced absorption of cyanocobalamin. Since leukocytosis as such is not associated with abnormal vitamin B$_{12}$ plasma absorption pattern, it is probably correct to assume that the abnormal absorption curves found in patients with myelogenous leukemia must in some way be associated with the leukemic process.

Serum vitamin B$_{12}$ concentrations of cyanocobalamin were measured in 20 of the 29 patients with leukemia as well as in the patients with non-leukemic leukocytosis. In 3 subjects with chronic myeloid leukemia the average value was 596 μμg/ml., whereas the average amount was 178 for 9 patients with chronic lymphatic leukemia, 632 for 8 patients with acute/subacute myeloid leukemia, and 433 for the 3 patients with non-leukemic leukocytosis. Increased serum vitamin B$_{12}$ concentrations have been found previously in both acute and chronic myelogenous leukemia. The values recorded in Table 46 were obtained at the time of the absorption tests, and, since most patients were tested while in remission, these values may not represent the patients' highest serum vitamin B_{12} levels. In fact, 2 of the subjects (J.M., Group I, and J.B., Group III) had a series of vitamin B_{12} determinations, and the highest values observed in these 2 patients were 2,354 and 1,156 $\mu\mu g$/ml., respectively. The fact that serum vitamin B_{12} is lowered when the patients are brought into clinical remission by therapy (443A) may be the reason why there is less of a difference between the values of control subjects and patients with acute and chronic myeloid leukemia in our series as compared with others (418, 443A).

The slightly lower than normal values for serum vitamin B_{12} found in the subjects with chronic lymphatic leukemia may be related to the decreased values for plasma absorption of cyanocobalamin from the gastrointestinal tract found in the same subjects.

The delayed peak in the plasma absorption curves in patients with chronic myeloid leukemia may be due to slower than normal absorption of cyanocobalamin but is more likely due to a more prolonged retention of the vitamin in the plasma of these patients (443B). A decreased plasma clearance of orally absorbed vitamin B_{12} could explain the increased concentration of cyanocobalamin in the plasma of patients with chronic myeloid leukemia. In order to prove this point, an oral test dose of 0.56 μg vitamin B_{12} containing 0.5 μc Co^{60} was given to one patient with chronic myeloid leukemia (subject J.M., Group I, Table 46). Three and seven days later a similar test dose was administered orally. One subject with chronic lymphatic leukemia (I.W., Group II, Table 46) and one non-leukemic control subject (J.A., Group IV, Table 46) were given test doses in a similar manner. From each of them blood samples were obtained at various time intervals up to two weeks from the day the first test dose was given. The results (Fig. 5) show that there was a much slower disappearance of radioactivity from the plasma of the patient with chronic myeloid leukemia than from the patient with lymphatic leukemia or the non-leukemic subject. Consequently, there was a much more rapid build-up of radioactivity in the plasma of the patient with chronic myeloid leukemia. Since it is believed that the radioactivity represents labeled vitamin B_{12} and there is no reason to believe that non-radioactive cyanocobalamin behaves differently, the phenomenon observed in this experiment is the most logical explanation for the high serum concentrations of vitamin B_{12} found in patients with myeloid leukemia.

Since the completion of this study, Weinstein and Watkin (646)

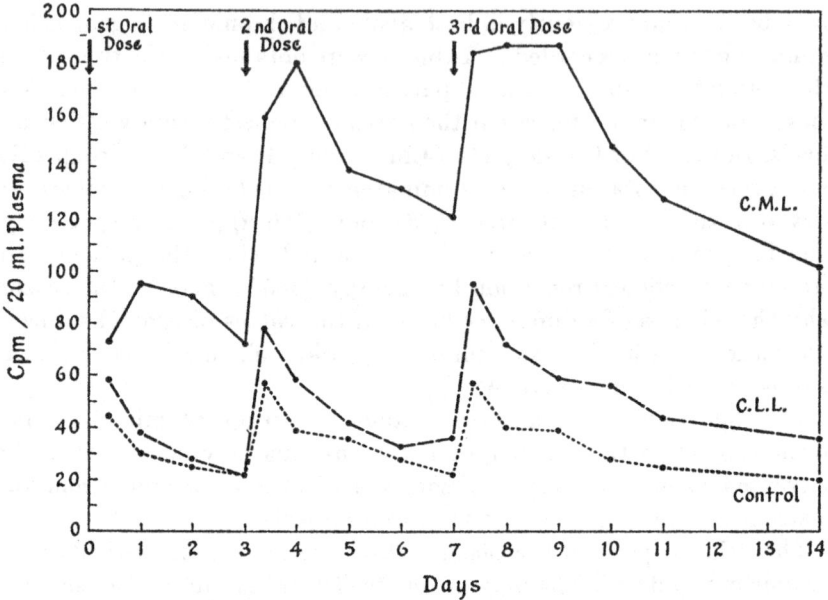

Figure 5. Radioactivity of plasma in 1 patient with chronic myeloid leukemia (C.M.L.),
1 patient with chronic lymphatic leukemia (C.L.L.), and 1 control subject; oral dose
0.56 µg B$_{12}$ (0.5 µc Co^{60}) given on the 1st, 3rd, and 7th day.

have reported on the plasma absorption of radiocyanocobalamin in 7
cases of chronic myeloid leukemia. Their finding is similar to that of
Mollin and Ross and that reported in this section.

Influence of Food on the Plasma Absorption of
Radiocyanocobalamin

When vitamin B$_{12}$ absorption tests are performed it is customary to
administer the oral test dose early in the morning after an overnight
fast and allow breakfast 2 hours later. The delayed plasma absorption
of the vitamin found under these experimental conditions has been commented upon earlier. Since it is also present in patients with pernicious
anemia when the oral test dose is administered together with intrinsic
factor, it must be assumed that lack of intrinsic factor on a fasting
stomach is not the cause for the delayed absorption of cyanocobalamin.
In order to rule out lack of some unknown food factor as the cause of
the unique absorption pattern, plasma absorption studies were carried
out on 16 control subjects; 6 subjects were given the test dose (0.56 µg
vitamin B$_{12}$, 0.5 µc Co^{60}) immediately before and 7 immediately after
an ordinary hospital breakfast, 3 received a similar test dose immediately before lunch. Blood was taken at various time intervals up to 24

hours from the time of the ingestion of the test dose. The results are shown in Fig. 6. The shaded area represents the normal variation found in 10 control subjects who were given similar test doses after an overnight fast and breakfast 2 hours later. It should be noted that food given either immediately before or after the oral test dose of labeled cyanocobalamin doesn't materially alter the shape of the plasma absorption curves. Thus the typical delay of absorption is present in all instances. Lack of a food factor is therefore not the cause for the delayed plasma absorption of cyanocobalamin.

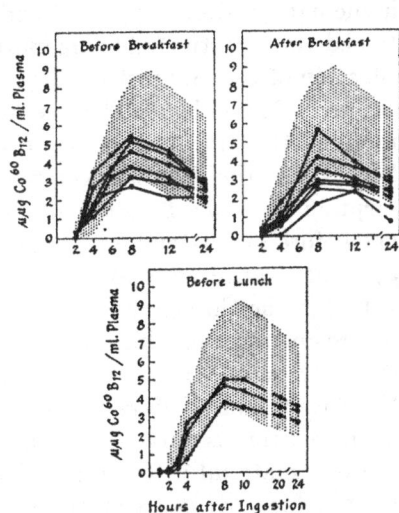

Figure 6. Radioactive B₁₂ of plasma in control subjects; oral dose 0.56 µg B₁₂ (0.5 µc Co⁶⁰) given immediately before or after breakfast or before lunch (solid lines) or 2 hours before breakfast (shaded areas).

The absorption curves in Fig. 6 indicate some decreased maximum plasma absorption values in subjects who received the test doses immediately after breakfast as compared with those who received the doses immediately before or 2 hours before breakfast was served. This might possibly mean some influence of food on the absorption of vitamin B₁₂. Earlier, Swendseid and associates (610) found an increased absorption of vitamin B₁₂ in 4 out of 7 normal subjects when a vitamin-B₁₂-free breakfast was administered together with small doses of the labeled vitamin. Recently, Deller and associates (144) found improved vitamin B₁₂ absorption in patients with partial gastrectomy when the labeled cyanocobalamin was administered together with a vitamin-B₁₂-free meal. This effect of food was not observed in normal subjects or patients with pernicious anemia. Gräsbeck and associates (252) found a decreased absorption of cyanocobalamin as judged by the Schilling test when the oral test dose was given after the evening meal. Prefed human subjects and rats had increased absorption of vitamin B₁₂ when a large unphysiologic test dose was administered in another study (581).

To learn more about the influence of food on the maximum plasma absorption values, it was decided to compare the 8-hour absorption values when the oral test dose was given immediately before or after breakfast or lunch: 6 patients received the oral dose before and 8 after breakfast; 9 were given the dose before and 9 after lunch. The influence of supper on the absorption was also tested in 18 control subjects. Half of this group received the test material immediately before, the rest immediately after supper. Blood samples in these subjects were obtained at 8 A.M. the following morning, 14 and 15 hours after the administration of the oral test doses respectively. The results of these studies are given in Table 53. The average absorption value in the group that received the oral dose before breakfast was 4.1 $\mu\mu$g/ml. (range 2.7–5.4). When the dose was given after breakfast the average 8-hour absorption value was 3.0 $\mu\mu$g/ml. (range 0.9–5.6). The corresponding values before and after lunch were 4.9 $\mu\mu$g/ml. (range 2.3–8.4) and 4.0 $\mu\mu$g/ml. (range 2.2–6.0). Thus, the average 8-hour plasma absorption values in the three groups that received the test material immediately before and after breakfast and immediately after lunch were lower than the average of 5.2 $\mu\mu$g/ml. value observed in the group that received the dose 2 hours before breakfast was served (Table 48). This latter average value is only slightly above that of the group which received the test material before lunch. Thus, giving the test material immediately before or after a meal seemed for the most part to have a slight depressing action on the average absorption values. This result is at variance with that described by Swendseid and associates (610) and Deller and colleagues (144). The reason for the observed discrepancy is probably differences in the experimental conditions. We allowed a normal hospital diet to be served, whereas previous investigators (144,

Table 53. Plasma Absorption of B$_{12}$ in 50 Control Subjects, with Oral Doses of 0.56 μg Co^{60}B$_{12}$ (0.5 μc), Given Immediately before or within 30 Minutes after Meals

Time of Oral Dose	Absorption in $\mu\mu$g/ml. Plasma									Average
Before breakfast* ...	2.7	5.4	4.6	3.2	3.8	5.1				4.1
After breakfast*	4.2	2.5	3.5	2.8	1.7	0.9	5.6	2.9		3.0
Before lunch*	4.0	8.4	6.9	4.7	4.7	3.8	5.0	4.3	2.3	4.9
After lunch*	5.4	3.5	3.8	4.1	6.0	2.2	2.6	2.2	5.8	4.0
Before supper†	2.8	4.0	3.6	4.9	5.1	4.4	3.2	3.9	2.1	3.8
After supper‡	6.8	4.2	4.5	6.4	3.9	5.4	5.3	4.0	4.8	5.0

* 8-hour plasma values.
† 15-hour plasma values.
‡ 14-hour plasma values.

610) served a vitamin-B_{12}-free meal. There are reasons to believe that dilution of the isotopically labeled vitamin B_{12} with "cold" cyanocobalamin occurred in the groups that received the oral test doses immediately before or after breakfast and after lunch; the reduction in the 8-hour plasma absorption values may be a reflection of this dilution.

The absorption values in subjects who received the oral doses immediately before and after supper are not completely comparable because of the one-hour difference in the administration of the oral dose (5 P.M. and 6 P.M.). Individual absorption values (Table 53) were generally of the same magnitude as the 8-hour absorption values observed in the 10 control subjects (Table 48). The impression is left that all of these subjects absorbed the labeled cyanocobalamin, and that there was very little, if any, interference with the absorption by the evening meal. This finding is somewhat at variance with that of Gräsbeck et al. (252) who found a decreased absorption of cyanocobalamin as judged by the Schilling test when the oral test dose was given after the evening meal. The discrepancy in the results may be due to the timing of the oral dose, since Gräsbeck et al. allowed 3 hours to elapse after the meals before the test was started, whereas none of our subjects received the oral test dose later than a half hour after supper.

Although meals to some extent may influence the absorption of cyanocobalamin, it is amazing to witness such a relatively good absorption of vitamin B_{12} throughout the day. In fact, only 1 of the 50 subjects included in this series given test doses immediately before or after meals had an abnormally low absorption value statistically, that is, a value below 1.7 $\mu\mu$g/ml. of plasma. This latter figure is equal to the average minus twice the standard deviation of the mean found in 100 control subjects who received the oral test doses two hours before breakfast (4.7 ± 1.5 $\mu\mu$g/ml. of plasma; see p. 114). The reduced absorption after meals, when it occurs, must therefore be short and temporary. This is in agreement with the findings of Abels et al. (2), who studied the absorption of radiocyanocobalamin before and 2 and 3 hours after an oral loading dose of 1 μg non-labeled vitamin B_{12}. The absorption was decreased 2 hours after the loading dose, but had returned to its preloading value by the time 3 hours had elapsed.

Results with Parenteral "Loading" Injections of Non-Labeled Vitamin B_{12}

In three previous sections it was shown that the plasma absorption of radio-labeled cyanocobalamin from the gastrointestinal tract was considerably increased when an injection of 1 mg. "cold" vitamin B_{12}

was administered shortly before the blood samples were withdrawn. Because the parenteral injections resulted in increased plasma values, it was decided to study this phenomenon in more detail. Consequently, the absorption curves in a group of control subjects were compared with those obtained following parenteral loading. The parenteral injections contained 30, 100, or 1,000 µg non-labeled cyanocobalamin. These intramuscular loading doses were administered simultaneously with or 4, 5, 6, or 7 hours after the oral test doses of 0.56 µg vitamin B$_{12}$ containing 0.5 µc Co^{60}. The control group consisted of 10 subjects, the experimental series of 31.

Table 48 shows the plasma absorption values in the control group. The average, as well as most of the individual absorption figures, shows their maximum values 8 hours after the oral test doses were administered. The average 24-hour value was 64.2 per cent of the average peak absorption value. The average 24-hour value was 65.4 per cent of the average 8-hour value. The corresponding figures for the 72-, 120-, and the 168-hour values were 40.4, 32.7, and 28.8 per cent respectively.

Fig. 7 shows the results in the 31 experimental subjects each of whom received a single "loading" injection at various time intervals after the oral dose. The shaded areas show the range observed in the 10 control subjects who were given no parenteral injections. A distortion in the appearance of the absorption curves was seen after parenteral "loading." The changes were more marked with 100 and 1,000 than with 30 µg parenteral doses of vitamin B$_{12}$. The alteration in the appearance of the individual curves was more pronounced when the "loading" doses were administered 4–7 hours after than simultaneously with the oral doses. The observed changes consisted of a rapid increase in radio-labeled vitamin B$_{12}$ in the plasma after the 4–7-hour injections and, following the peak concentrations, a faster than normal decline of the absorption curves.

In the experimental subjects the average maximum plasma absorption values were 6.8, 7.9, and 8.6 µµg/ml. of plasma in the 3 groups receiving 30, 100, and 1,000 µg parenteral loading doses respectively, while the average peak value for the entire 31 subjects was 7.8. Excluding the 7 subjects who received the parenteral injections at the time of the oral dose, the average maximum value was 8.2 µµg/ml. of plasma. The difference between the average peak of 7.8 µµg/ml. in the experimental group and the corresponding figure of 5.3 in the 10 control subjects (Table 48) is statistically significant (p < 0.01).

The 24-hour plasma values in the experimental series, although usually within the normal limits, were most often found in the lower part of the normal range. The average 24-hour values were 3.0, 2.7, and 2.3

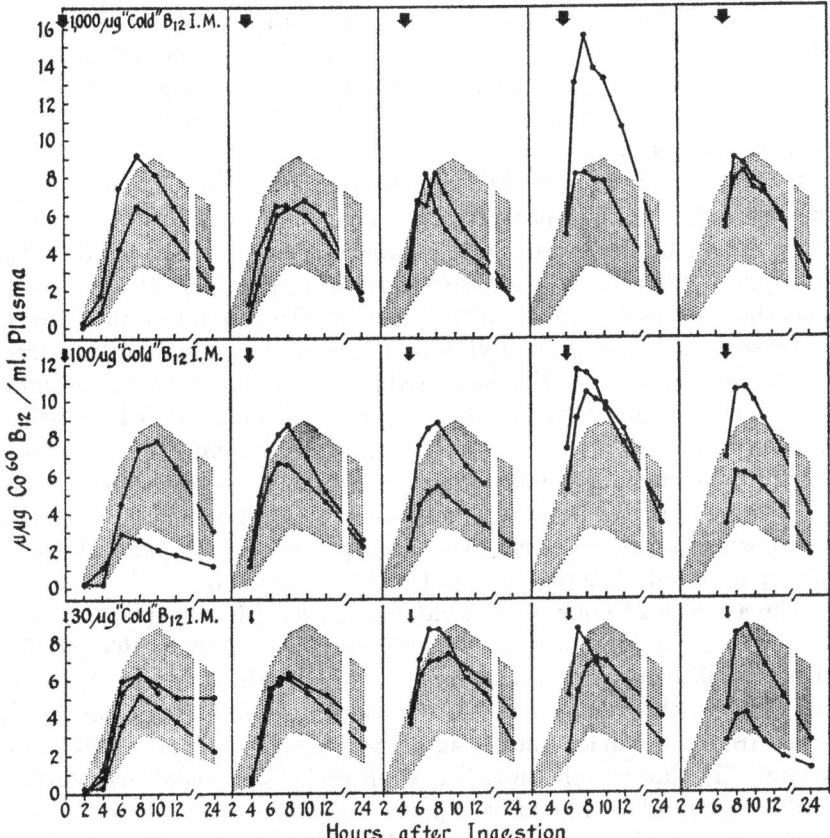

Figure 7. Radioactive B₁₂ of plasma in 10 control subjects without "flushing" injections (shaded areas) and in 31 control subjects; varying parenteral doses of "cold" B₁₂ given at differing time intervals (solid lines); oral dose 0.56 μg B₁₂ (0.5 μc Co⁶⁰).

$\mu\mu$g/ml. of plasma in the three groups receiving 30, 100, and 1,000 μg loading doses respectively, while the corresponding value was 2.7 for the entire 29 experimental subjects who had blood samples drawn at 24 hours. These values should be compared with the figure of 3.4 $\mu\mu$g/ml. observed in the 10 control subjects (Table 48). The difference was not statistically significant between the average 24-hour absorption value in the control group and that of the entire experimental series ($0.5 < p < 0.1$) or the group that received the largest parenteral injection ($0.05 < p < 0.1$).

The average 24-hour figures were 44.1, 34.2, and 26.7 per cent of the average peak absorption values for the three groups receiving 30, 100, and 1,000 μg parenteral doses of vitamin B₁₂ respectively; the corresponding figure was 34.6 per cent for all the experimental subjects together. These figures should be compared with the corresponding value of 64.2 per cent observed in the 10 control subjects. The difference between this index (100 $\times$ average 24-hour value/average peak value) in the control group and in the experimental subjects is statistically significant (p $<$ 0.001).

It is interesting to note that parenteral injections of cyanocobalamin increased the average peak concentration of $Co^{60}B_{12}$ in the plasma. Since large parenteral doses of non-labeled cyanocobalamin reduce the total amount of vitamin B_{12} absorbed from the gut (20, 82) it is evident that the increased plasma $Co^{60}B_{12}$ concentration is not an indicator of increased total absorption of vitamin B_{12} from the gastrointestinal tract under these conditions. The increased amount of labeled vitamin in the plasma shortly after the parenteral injections could result from an increased rate of absorption of the vitamin from the intestine, a reduced rate of removal from the blood stream, or a combination of both. From the figures presented here it is not possible to tell which mechanism is responsible for the raised plasma concentration of radiocyanocobalamin after parenteral "loading" doses of "cold" vitamin B_{12}.

The average 24-hour plasma values decreased in a stepwise manner when the parenteral loading doses were raised from 30 to 100 and, further, to 1,000 μg. With the number of subjects included in the series, the changes observed in the 24-hour values were not significantly different from those in the control subjects. The urinary loss of radioactive vitamin B_{12} that accompanies the parenteral injections of large doses of "cold" cyanocobalamin may explain the observed stepwise decrease in the 24-hour plasma values of $Co^{60}B_{12}$. Thus, in a previous section it was shown that the average 24-hour urinary loss of radioactivity was 5.6 per cent of the oral test dose when the parenteral injection contained 100 μg vitamin B_{12}, but that this figures rose to 28.9 per cent when the dose was raised to 1,000 μg. Even in the subjects who received parenteral doses of 30 μg a slight decrease in the average 24-hour plasma value was observed as compared with the control group. Since an insignificant amount of a parenteral dose of this magnitude is excreted in the urine (122, 442, 595, 631, 632) it is believed that the "flushing" effect of the 30 μg injections of vitamin B_{12} was also negligible. Consideration should therefore be given to the idea that the parenteral injections speeded up the removal of cyanocobalamin from the blood stream, including that which had been absorbed from the gut. It remains, however, for future studies to definitely prove that parenteral doses of "cold" vitamin B_{12} will speed up the removal from the blood stream of radiocyanocobalamin absorbed from the gut with subsequent deposition in the storage organs.

A Dual Mechanism of Vitamin B_{12} Plasma Absorption *

Recent reports have described two types of plasma absorption curve after the oral administration of vitamin B_{12}. With microbiological assay methods, after massive doses of vitamin B_{12} early significant plasma levels have been found indiscriminately in both pernicious anemia patients and control subjects (551, 632). On the other hand, two independent laboratories, using radio-labeled cyanocobalamin, have successfully determined plasma absorption curves after the oral administration of only 0.46 to 1.0 μg doses (60, 162–164). With these small amounts of vitamin B_{12} a distinctly different kind of absorption curve was found in normal subjects and in patients with Addison's pernicious anemia when intrinsic factor was added. This curve was characterized by little or no plasma radioactivity during the first 4 hours of the test and a peak concentration in the 8- to 12-hour interval. Furthermore, there was clear differentiation between control subjects and patients with pernicious anemia, because at these dosage levels the latter, without added intrinsic factor, showed insignificant plasma radioactivity.

In this investigation, plasma absorption curves were obtained in pernicious anemia patients with and without intrinsic factor, as well as in control subjects after the oral administration of test doses of radiolabeled cyanocobalamin which ranged from 0.56 to 500 μg. This included a dosage range not previously examined.

The cobalt[58]-labeled vitamin B_{12} used in this study had an initial specific activity of 1,137 μc per mg., while that of the Co^{60}-labeled vitamin B_{12} used was 893 μc per mg. When used, IFC was added in 100 or 200 mg. amounts to the solution of vitamin B_{12}, which is equal to 1 or 2 USP units. This material had been found active in pernicious anemia patients when tested by the method of Heinle et al. (289) and that of Schilling (557). Blood was withdrawn at different time intervals after the test dose. A preset count of 32,000 was used throughout this study. Generally, for each patient a pretest plasma sample was used for background count. Altogether, eight tests were carried out in 8 control subjects and twelve tests in 8 patients with Addison's pernicious anemia in remission. The diagnosis in each of the latter had been substantiated by absorption tests with and without the addition of IFC. External monitoring over the liver area was carried out one to two weeks after the tests were given according to the method of Glass et al. (221).

Two male patients with pernicious anemia, aged 61 and 64, were given

* This section appeared in slightly different form in Doscherholmen and Hagen, J. Clin. Invest., 36:1551, 1957, American Society for Clinical Investigation (158). An abstract of the section appeared in J. Clin. Invest., 36:884, 1957, American Society for Clinical Investigation (157B).

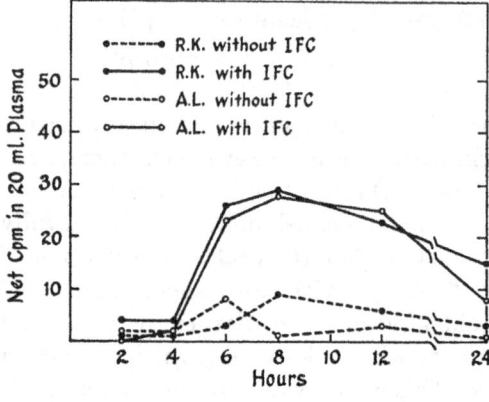

Figure 8. Radioactivity of plasma in 2 patients with pernicious anemia in remission after oral dose of 0.56 μg B$_{12}$ (0.5 μc Co^{60}), with and without intrinsic factor concentrate. (From Doscherholmen and Hagen: A dual mechanism of vitamin B$_{12}$ plasma absorption. J. Clin. Invest., 36: 1551, 1957.)

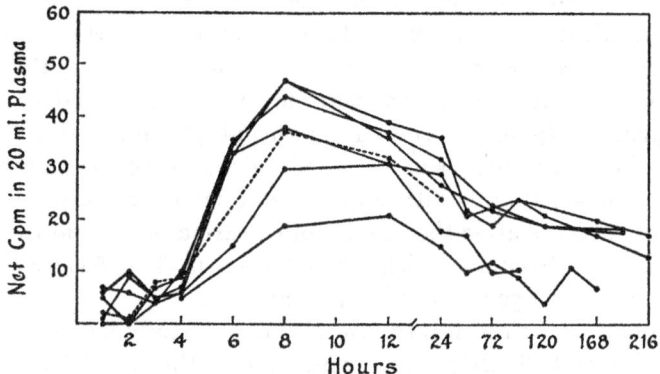

Figure 9. Radioactivity of plasma in 6 control subjects (solid lines), oral dose 0.46 μg B$_{12}$ (0.5 μc Co^{60}), and in 1 patient with Laennec's cirrhosis of the liver after a portacaval shunt operation (broken line), oral dose 0.56 μg B$_{12}$ (0.5 μc Co^{60}). (From Doscherholmen and Hagen: A dual mechanism of vitamin B$_{12}$ plasma absorption. J. Clin. Invest., 36: 1551, 1957.)

oral test doses of 0.56 μg (0.5 μc Co^{60}) first without and later with the addition of IFC. Four weeks elapsed between the repeated tests. Fig. 8 shows that there was but little radioactivity in the plasma unless intrinsic factor was given with the test dose. When IFC was added, absorption curves were similar to those found in control subjects given test doses of like amounts (Fig. 9); negligible radioactivity appeared in the plasma during the first four hours of the test, and peak concentrations in the plasma were not attained until 8 hours following dosage.

Differing absorption curves were observed in 5 of 6 pernicious anemia subjects given from 50 to 300 μg doses of radiocyanocobalamin without IFC. The results are summarized in Table 54 and are shown graphically in Fig. 10. One patient with the 50 μg test dose had little plasma radio-

Table 54. Radioactivity in cpm in 20 ml. Plasma at Different Hours after Various Oral Doses of $Co^{58}B_{12}$ (all patients male)

Patient	Age	Diagnosis	Dose of $Co^{58}B_{12}$ μg	Dose of $Co^{58}B_{12}$ μc	cpm at Different Hours after Oral Dose 1	2	3	4	5	6	8	10	12	24	36	Max. Calculated Amount Labeled B_{12} (μμg/ml plasma)	Radioactivity over the liver (net cpm)
H.M.	23	healthy	10	5.0	8	8	8	13		38	66		56		31	16	
G.B.	21	healthy	50	8.0	7	9	11	11	15	25	34	32	20	23		26	1,125
R.R.	40	psychoneurosis	50	8.0	3	7	6	9	15	23	24			16		18	
E.J.	25	appendicitis	100	8.0	1	2	4	9	12	14	16		14	11		24	
E.E.	59	essential hypertension	100	8.0	13	9	17	20		20	24		23	21		51	
A.H.	58	emphysema	200	16.0	11	15	19	26		27	36		33	26		54	1,123
M.F.	44	duodenal ulcer	300	16.0	14	21	20	17	20	22	25		27	21		61	
G.G.	40	bronchial asthma, diabetes	500	16.0	7	15	19	18	19	22	21		21	19		83	
A.O.*	60	pernicious anemia	50	8.0	6	16	19	24		21	21		21	15		18	670
L.B.*	63	pernicious anemia	50	8.0	2	3	5	2		0	1		-2	1		4	118
C.L.*	64	pernicious anemia	50	8.0	3	10	15	15		16	18		12	10		14	254
C.L.*†	64	pernicious anemia	50	8.0	2	3	4	6		8	14		21	14		16	721
A.B.	68	pernicious anemia	100	9.8	16	45	55	58		62	51		41	30		76	760
A.B.†	68	pernicious anemia	100	8.9	5	4	6	10		15	20		22	11		30	946
J.P.	45	pernicious anemia	200	16.0	12	13	21	22		23	17		12	9		85	170
P.E.	66	pernicious anemia	300	16.0	17	21	28	32		28	19		20	15		72	370

(From Doscherholmen and Hagen: A dual mechanism of vitamin B_{12} plasma absorption. J. Clin. Invest., 36:1551, 1957.)
* Approximately 4.0 μc $Co^{60}B_{12}$ included.
† 200 mg. intrinsic factor concentrate added.

141

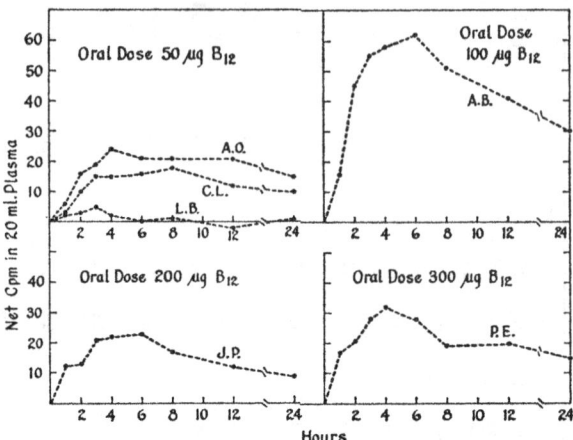

Figure 10. Radioactivity of plasma in 6 patients with pernicious anemia after oral doses of 50, 100, 200, and 300 μg of radioactive B₁₂. (From Doscherholmen and Hagen: A dual mechanism of vitamin B₁₂ plasma absorption. J. Clin. Invest., 36:1551, 1957.)

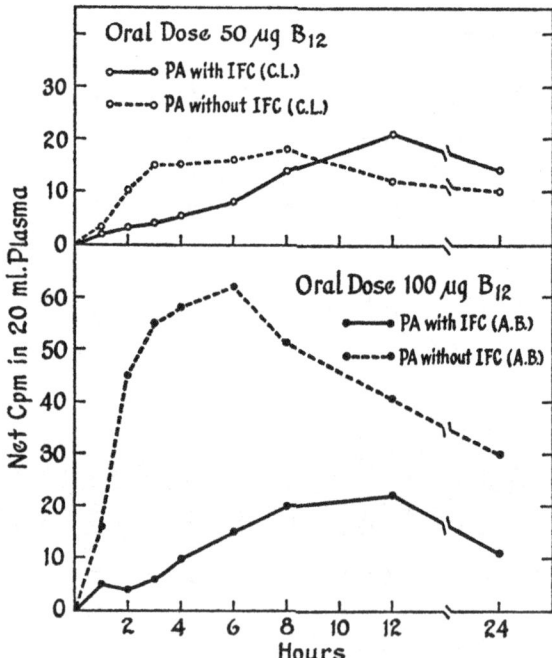

Figure 11. Radioactivity of plasma in 2 patients with pernicious anemia after oral doses of 50 and 100 μg of radioactive B₁₂ with and without intrinsic factor concentrate. (From Doscherholmen and Hagen: A dual mechanism of vitamin B₁₂ plasma absorption. J. Clin. Invest., 36:1551, 1957.)

activity, but each of the other 5 had relatively high values by 3 hours with peak concentrations usually in 4 to 6 hours.

Two of these patients were retested with the same doses of vitamin B_{12}, but with the addition of 200 mg. IFC. The early rise in plasma radioactivity was abolished in each case (Fig. 11). Instead there was a gradual rise in radioactivity to peak values at 12 hours. While there was inhibition of that phase of absorption not mediated by intrinsic factor, radioactivity measurements over the livers after IFC showed higher counts in each instance (Table 54).

Fig. 12 depicts the absorption curves in 8 control subjects given 10 to 500 μg test doses of radiocyanocobalamin. Three kinds of curve were obtained: the familiar delayed type; a new, somewhat biphasic, plateau-shaped configuration; and curves intermediate between these two. None of the curves was the same as that found with comparable dosages of vitamin B_{12} without addition of IFC in patients with pernicious anemia. The early, proportionately large amount of radioactivity in the plasma found in pernicious anemia was not obvious until the 200 to 300 μg dosage. Then, in contrast to the continued falling away after the early peak in the pernicious anemia patients, a second phase was observed in the control subjects, in which plasma radioactivity increased and persisted for many hours. At dosage levels of 50 to 100 μg intermediate types of curve were found.

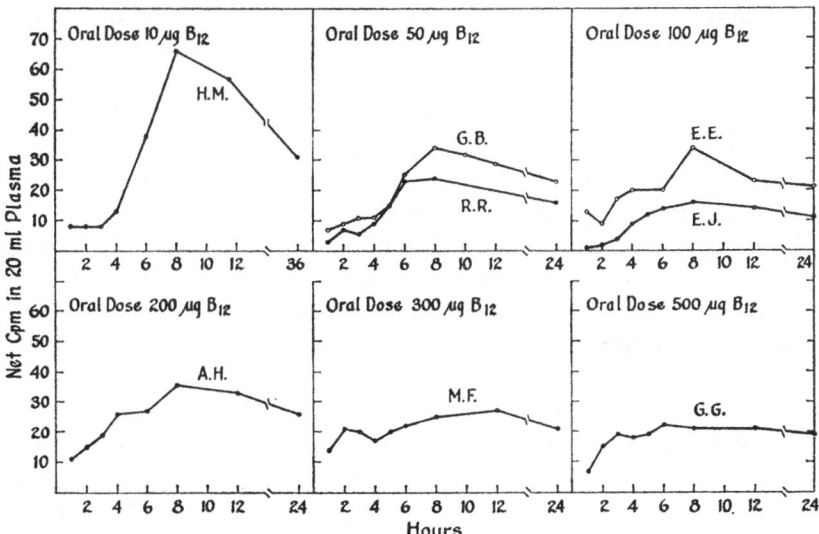

Figure 12. Radioactivity of plasma in 8 control subjects after oral doses of 10, 50, 100, 200, 300, and 500 μg radioactive B_{12}. (From Doscherholmen and Hagen: A dual mechanism of vitamin B_{12} plasma absorption. J. Clin. Invest., 36:1551, 1957.)

Table 54 includes the maximum amounts of vitamin B_{12} absorbed into the plasma. Sixteen $\mu\mu g$ per ml. of plasma were found when the 10 μg test dose was given to a control subject. In general, with increasing size of test dose larger amounts of cyanocobalamin were found, 83 $\mu\mu g$ per ml. being observed in the subject who received the 500 μg test dose. This same tendency was seen in the 6 pernicious anemia patients to whom IFC was not given. However, the individual results showed wide variation.

The results of measurements of radioactivity over the liver one to two weeks after dosage are recorded in Table 54. Consistently higher values were observed in normal subjects and in patients with pernicious anemia when IFC accompanied the test dose, than in patients with pernicious anemia without IFC. This was true even when higher peak plasma radioactivity had been found in the latter. The effect of intrinsic factor can be illustrated by comparison of ratios of liver radioactivity to the peak radioactivity of 20 ml. of plasma. The average ratio was 16 in 6 patients with pernicious anemia without the addition of IFC to the test dose (range 7 to 28). On the other hand, the ratio was raised to 34 and 43 in two pernicious anemia patients retested with added IFC, and was 31 and 33, respectively, in 2 normal subjects.

These studies show that patients with pernicious anemia absorb significant amounts of radio-labeled cyanocobalamin in the dosage range of 50 to 300 μg of the vitamin. The resulting plasma absorption curves were unique, with rapid rises in plasma radioactivity to peaks, usually in 4 to 6 hours. The peaks were followed by declines of radioactivity relatively more rapid than those in control subjects given comparable dosages. For example, in the pernicious anemia patients the average plasma concentration after 24 hours was 45.4 per cent of the peak plasma level, compared with 71.6 per cent in control subjects. The difference is statistically significant ($p < 0.01$).

Of particular interest was the finding that IFC abolished this early type of absorption curve and gave rise instead to gradual increases of radioactivity in the plasma with delayed peaks (Fig. 11) such as were found with smaller test doses with intrinsic factor present. Although excessive amounts of intrinsic factor can inhibit the absorption of small test doses (e.g., 0.5 μg) of vitamin B_{12} (81, 227), inhibition of the absorption of larger test doses has rarely been found (113). The retarded absorption presently observed might be due to interference with absorption by some non-specific material in the IFC (227). However, the intrinsic factor may have been responsible, because the resulting absorption curves were similar to those observed in control subjects given comparable amounts of cyanocobalamin. Moreover, the addition of

IFC resulted in each instance in higher hepatic radioactivity. This suggests that more, rather than less, cyanocobalamin was absorbed in spite of the change in the contour of the absorption curves.

Another possibility must be considered to explain the delayed rise of radioactivity in peripheral blood samples in the presence of intrinsic factor. With intrinsic factor there could be early removal of the absorbed vitamin B_{12} by peripheral tissues or organs such as the liver. Simultaneous radioactivity measurements of blood samples from the portal vein would be most helpful to place the cause of the slower rise in plasma radioactivity. Such studies are not available. But Booth and Mollin (60) found maximum radioactivity in the plasma 8 to 12 hours after dosage, whereas the highest counts over the liver were not obtained until 2 to 6 days later. On the other hand, we have observed a plasma absorption curve in 1 patient with an effective portacaval shunt. The subject, a 46-year-old man with Laennec's cirrhosis, was studied 17 months after operation. As seen in Fig. 9, there was a delay in the peak of radioactivity in the plasma identical with that found in normal subjects. These observations make it unlikely that the liver immediately removes cyanocobalamin from the blood under the influence of intrinsic factor and thereby causes the delay in the rise of radioactivity in the plasma. Moreover, we are not aware of any evidence that peripheral tissues selectively remove and temporarily store newly absorbed vitamin B_{12} after oral administration. It therefore seems more likely that the intestine is in some way responsible for the slower rise in radioactivity in the plasma in the presence of intrinsic factor. This view is in agreement with that suggested by Booth and Mollin (60).

Tests in control subjects showed that the inhibition of the early rise of radioactivity in the plasma could be overcome by larger doses of vitamin B_{12}. Examination of Fig. 12 shows that in one of two control subjects given 100 μg and in the subjects tested with 200 μg there was considerable plasma radioactivity after 4 hours had elapsed, as compared with the results at the 10 and 50 μg levels. With 300 and 500 μg doses relatively high plasma radioactivity was found after 2 and 3 hours. Then, in contrast to the results in patients with pernicious anemia, the peak was followed by a plateau-like curve. This prolongation was probably due to the superimposition of absorption mediated by intrinsic factor.

The results of these studies lend support to the hypothesis that there are two modes of intestinal absorption of cyanocobalamin: one, mediated by intrinsic factor, is characterized by more gradual and prolonged plasma absorption curves; the other, found with much larger doses of cyanocobalamin, is characterized by early rises in plasma levels of vitamin B$_{12}$, as indicated by measurements of radioactivity. It has been suggested that this latter mechanism is due to a passive diffusion across the intestinal barrier (633). However, in pernicious anemia the peak radioactivity in plasma was observed from 4 to 6 hours after the oral doses were given (Fig. 10), later than would be expected from a process of simple diffusion. The particular curves can be compared to the plasma absorption curves of iron which are believed to be related to an active process of absorption. Oral administration of iron results in peak plasma concentrations 2½ to 5 hours after test doses (451). Until more details are known it is perhaps best to refer to the two mechanisms of absorption of vitamin B$_{12}$ as the one mediated by intrinsic factor, and the other as absorption independent of this factor.

Recently, it has been estimated that 100 gm. of undried beef liver may contain 60 to 118 μg of vitamin B$_{12}$ (555, 578). Fig. 10 includes plasma absorption curves with dosages in this general range. Such absorption suggests the possibility that the success of the dietary liver therapy of Minot and Murphy (429) was due to the cyanocobalamin content itself and not necessarily to other factors present in the liver which may have promoted hematopoiesis or vitamin B$_{12}$ absorption.

Clinical experience has indicated a wide variation in results in the treatment of pernicious anemia patients with oral doses of cyanocobalamin. Whereas some may show an almost optimal response to daily doses of 5 to 15 μg (181, 434) and some can be successfully treated with daily oral doses of 50 to 150 μg (70, 101, 102, 300, 391), failures or poor response have been reported with daily oral doses of varying amounts even up to 250 μg (263, 408, 408A, 597). This great variation in response is believed to be caused by variation in the absorption of the vitamin which is well illustrated in Fig. 10 at the 50 μg dose. Two patients had significant plasma absorption curves and hepatic radioactivity (Table 54), while a third patient showed little absorption and only a half to a sixth of the liver radioactivity of the other two. These findings suggest great individual variation in the absorption gradient in patients with pernicious anemia for doses of vitamin B$_{12}$ above the physiologic range. Such a variation in the absorption gradient is well known also for test doses of a more physiologic magnitude, when a source of intrinsic factor is added (20).

The plasma absorption curves determined by bioassay of vitamin B$_{12}$ after the administration of massive doses of the vitamin have shown peak plasma concentrations 1 to 24 hours after the administration of the tests, and no definite separation between patients with pernicious anemia and control subjects has been claimed (551, 632). This is in contrast to the definitive results when test doses of 50 to 300 μg were given. However, with the larger test doses there was less difference between the absorption curves of pernicious anemia patients and normal subjects, probably because as the test doses were increased, the absorption mechanism independent of intrinsic factor gradually became the more dominant also in the control subjects.

The calculated maximum amount of vitamin B_{12} absorbed was found to range from about 18 $\mu\mu g$ per ml. of plasma in a control subject given the 50 μg test dose to 83 $\mu\mu g$ per ml. of plasma when 500 μg were administered. The figures were not very different in the patients with pernicious anemia, except in the patient who absorbed only a minor amount when the 50 μg test dose was given. Our data are too few to make a more detailed comparison between the amounts calculated to have been absorbed in each group.

Because such small amounts of cyanocobalamin were absorbed it is understandable that bioassay has failed to reveal definite changes in the concentration of vitamin B_{12} in the serum after single oral test doses of less than 500 μg (434, 633). Tracer techniques, being more sensitive, have the further advantage that they can determine absorption without measurable changes in the total amount of vitamin B_{12} in the serum.

Delay of Absorption of Radio-Labeled Cyanocobalamin in the Intestinal Wall in the Presence of Intrinsic Factor *

When radio-labeled vitamin B_{12} was given in physiologic test doses to control subjects, no or negligible radioactivity was observed in the plasma during the first 3 to 4 hours of the tests. Subsequently a rapid rise in plasma activity occurred, with peak concentrations in the 8–12-hour interval (60, 158, 162, 163). The same pattern of absorption was found in patients with Addison's pernicious anemia when IF was administered together with the labeled cyanocobalamin (60, 158).

The results of radioactivity measurements over the abdomen and liver (60, 232), as well as studies of the urinary excretion of radioactivity (39), and of the plasma absorption patterns of peripheral venous blood (60, 162) have all been interpreted as being consistent with a slow absorption of vitamin B_{12} through the intestinal wall. But alternative explanations such as rapid absorption from the intestine with temporary storage in the liver or other extragastrointestinal organs (39, 60,

---

* This section is taken with minor changes and additions from Doscherholmen and Hagen, J. Lab. Clin. Med., 54:434, 1959, published by the C. V. Mosby Company, St. Louis (160). An abbreviated version appeared in Proc. 7th Congr. Internat. Soc. Hemat., Rome, 1958, Grune & Stratton, New York, 2:1419, 1960 (160A), and an abstract appeared in J. Clin. Invest., 37:888, 1958, American Society for Clinical Investigation (159A).

162, 232) or an effect of gastrointestinal transit time (60, 162, 232) were not entirely ruled out.

The purpose of the present study was to determine the approximate locus of the delay of the absorption into the plasma of radio-labeled cyanocobalamin in the presence of IF.

The observed delay in the rise of radioactivity in peripheral blood could result from slow absorption from the intestine or from an effect of the liver, lungs, or peripheral tissues. To circumvent the possible role of the liver, the plasma radioactivity patterns were determined in 5 patients with portacaval shunts. All 5 had Laennec's cirrhosis of the liver; the portacaval shunting procedure had been performed 2–56 months before the absorption tests. In all 5 the radioactivity curves of the plasma after the ingestion of 0.56 μg vitamin B$_{12}$ containing 0.5 μc Co^{60} were similar to those of 10 control subjects (Fig. 13). If the livers were effectively bypassed by the portacaval shunts, these results meant that the liver did not cause the delay in the rise in the plasma radioactivity. One of the 5 patients (K.H.) has died since the test was performed and autopsy revealed a widely patent portacaval shunt; the clinical courses of the other 4 indicated well-functioning shunts.

In order to exclude the liver more definitely, and at the same time exclude possible effects of the lungs and peripheral tissues, serial blood

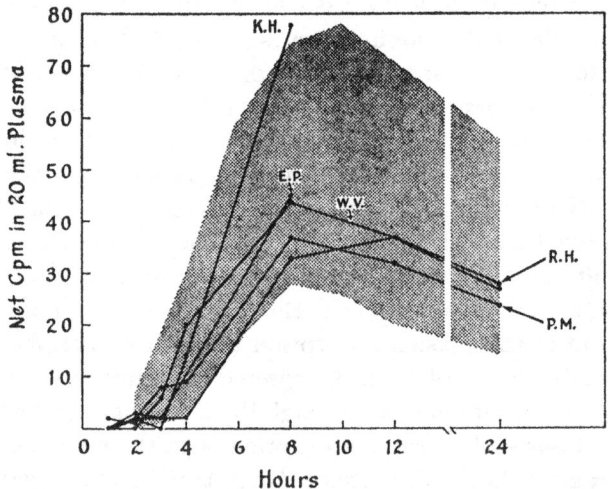

Figure 13. Radioactivity of plasma in peripheral vein blood in 10 control subjects (shaded area) and in 5 patients having functional portacaval shunts (solid lines); oral dose 0.56 μg B$_{12}$ (0.5 μc Co^{60}). (Taken, with slight changes, from Doscherholmen and Hagen: Delay of absorption of radiolabeled cyanocobalamin in the intestinal wall in the presence of intrinsic factor. J. Lab. Clin. Med., 54: 434, 1959, published by the C. V. Mosby Company, St. Louis.)

Figure 14. Radioactivity of plasma in portal vein blood (solid dots and crosses) and in peripheral vein blood (circles); oral dose 0.56 μg B₁₂ (0.39 μc Co⁶⁰). (Taken, with slight changes, from Doscherholmen and Hagen: Delay of absorption of radiolabeled cyanocobalamin in the intestinal wall in the presence of intrinsic factor. J. Lab. Clin. Med., 54:434, 1959, published by the C. V. Mosby Company, St. Louis.)

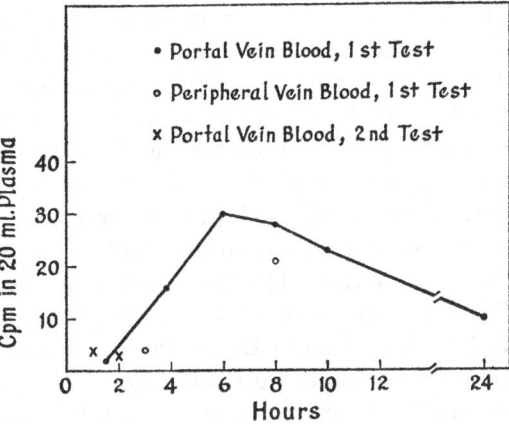

samples were obtained by catheter directly from the portal vein in 1 subject, a 29-year-old man with cirrhosis of the liver of unknown etiology. Because of hemorrhage, apparently from esophageal varices, a portacaval shunt operation was contemplated; but at laparotomy the portal venous pressure was found only mildly elevated (25 cm. of water) and the shunt procedure was not carried out. A catheter was left in the portal vein for several days to record variations in pressure. On the fifth post-operative day when the patient's gastrointestinal functions had returned to normal, an absorption test was performed with an oral test dose of 0.56 μg vitamin B₁₂ containing 0.5 μc Co⁶⁰. Six samples of blood were taken serially from the portal vein by means of the indwelling catheter and two from a peripheral vein. X-ray examination before and upon completion of the absorption studies showed the catheter correctly placed. There was a delay in the rise of the plasma radioactivity in the portal vein with highest values at 6 and 8 hours (Fig. 14). The two peripheral blood samples showed low activity after 3 hours and higher activity after 8 — a normal pattern of absorption. To double check the possibility of an early influx of radioactivity into the portal vein, the absorption test was repeated the next day. Portal vein blood samples were withdrawn immediately before the repeat oral test for a background count and 1 and 2 hours after the dose. These samples confirmed that there was slow absorption into the portal system, demonstrating that slow absorption from the intestine caused the delay of the rise of radioactivity found in the peripheral blood. The observations in the patients with portacaval shunts were in agreement with this conclusion.

The peak of radioactivity of the portal vein blood was at 6 hours, whereas it is usually found in the 8-12-hour interval in the peripheral blood. However, there were only 2 cpm difference between the 6- and 8-hour samples of portal blood, a difference not statistically significant. Moreover, 1 of the 10 control subjects had equal radioactivity values in the 6- and 8-hour peripheral samples (Table 48). The most important characteristic, i.e., the absence of radioactivity during the first hours of the tests, was similar for both portal and peripheral blood curves.

Of interest was the fact that the portal vein blood radioactivity was significantly higher than that found in a peripheral blood sample taken at the same time. This discrepancy has also been found in dogs (546). The difference may result from deposition or utilization of some of the radioactive vitamin B_{12} in the liver, lungs, or peripheral tissues or it may result simply from a dilution effect, since the portal venous blood volume is much smaller than the total blood volume of the body.

Slow absorption from the intestine could result either from a delay in transit of the test dose to an area or areas of the intestine where absorption occurs, or from slow transport through the intestinal wall itself. To determine which mechanism prevails, absorption studies were performed in 3 patients who had ileostomies because of total colectomy for ulcerative colitis (Fig. 15) after the oral test dose of 0.56 μg B_{12} containing 0.5 μc Co^{60}. In each case the peripheral blood showed the usual delay of rise in the plasma radioactivity. In all instances, however, the bulk of the radioactivity which was excreted had already passed through

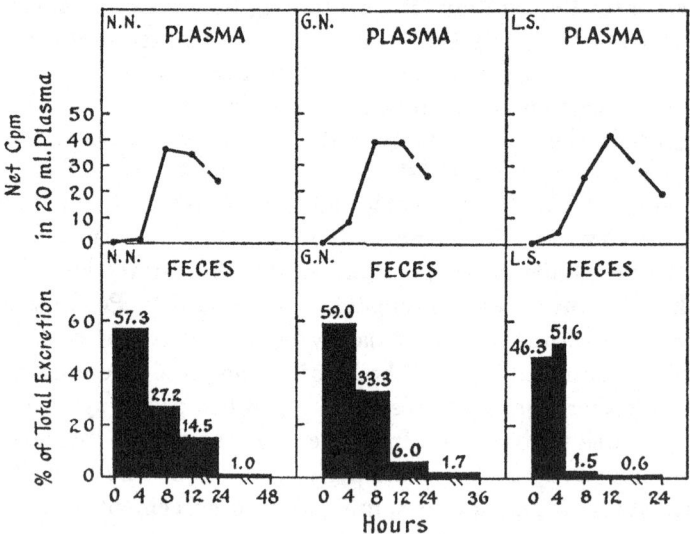

Figure 15. Radioactivity of feces in 3 patients with total colectomy and ileostomy, and simultaneous radioactivity of plasma from peripheral vein blood; oral dose 0.56 μg B_{12} (0.5 μc Co^{60}).

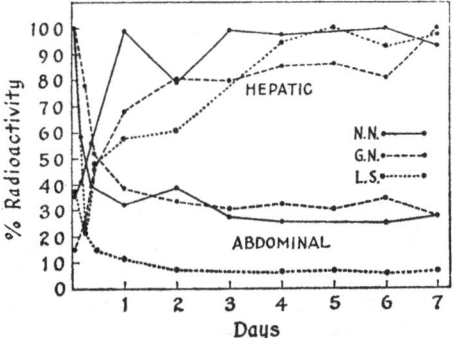

Figure 16. In-vivo radioactivity over the hepatic and abdominal areas in 3 patients with total colectomy and ileostomy; abdominal radioactivity is the average count over the upper and lower left quadrants; oral dose 0.56 μg B_{12} (0.5 μc Co^{60}).

the entire small bowel and into the ileostomy bag within the first 5 hours.

In-vivo hepatic radioactivity measurements were made in these 3 patients and the results are shown in Fig. 16. After the rather rapid evacuation of radioactivity into the ileostomy bags during the first day, in each patient there was persistence of radioactivity over the abdomen with only a gradual rate of fall. During this time hepatic radioactivity increased.

Although these observations do not reveal the specific site or sites of absorption, they eliminate transit time as the factor responsible for delayed absorption. At the same time, the observation of persistence of abdominal radioactivity with a slow increase in hepatic radioactivity is consistent with temporary storage of cyanocobalamin in the intestinal wall resulting in delayed and prolonged release to the blood.

Transit time as cause for the delayed absorption of cyanocobalamin was also ruled out in a different manner. In 2 control subjects a Miller-Abbott tube was passed into the midportion of the small intestine and

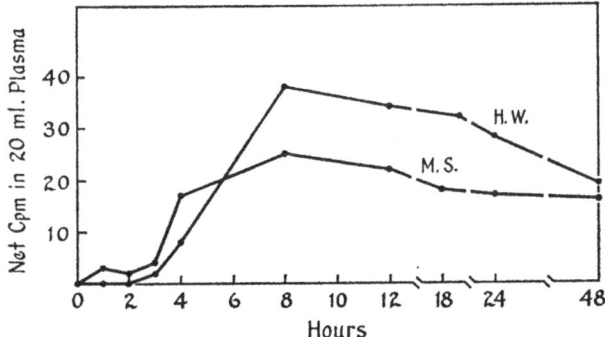

Figure 17. Radioactivity of plasma from antecubital veins in 2 control subjects; 0.56 μg B_{12} (0.5 μc Co^{60}) inserted through a Miller-Abbott tube into the midportion of the small intestine.

the labeled vitamin, 0.56 μg B$_{12}$ containing 0.5 μc Co^{60}, was inserted through the tube with 1 USP unit of intrinsic factor. The tube was rinsed with water to flush out the inserted material, and removed. Peripheral venous blood samples were obtained serially. The results (Fig. 17) show a delayed absorption similar to that observed after oral ingestion of the test dose.

These studies provide more direct evidence than heretofore available concerning the delay of absorption of small doses of radio-labeled cyanocobalamin in the presence of intrinsic factor. They show that under these conditions cyanocobalamin is stored temporarily in the intestinal wall with slow release to the blood stream.

4 | ABSORPTION, EXCRETION, DISTRIBUTION, AND KINETICS OF INGESTED RADIO-CYANOCOBALAMIN

Investigation of the Basic Mechanism of the Schilling Test *

DESPITE the widespread use of the urinary excretion test over a period of years, there is a virtual absence of detailed or factual information as to the basic mechanism of this test. For example, nobody knows the exact mode of action of the parenterally injected vitamin B_{12}. Schilling hypothesized that either the radioactivity was in a molecule which was in competition with the non-radioactive vitamin B_{12} for the renal reabsorption mechanism, or that the non-labeled cyanocobalamin saturated the binding capacity for vitamin B_{12} in the plasma so that the labeled cyanocobalamin absorbed from the gut would not be protein-bound, leading to its appearance in the glomerular filtrate. Although the phrase "saturating" injection would have been a most logical descriptive name according to the latter hypothesis, the preferred terms in the literature have been "flushing" (234, 379, 415, 509, 559) and "flooding" (82, 560) injection. Because experimental evidence to support any claim as to the mode of action of the parenteral dose seems to be lacking, it was decided to investigate in detail the basic mechanism of the urinary excretion test. To this end various experiments were carried out in vivo in control subjects as well as in vitro, as described in more detail in the following paragraphs.

Two normal subjects were given oral test doses of 1.12 μg vitamin B_{12} containing 3.3 μc Co^{57}. One of them (C.S.) received 1 mg. "cold" cyanocobalamin intramuscularly 2 hours after the oral dose while the other (L.P.) served as a control. The radioactivity was determined in

* Brief abstracts from this section appeared in Doscherholmen, J. Lab. Clin. Med., 58:813, 1961, published by the C. V. Mosby Company, St. Louis (152A); in Fed. Proc., 21:472, 1962, Federation of American Societies for Experimental Biology (155A); and in Proc. 9th Congr. Internat. Soc. Hemat., Mexico City, 1962, Grune & Stratton, New York, in press (155B).

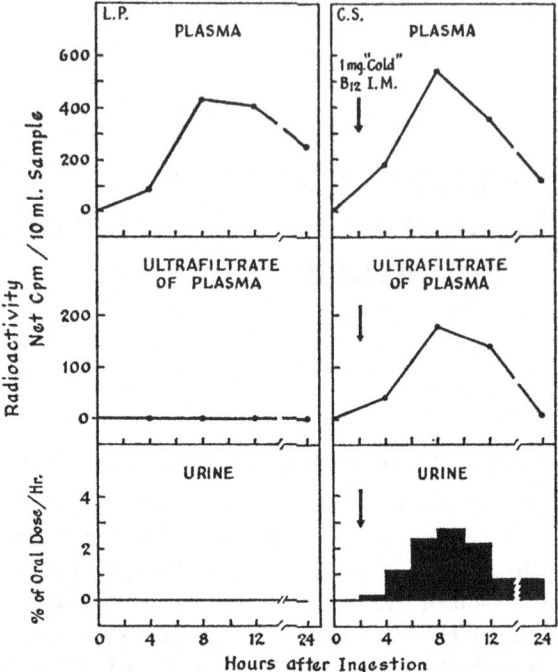

Figure 18. Radioactivity in plasma, ultrafiltrates of plasma, and fractionated urine collections in 2 normal subjects; oral dose 1.12 μg B$_{12}$ (3.3 μc Co^{57}); 2 hours after oral dose 1 mg. "cold" B$_{12}$ given intramuscularly to C.S. only.

serially obtained samples of plasma, ultrafiltrates of plasma, and fractionated urine samples. The ultrafiltrates were prepared at temperatures of 2–5°C. Fig. 18 shows that the plasma absorption curves were similar to those observed previously under identical experimental conditions. Thus, peak absorption values were found 8 hours after the administration of the oral test doses. Furthermore, as would be expected, the peak absorption figure was higher and the 24-hour plasma value was lower with than without parenteral injection of non-labeled cyanocobalamin.

In the control subject there was no radioactivity in the ultrafiltrates of plasma and only traces of radioactivity appeared in the urine samples. The entire 24-hour urine collection contained only 0.15 per cent of the orally administered test dose. In the subject who received the parenteral injection, on the other hand, there was some radioactivity in the ultrafiltrate of plasma after 4 hours, and much more 8 and 12 hours after the administration of the test material. After 24 hours practically no ultrafiltrable radioactivity was found in the plasma. The maximum amount of ultrafiltrable radioactivity was 32.9 per cent of the simultaneously observed plasma value. In the fractionated urine collections, radioactivity started to appear in considerable amount in the sample collected between 4 and 6 hours after the oral dose was administered, whereas the peak 2-hour urinary radioactivity was found in the 8-10-hour collection period. The total 24-hour urinary radioactivity amounted to 26.9 per cent of the oral test dose.

These observations showed that the parenterally injected vitamin B_{12} made some of the radio-labeled vitamin in the plasma appear in an ultrafiltrable form. Furthermore, the urinary radioactivity reflected the ultrafiltrable radioactivity in the plasma rather than the plasma radioactivity. That there was practically no ultrafiltrable radioactivity left in the plasma after 24 hours explains why so little radioactivity is regained in the urine after the first 24 hours unless another "flushing" injection is administered.

When the parenteral injection of the "cold" vitamin B_{12} is administered at the height of the absorption of the radioactivity into the blood stream, there is an immediate appearance of a considerable amount of radioactivity in the first 2-hour post-injection urine sample. However, the maximum rate of urinary excretion of radioactivity is not found until several hours later (60, 165A); the reason for this delay is not known (60). From previous experience it might be expected that the ultrafiltrable radioactivity in the plasma in these instances reaches its peak value some hours after the injection. To test this supposition, an experiment was carried out on a normal subject who received 0.56 μg vitamin B_{12} containing 5.0 μc Co^{57}. The radioactivity was determined in serially obtained samples of plasma, ultrafiltrates of plasma, and fractionated urine collections (Fig. 19). Immediately after the withdrawal of the 8-hour blood sample, one mg. "cold" vitamin B_{12} was injected subcutaneously. Traces of radioactivity were found in the urine only up to the time of the parenteral injection. As expected, a considerable amount of radioactivity appeared in the urine immediately after the injection. The maximum rate of urinary excretion of radioactivity took place in the 10-12-hour collection period. It should, however, be noted that even in the 12-14-hour period there was more urinary radioactivity than in the immediate 2-hour post-injection collection period. The plasma radioactivity rose steeply after the subcutaneous injection, reaching a peak value at 5 P.M. or an hour after the injection. Thereafter a rapid decline ensued. No measurable ultrafiltrable radioactivity was present in the plasma after 4 hours and an insignificant amount was present after 8. After the "cold" vitamin B_{12} was administered there was a rapid appearance of ultrafiltrable radioactivity, with a peak 3 hours after the injection. The curve of the ultrafiltrable

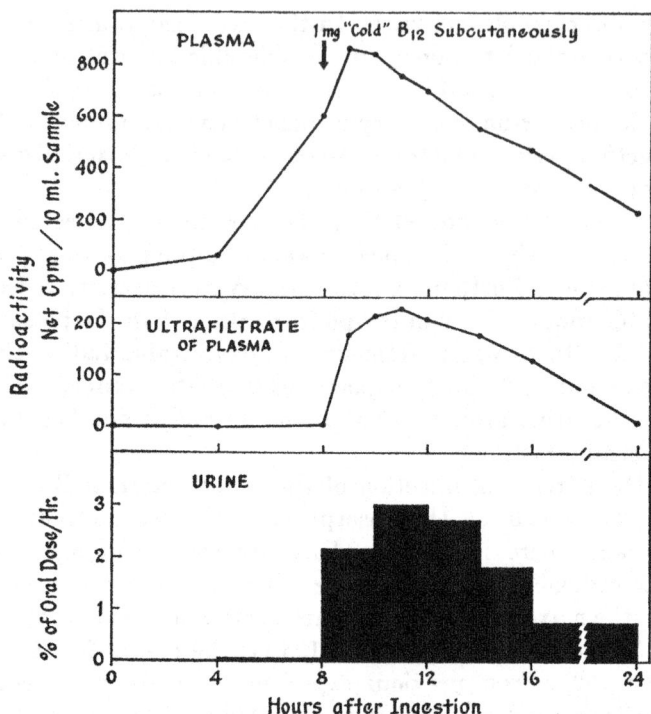

Figure 19. Radioactivity in plasma, ultrafiltrates of plasma, and fractionated urine collections in a control subject; oral dose 0.56 μg B$_{12}$ (5.0 μc Co^{57}); 1 mg. "cold" B$_{12}$ given subcutaneously 8 hours after the oral dose.

radioactivity was more sustained and showed a less steep decline than the corresponding curve depicting the plasma radioactivity. Thus at 8 P.M. the ultrafiltrable radioactivity had declined only 8.3 per cent from its peak value while at the same time plasma radioactivity had declined 18.6 per cent. The corresponding figures at 10 P.M. were 21.5 and 35.6 per cent, respectively. As expected, the urinary excretion of radioactivity reflected the radioactivities in the ultrafiltrates of plasma much closer than those of the plasma.

Patients with kidney disease and uremia are often found to excrete smaller than normal amounts of radioactivity in the first 24-hour urine collection after a single injection of "cold" cyanocobalamin given shortly after the oral test material (73, 169, 415, 516, 517). But in contrast to normal subjects (41, 73) the uremic patients continue to excrete radioactivity in the urine for several days (73, 516, 517). If the claim as to the function of the parenteral vitamin B$_{12}$ is correct, the uremic patients would be expected to have more ultrafiltrable radioactivity in their plasma after the first 24 hours than normal subjects. To test this assumption, 1 patient with chronic glomerulonephritis (blood urea nitrogen 54 mg./100 ml. of blood) and 1 normal subject ingested oral doses of 0.56 μg vitamin B_{12} containing 5.0 μc Co^{57}. The parenteral injections were administered 2 hours later. Urine collections were begun immediately after the injections and three successive 24-hour collections were made in both cases. The radioactivity was determined on urine, serially obtained samples of plasma and ultrafiltrates of plasma. The urinary radioactivities in the uremic patient were 15.16, 10.21, and 3.63 per cent of the oral test dose on the first, second, and third days, respectively; the corresponding figures in the normal control subject were 38.18, 0.24, and 0.05 per cent (Fig. 20). Differences were observed in the curves depicting the radioactivities in both plasma and ultrafiltrates of plasma. In both subjects the peak plasma radioactivity was observed 8 hours

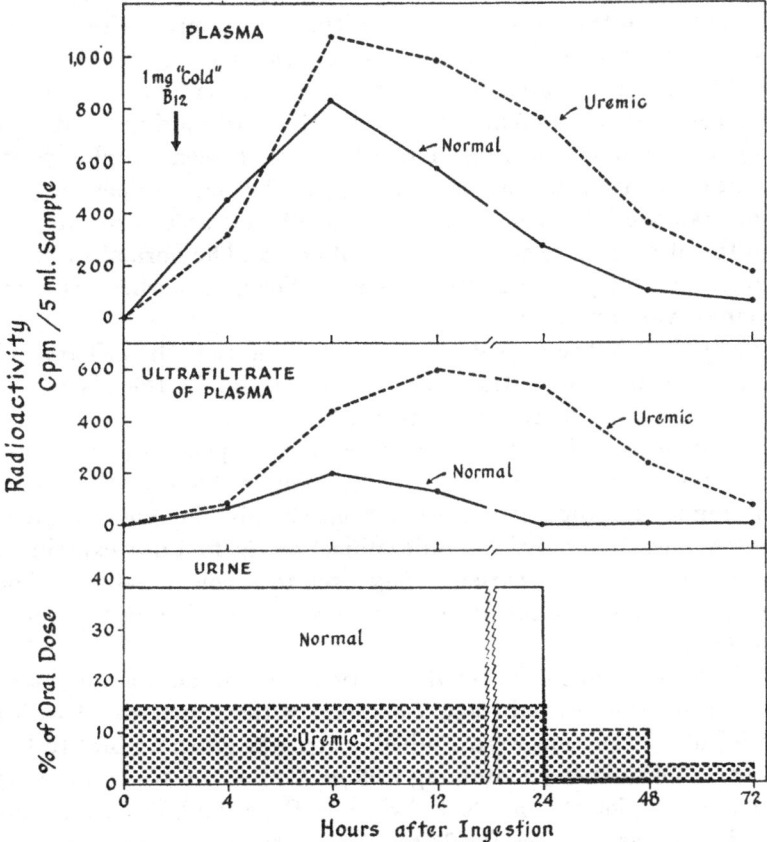

Figure 20. Radioactivity in plasma, ultrafiltrates of plasma, and urine in 1 normal subject and 1 patient with uremia; oral dose 0.56 µg B_{12} (5.0 µc Co^{57}); 1 mg. "cold" B_{12} given intramuscularly 2 hours after oral dose.

after the oral test doses were administered, but the maximum radio-activity value in the uremic patient was 29.6 per cent higher than in the normal subject. Furthermore, the former showed a much slower decline in his plasma activity as compared with the normal subject. For example, the 24-hour plasma value in the uremic patient was 70.7 per cent of his peak absorption value whereas the corresponding figure for the normal subject was 33.5 per cent.

The maximum ultrafiltrable radioactivity in the plasma in the normal subject occurred 8 hours after the test material was administered; in the uremic subject the peak was not reached, however, until 12 hours after. Furthermore, in the uremic patient the maximum ultrafiltrable radioactivity was three times higher than in the normal. Ultrafiltrable radioactivity had practically disappeared from the plasma in the normal subject by 24 hours, but in the uremic patient there was a very slow decline of the ultrafiltrable radioactivity. For example, after 48 hours the uremic patient had more ultrafiltrable radioactivity in the plasma than the normal exhibited at 8 hours, and even after 72 hours there was still a considerable amount of ultrafiltrable radioactivity left in the plasma of the uremic patient. The latter also showed a higher relative amount of ultrafiltrable radioactivity in the plasma: 60.7 per cent of his plasma radioactivity was present in an ultrafiltrable form at a time when the ultrafiltrable activity was at its peak. The normal subject exhibited only 23.7 per cent ultrafiltrable radioactivity when his absorption curve was at its peak.

The findings in these 2 subjects again showed that the urinary radioactivity mirrored the ultrafiltrable radioactivity in the plasma. The presence of a considerable amount of ultrafiltrable radioactivity in the plasma of the uremic patient for several days explains the excretion of radioactivity in the urine beyond the first day in this and other patients with uremia. The high absolute and relative value for the ultrafiltrable plasma radioactivity of the uremic subject on the first day explains why this and other similar patients may excrete a considerable, although often subnormal, amount of radioactivity in the urine on the first day of the test.

To learn the mode of the renal excretion of the radiovitamin absorbed from the gastrointestinal tract, 7 subjects with normal and 3 with impaired kidney function were studied. Each was given an oral test dose of 1.12 μg vitamin B_{12} containing 2.63 μc Co^{57} at 8 A.M., and the intramuscular injection of 1 mg. "cold" vitamin B_{12} was administered 2 hours later. Urine was collected for 24 hours after the injections, and a quantitative 30-minute urine sample was taken between 4 and 4:30 P.M. for clearance studies, at a time interval when the radioactivity in the plas-

Table 55. Radioactivity in Plasma and Ultrafiltrates of Plasma: Oral Dose 1.12 µg Co⁵⁷B₁₂ (2.63 µc), with 1 mg. "Cold" B₁₂ Given 2 Hours after Oral Dose

	Radioactivity, cpm/10 ml. Sample					
	Plasma			Ultrafiltrates of Plasma		
Patient	4 P.M.	4:15 P.M.	4:30 P.M.	4 P.M.	4:15 P.M.	4:30 P.M.
T.N.	460	455	456	132	130	136
C.P.	320	315	315	112	113	112
A.N.	311	304	310	118	118	123
W.T.	400	382	388	132	134	136
K.O.	546	528	521	220	219	207

ma and ultrafiltrates of plasma was at a constant level (Table 55). Because there was no real difference between the radioactivities in the plasma and in the ultrafiltrates of plasma at 4, 4:15, and 4:30 P.M., the samples collected at 4:15 P.M. were used for the clearance studies. The endogenous creatinine clearance was determined simultaneously with the vitamin B₁₂ clearance in each instance and used as a measure for the glomerular filtration rate. Table 56 shows the statistical data from this study. It is evident that in uremia there is an impaired urinary excretion of radioactivity, especially in the 30-minute urine sample. The amounts of radioactivity excreted in the 30-minute urine samples were correlated with the radioactivities in the samples of plasma and ultrafiltrates of plasma, the glomerular filtration rate, and the filtered load of radioactivity in the kidneys (Table 57). There was no correlation between the urinary radioactivity and the radioactivity in the plasma or the ultrafiltrates of plasma in this heterogeneous group of patients, but

Table 56. Urinary Radioactivity, Ultrafiltrable Plasma Radioactivity, and Clearances for Creatinine and Co⁵⁷B₁₂ in 10 Subjects: Oral Dose 1.12 µg Co⁵⁷B₁₂ (2.63 µc), with 1 mg. "Cold" B₁₂ Given after 2 Hours, 30-Minute Urine Sample Collected between 4 and 4:30 P.M.

	Urinary Radioactivity, % of Oral Dose		Ultrafiltrable Radioactivity in Plasma	Creatinine Clearances	B₁₂ Clearances	
					Uncorrected	Corrected
Patient	30 Min.	24 Hr.	(cpm/10 ml.)	(ml./min.)	(ml./min.)	(ml./min.)
K.O.	2.5		219	155	153	107
L.S.	1.4	25.2	230	115	131	91
R.J.	1.4	25.6	201	119	138	97
A.N.	1.2	21.6	118	153	102	71
W.T.	1.4	23.3	156	127	90	63
S.Z.	0.8	23.2	135	102	125	87
T.N.	1.2	15.2	130	104	83	58
L.O.	0.4	18.4	254	21	29	20
R.P.	0.3	28.4	138	36	21	15
V.K.	0.1	7.8	229	9	8	6

Table 57. Correlation between Urinary Radioactivity and Radioactivity of Plasma and Ultrafiltrates of Plasma, Glomerular Filtration Rate, and the Filtered Load of Radioactivity in the Kidneys

Urinary Radioactivity	r-Value
Versus plasma radioactivity	−0.08
Versus ultrafiltrable radioactivity	0.08
Versus glomerular filtration rate	0.87
Versus filtered load of radioactivity	0.97

a good correlation was found between the urinary radioactivity and the glomerular filtration rate and an even better correlation between the urinary radioactivity and the filtered load of radioactivity in the kidneys, i.e., the glomerular filtration rate times the ultrafiltrable radioactivity. The urinary excretion of radioactivity depends, then, mainly on two factors: the amount of ultrafiltrable radioactivity present in the plasma and the glomerular filtration rate. In this respect it is interesting to note that after saturation of the body's B_{12}-binding capacity by large amounts of cyanocobalamin, the free portion of B_{12} in the blood is also excreted by glomerular filtration (458A, 642A).

The data for the ultrafiltrable radioactivities in the plasma samples were used to calculate the actual clearances of the radio-vitamin. The results recorded in Table 56 show that these clearance values for vitamin B_{12} are in the same general range as those for the endogenous creatinine. It is, however, quite possible that the clearance for radiocyanocobalamin is smaller than calculated from the raw data for the ultrafiltrable radioactivities in the plasma samples. The reason for this is inherent in the method used for the ultrafiltration: when radiocyanocobalamin is dissolved in normal saline and subjected to the ultrafiltration procedure, approximately two thirds or roughly 70 per cent of the radioactivity is recovered in the ultrafiltrates (Table 58). Similar results are obtained when the labeled vitamin is dissolved in tap water or an ultrafiltrate of plasma. Nabet and Wolff have also found that free vitamin B_{12} is partially retained by ultrafiltration in a cellophane bag (456A). Assuming that free radiocyanocobalamin in the plasma behaves as it does in water, normal saline, or an ultrafiltrate of plasma, the observed values for the ultrafiltrable or free radio-B_{12} in the plasma samples represent approximately 70 per cent of the true value for free radiocyanocobalamin in the samples. The kidney clearances for radiocyanocobalamin were, therefore, recalculated from the corrected values for the ultrafiltrable radioactivities (Table 56). The corrected vitamin B_{12} clearance values were about 30 per cent smaller than the values for the endogenous creatinine clearances. This could mean that a propor-

Table 58. Ultrafiltration Studies of Control Saline Solutions Containing Various Concentrations of $Co^{60}B_{12}$, the Radioactivity Expressed as Percentages of the Various Saline Concentrations of $Co^{60}B_{12}$

$Co^{60}B_{12}$ in Solution ($\mu\mu g/ml.$)	Percentage of Ultrafiltrable Radioactivity
500	67.3
1,000	64.7
2,000	64.7
3,000	66.2
4,000	66.2
5,000	66.9
10,000	65.8
15,000	67.9

Table 59. Comparison of the Radioactivity of Urine Samples and Their Corresponding Ultrafiltrates

Patient	Radioactivity, cpm/20 ml.		
	Urine (A)	Ultrafiltrate of Urine (B)	B/A × 100
M.B.	20	12	60.0
	183	116	63.4
V.O.	216	155	71.8
	845	509	60.2
H.K.	311	248	79.7
	567	469	82.7
L.S.	156	123	78.8
	697	558	80.1
R.V.	832	536	64.4
	434	307	70.7
C.L.	1029	673	65.4
	263	187	71.1
Average			70.7

tionately smaller amount of radiocyanocobalamin than of creatinine was filtered through the glomeruli per unit of time or that some of the vitamin was reabsorbed by the tubuli. Still another possibility to be considered is that the endogenous creatinine clearance might be higher than the true glomerular filtration rate because of tubular secretion of creatinine (498A, 526A).

Ultrafiltrates were made of 12 samples of urines from 6 subjects. The radioactivities of 20 ml. of urines and their corresponding ultrafiltrates are recorded in Table 59, with radioactivity expressed as a percentage of the activity in a similar amount of the corresponding urine sample. The individual percentages ranged from 60.0 to 82.7, with an average value of 70.7. Because of the similarity between the average percentage figures of the ultrafiltrates of urine and of saline solutions of radiocyanocobalamin it is believed that all of the radio-B_{12} activity in the urine was present in a free or ultrafiltrable form. In normal subjects vitamin B_{12} has previously also been found to be present in a free or dialyzable form (417). Our findings are in agreement with this claim.

The question arose next as to how the parenteral injection could make radiocyanocobalamin appear in the plasma in an ultrafiltrable or free form. Two possibilities come to mind. The radio-vitamin may be discharged from the intestinal mucosal cells into the blood stream in either a free or a bound form. If it is absorbed in a free form, it will immediately become bound to the specific vitamin B_{12} binding protein in the plasma. Saturation of this binding protein with parenterally injected "cold" vitamin B_{12} would leave the absorbed radiocyanocobalamin no binding sites to become attached to, and consequently it would appear in an ultrafiltrable or free form in the plasma. On the other hand, if the radiocyanocobalamin is absorbed into the blood stream in a bound form, the parenterally injected "cold" vitamin B_{12} must in some way bring about release of this radio-vitamin so that it will appear in the plasma in an ultrafiltrable form. Investigations related to both of these possibilities were carried out.

In order to learn whether saturation of the binding sites for vitamin B_{12} occurs when a large injection of the vitamin is administered, in-vitro saturation studies were performed on plasma secured before and at various time intervals after the intramuscular injection of 1 mg. "cold" vitamin B_{12}. Radiocyanocobalamin was added in a concentration of 1,000 $\mu\mu g$ per ml. of plasma. After 30 minutes of incubation the mixtures were subjected to ultrafiltration and the radioactivity both of the whole mixtures and the ultrafiltrates was determined. A control mixture contained normal saline instead of plasma. The results (Table 60) show that up to 4 hours after the injection, plasma had no more binding power for radiocyanocobalamin than had a solution of normal saline. Starting with the 8-hour plasma sample there was a gradual restoration

Table 60. In-Vitro B_{12}-Binding Power of Plasma before and after Intramuscular Injection of 1 mg. "Cold" B_{12}: Plasma Was Mixed with Equal Amounts of Saline Solution Containing 1,000 $\mu\mu g$ $Co^{60}B_{12}$ per ml. and Subjected to Ultrafiltration

Patient	Before Injection	Percentage of Ultrafiltrable Radiocyanocobalamin, Plasma at Specified Hours after Intramuscular Injection					Saline Control
		2	4	8	12	24	
E.S.	0.9	73.4	74.7	66.4	58.0	33.4	73.9

of the binding capacity for cyanocobalamin, but even 24 hours after the injection it was still not back to the pre-injection level.

These studies showed that the injected cyanocobalamin did indeed saturate the binding sites for the vitamin in the plasma. Presumably other binding sites in the body were also saturated. If free radiocyanocobalamin then enters the blood stream shortly after the injection of the "cold" B_{12}, it must be presumed to circulate in a completely ultrafiltrable form.

In-vitro studies were performed to learn whether an exchange takes place between the non-ultrafiltrable radiocyanocobalamin absorbed from the gastrointestinal tract and added "cold" vitamin B_{12}. Each of several control subjects was given an oral test dose of 0.56 μg cyanocobalamin containing 3.42 μc Co^{57}. Plasma from two subjects was usually needed for each study. Plasma was mixed with a solution containing the desired amounts of crystalline vitamin B_{12} or an equal amount of saline as control. The radioactivities of 20 ml. of the mixtures were determined and they were then incubated for 1 to 4 hours in a shaking water bath at 37°C. After termination of the incubation period the mixtures were subjected to the ultrafiltration procedure at room temperature and the amounts of radioactivity in the ultrafiltrates determined. Table 61 shows that there was no radioactivity in the ultrafiltrates in any of the five experiments when saline was added to the plasma. However, when non-labeled cyanocobalamin was added, definite radioactivity appeared in the ultrafiltrates, and more radioactivity was recovered after 4 than after 1 hour of incubation. In the first two experiments an amount of vitamin B_{12} was added which was equal to 25 μg per ml. of plasma. It was realized that this amount was far in excess of that which is attained in the human body after the injection of 1 mg. non-labeled cyanocobalamin. Subsequently an amount of vitamin B_{12}

Table 61. Exchange between Protein-Bound Radiocyanocobalamin Absorbed from the Gastrointestinal Tract and Crystalline Non-Labeled B_{12} Added to Plasma in Vitro

Experiment Number	B_{12} Added (μμg/ml. Plasma)	Control*	Radioactivity, cpm/20 ml. Sample Ultrafiltrate			
			1 Hr. Incubation		4 Hr. Incubation	
			With B_{12}	With Sal.†	With B_{12}	With Sal.†
1	25,000,000	473	63	1	—	—
2	25,000,000	325	76	0	174	2
3	50,000	297	44	0	114	0
4	50,000	259	86	2	135	1
5	50,000	309	60	—	120	2

* Plasma with saline before ultrafiltration was performed.
† Normal saline.

equal to 50,000 $\mu\mu$g per ml. of plasma was added, an amount attained in the blood in vivo after the injection of the "flushing" dose in the Schilling test. This smaller amount of cyanocobalamin effected only a slight decrease in the average amount of radioactivity found in the ultrafiltrates. The concentrations of vitamin B$_{12}$ attained in vivo after the parenteral "flushing" procedure have, therefore, a definite exchange effect in vitro.

These experiments clearly demonstrate that the binding of radio-cyanocobalamin in the plasma can be influenced by the addition of non-labeled vitamin B$_{12}$ in vitro, thereby creating an exchange effect. There is every reason to believe that the same phenomenon also occurs in vivo. If radiocyanocobalamin is absorbed in a bound form, the injected "cold" vitamin B$_{12}$ affords an in vivo mechanism for the release of this radio-B$_{12}$. The binding of cyanocobalamin in the plasma is probably not a static but a dynamic process; the fact that exchange in vitro is possible is best explained by such an assumption. The phenomenon of exchange as here described should be investigated more closely, especially in conditions where vitamin B$_{12}$ binding abnormalities have been found in the plasma.

Table 62. Ultrafiltrable Radioactivity in Homogenates of Rat Liver with and without "Cold" B$_{12}$: Rats Were Given 0.4 or 0.7 μg B$_{12}$ Containing 0.9 or 2.7 μc Co^{57} Subcutaneously 1 Week Prior to Sacrifice

	Hours of Incubation	Radioactivity, cpm/20 ml. Sample		
		Homogenate	Ultrafiltrates	
			Warm Incub.	On Ice
Experiment 1				
Homogenate + B$_{12}$	4	7,818	1,162	706
Homogenate + buffer			530	194
Experiment 2				
Homogenate + B$_{12}$	4	39,150	2,813	1,971
Homogenate + buffer			2,767	479
Homogenate + B$_{12}$	½		1,377	
Homogenate + buffer			894	

If free vitamin B$_{12}$ can penetrate into body cells, there may even be some exchange between the "cold" vitamin B$_{12}$ in the plasma and the intracellularly located protein-bound radiocyanocobalamin. Experiments performed on rat liver homogenates seem to bear this out. Rats were given 0.4 or 0.7 μg vitamin B$_{12}$ containing 0.9 or 2.7 μc Co^{57} subcutaneously one week before being sacrificed. The livers were homogenized in phosphate buffer with a pH of 7.4 and incubated at 37°C. or on ice with and without the addition of 1,000 μg "cold" vitamin B_{12} per 50 ml. of homogenate. Control mixtures contained phosphate buffer instead of vitamin B_{12} solution. Table 62 shows that radio-vitamin B_{12} could be released from its bound form in the liver homogenates by incubation and, furthermore, that the process was accelerated by the addition of large amounts of "cold" cyanocobalamin.

Since there is very little "flushing" effect of delayed injections of "cold" vitamin B_{12} in vivo, this type of exchange between free cyanocobalamin in the plasma and protein-bound vitamin B_{12} in the cells is not of much importance in the Schilling test. This is borne out by the following experiment: A control subject received a test dose of 0.56 μg vitamin B_{12} containing 5.0 μc Co^{57}. A complete plasma absorption curve showed normal absorption. The 24-hour urinary radioactivity during the first day of the test amounted to 7,664 cpm (0.10 per cent of the oral dose). On the ninth and again on the fifteenth day a "flushing" dose of 1 mg. "cold" vitamin B_{12} was given intramuscularly at 8 A.M. Twenty-four-hour urine collections were made for radioactivity measurements on the days of these injections as well as on the days immediately preceding and following them. Plasma samples were also obtained for radioactivity measurements on each of these days at 8 A.M. Table 63

Table 63. "Flushing" Effect of Delayed Parenteral Injections of 1 mg. "Cold" B_{12} in a Control Subject: Oral Dose 0.56 μg $Co^{57}B_{12}$ (5.0 μc)

Day	"Cold" B_{12} I.M. μg	Urinary Radioactivity		Plasma Radioactivity (cpm/20 ml.)
		Cpm	% of Oral Dose	
1	0	7,664	0.10	983
8	0	2,048	0.03	338
9	1,000	50,693	0.69	291
10	0	3,381	0.05	268
14	0	1,785	0.02	184
15	1,000	28,436	0.39	179
16	0	4,133	0.06	165

shows the results. During the days of the "flushing" injections the 24-hour urine collections contained 50,693 and 28,436 cpm, respectively. The corresponding values on the preceding days were 2,048 and 1,785 cpm, and on the following days 3,381 and 4,133 cpm. A small but definite "flushing" effect from delayed parenteral injections is hereby established. Assuming a normal plasma volume (3,000 ml.), the decline in the plasma radioactivity during the two days of "flushing" amounted to 6.8 and 7.4 per cent of the excreted urinary radioactivity. The major portion of the urinary radioactivity must therefore have come from the tissues. It is reasonable to assume that the injected "cold" vitamin B_{12} was in some way exchanged with tissue-bound radiocyanocobalamin. Experience with multiple injections of "cold" cyanocobalamin support this viewpoint (165).

The experiments cited so far show that if radiocyanocobalamin is given orally, the parenterally injected non-radioactive vitamin B_{12} will provide a mechanism for the radiocyanocobalamin to appear in the blood in an ultrafiltrable form whether the vitamin is absorbed from the gastrointestinal tract in a free or a bound form. They do not, however, provide any actual information about the form in which the vitamin is discharged from the gut into the blood stream. Another type of experiment was therefore designed in the hope that it might shed some light on this question. It has been noted that there is a rapid increment in plasma radioactivity after an intravenous injection of "cold" vitamin B_{12} administered at the height of the plasma absorption. It was therefore decided to analyze the changes that take place in the plasma immediately after such injections. Three control subjects were given oral test doses of 1.12 μg vitamin B_{12} containing 3.3 μc Co^{57}. An intravenous injection of 1 mg. "cold" vitamin B_{12} was administered to each of them 8 hours later. Blood was obtained immediately before and 5 and 10 minutes after the injections. The blood was immediately put into iced water and its temperature brought down to 7°C. within 3 minutes. The formed elements were spun down at 2–5°C. and the plasma removed with and into glassware that had been kept in the deepfreeze. The ultrafiltrates were prepared at 2–5°C. In these experiments it is important to keep the temperature of the blood and the plasma low to avoid the in-vitro exchange effect of the large amount of free non-radioactive vitamin B_{12} circulating in the blood after the intravenous injections. A separate experiment showed that there was no in-vitro exchange at low temperatures, at least up to 7°C. (Table 64). The results from the 3 experiments are shown in Table 65. Five minutes after the intravenous injections, plasma radioactivity increased on an average of 24.2 per cent (range 15.7 to 29.2 per cent) over and above the pre-injection levels. Ten minutes after the injections, the corresponding average value was 40.0 per cent (range 29.0 to 52.5 per cent). Before the injections there was no or very little ultrafiltrable radioactivity in the plasma. Five and ten minutes after the injections this picture had changed, because now plasma contained on the average 4.4 and 7.0 per cent ultrafiltrable radioactivity. These two figures correspond to an average of 25 per cent of the increment in the plasma radioactivity over and above the pre-injection values. A correction should be made for the fact that only approximately 70 per cent of free radiocyanocobalamin in a solution is ultra-filtrable by the present method. With such a correction an average of 6.3 per cent and 10.0 per cent of the 5- and the 10-minute post-injection radiocyanocobalamin was ultrafiltrable, respectively. These two figures correspond to 35.8 and 37.4 per cent of the increment in the plasma radioactivities over and above the pre-injection levels.

Table 64. Exchange Experiment in Vitro: 50,000 μμg per ml. "Cold" B_{12} Added to Plasma Containing Radiocyanocobalamin Absorbed from the Gastrointestinal Tract, Saline Added in Equal Amount to the Control; after Incubation for 4 Hours at 37°C. or 7°C. Mixtures Were Subjected to the Ultrafiltration at 2–5°C.

	Radioactivity, cpm/10 ml. Sample
Plasma with saline	641
Ultrafiltrate of plasma with saline after incubation at 37°C.	0
Ultrafiltrate of plasma with "cold" B_{12} added after incubation at 37°C.	47
Ultrafiltrate of plasma with "cold" B_{12} added after incubation at 7° C.	0

Table 65. Radioactivity in Samples of Plasma and Ultrafiltrates of Plasma Immediately before and 5 and 10 Minutes after the Intravenous Injection of 1 mg. "Cold" B_{12}: Parenteral Dose Administered 8 Hours after Oral Dose of 1.12 μg $Co^{57}B_{12}$ (3.3 μc)

	Radioactivity, cpm/10 ml. Sample					
	Plasma			Ultrafiltrate of Plasma		
Patient	4 P.M.	4:05 P.M.	4:10 P.M.	4 P.M.	4:05 P.M.	4:10 P.M.
O.F. 338	391	436	0	21	34	
O.B. 395	504	547	4	28	41	
M.F. 455	588	694	0	18	39	

These experiments showed that a considerable increment in the plasma radioactivity occurred immediately after the intravenous injections of "cold" vitamin B_{12} given at the height of the absorption. It is reasonable to assume that this influx of radioactivity into the blood stream came from the gut, an assumption supported by the fact that no immediate increment in plasma radioactivity took place when the intravenous "flushing" was undertaken 11 days after the administration of the oral test material, i.e., at a time when the absorption of radiocyanocobalamin had been completed (Table 66). Most of the increment was found to be present in the plasma in a non-ultrafiltrable form 5 and 10 minutes after the injections. It must be assumed that this part of the increment was discharged from the intestinal mucosal cells into the blood stream in a non-ultrafiltrable form. The amount of radiocyanocobalamin that was found ultrafiltrable or free after the injections might have been discharged from the gut into the blood stream in a free form.

On the other hand, it might also have been released from its binding in the blood stream between the time of the intravenous injections and the time the blood was withdrawn and reached a temperature so low that the exchange between the free "cold" vitamin B$_{12}$ and the bound radiocyanocobalamin was abolished. These time intervals were at the most 10 and 15 minutes for the two post-injection blood samplings (waiting period from the time of the injections, time for withdrawal of the blood samples, and time for the cooling of the blood). It is not known for certain whether this much exchange can take place in vivo in such a short time. In an in-vitro exchange experiment (Table 64) it took 4 hours to release 7.3 per cent of the plasma radioactivity (corrected value 10.4). This figure is in the same general range as those

Table 66. Plasma Radioactivity Immediately before and 10 Minutes after a "Flushing" Intravenous Injection of 1 mg. "Cold" B$_{12}$, Parenteral Dose Given 11 Days after Oral Dose of 0.56 μg Co^{57}B$_{12}$ (5.0 μc)

	Plasma Radioactivity, cpm/20 ml. Sample	
Patient	Before Intravenous Injection	After Intravenous Injection
W.S.	204	195
A.S.	114	116

found 10 minutes after the intravenous injections. Unless the exchange in vivo proceeds at a much faster speed than that observed in vitro (and this possibility is not yet excluded), it is not unlikely that some of the radiocyanocobalamin observed in an ultrafiltrable form in the plasma after the injections entered the blood stream in a free form. Under the conditions of these experiments, however, most of the radiocyanocobalamin seemed to be absorbed from the intestine in a bound form, but it is not impossible that some smaller portion could have entered the blood stream in a free or ultrafiltrable form.

Absorption or transport through cell membranes is still poorly understood. The part of radiocyanocobalamin that is found to enter the blood stream in a bound form after the intravenous injections is most likely absorbed through an active process. If some smaller portion enters the blood stream in an ultrafiltrable form it is most likely that this is a passive form of absorption. If free radioactive vitamin B$_{12}$ exists inside the mucosal cells of the small intestine and the mucosal cells are permeable for the free non-labeled vitamin B$_{12}$, the parenteral injection might well have resulted in a discharge into the blood stream of some free radiocyanocobalamin from the mucosal cells. This could have happened in the following way: Immediately after the injections the concentration of free "cold" B_{12} outside the intestinal mucosal cells would increase greatly. The non-labeled vitamin B_{12} would move into these cells until an equilibrium was established, but the concentration outside the cells would fall rapidly because of the rapid urinary excretion of free cyanocobalamin. The gradient between the mucosal cells and the extracellular fluid would be reversed and the vitamin would move out of these cells again. The amount of radiocyanocobalamin moving out of the cells would then depend on the relative amount of free non-labeled vitamin B_{12} and radio-B_{12} present in the cells. This hypothesis is based on two premises: (1) That an intracellular mechanism exists for the release of cyanocobalamin from the intrinsic factor or the cellular binding protein which is responsible for bringing the vitamin into the mucosal cells. Recently it has been found that cyanocobalamin bound in the intestinal wall can be released from its binding under appropriate conditions, presumably by an enzymatic process (155). It has also been shown that extracts (126) or homogenates (155) of small intestine can release vitamin B_{12} from its binding to the intrinsic factor. The intestinal mucosal cells therefore seem to possess the mechanism for building up a concentration of free vitamin B_{12} inside the cells. (2) That vitamin B_{12}, given parenterally in excessive amounts, has the ability at least to some extent to penetrate the mucosal cells of the small intestine. These cells are permeable for cyanocobalamin when the vitamin is present in high concentrations in the intestine (158). This kind of absorption is not dependent on the presence of intrinsic factor. It is generally believed to come about through a process of simple diffusion across the intestinal membrane (633). There is no reason to believe that this diffusion process, if it exists, is unidirectional. Uptake of vitamin B_{12} by body cells may be enhanced by the presence of intrinsic factor in vivo (477) and in vitro (10, 166, 302, 304, 307, 312, 334, 361, 426). This phenomenon of cellular uptake of B_{12} in the presence of intrinsic factor does not, however, preclude the possibility that some of the B_{12} can enter body cells in the absence of such a factor, i.e., in a free form. This may be especially true if the vitamin is present in excessive amounts.

If free vitamin B_{12}, present in excessive amounts in the body fluids, doesn't enter the mucosal cells of the small intestine from the blood stream, it will be difficult to explain the absorption of free radiocyanocobalamin from the mucosal cells under the present experimental conditions. Such an absorption would then take place against a positive gradient and could only occur in the presence of an active "vitamin B_{12} pump."

Distribution of Radioactivity in Man after the Oral Ingestion of Small Test Doses of Radiocyanocobalamin *

In another part of this book (pp. 147–152) it was concluded that the wall of the small intestine serves as a temporary storage organ for vitamin B_{12} after the ingestion of small test doses of radiocyanocobalamin in the presence of intrinsic factor. Since this conclusion was drawn from indirect laboratory evidence the purpose of the present study was to observe directly the distribution of radioactivity at differing time intervals after the oral administration of small doses of radio-labeled cyanocobalamin in the presence of IF. The test doses were administered to seriously ill patients and whenever postmortem examinations were made the distribution of radioactivity in the gastrointestinal tract and other organs was measured by direct counting. Particular attention was directed to details of the distribution of radioactivity in the small intestine. Results were obtained in 11 subjects who died from 2 hours to 113 days following the ingestion of the radio-labeled vitamin.

The oral test dose of 0.56 μg vitamin B_{12} containing 0.5 μc Co^{60} was administered in 20 ml. of water after an overnight fast in 5 patients and between breakfast and noon in 6. Because the status of IF production was unknown in these subjects, one USP unit of IFC was always added to the labeled cyanocobalamin immediately before the tests. The radioactivity was determined on weighed samples of liver, spleen, kidney, pancreas, lung, heart muscle, pectoralis muscle, and rib. The wet tissue samples were placed in 20 ml. disposable vials and counted in a well-type scintillation detector employing a preset count of 12,800. Total organ activity was calculated from the activity of the samples and the wet weights of the respective organs. In the case of the skeleton and skeletal musculature, however, the activity was calculated from their estimated weights, namely 13.2 per cent of the body weight for the skeleton and 39.7 per cent for the musculature (453). The gastrointestinal tract was rinsed with running tap water and, starting from the pylorus, the small intestine was cut into one-foot segments which were counted individually. The total radioactivity of the small intestine was the sum of the counts of these segments. In some instances the activities of the stomach and one-foot segments of ascending, transverse, and sigmoid colon, respectively, were obtained in a similar manner.

Table 67 summarizes the results of the studies. Comparison of the radioactivity of the small intestine with the total visceral radioactivity

---

* This section is taken with minor changes from Doscherholmen, Finley, and Hagen, J. Lab. Clin. Med., 56:547, 1960, published by the C. V. Mosby Company, St. Louis (156). An abbreviated version appeared in Proc. 7th Congr. Europ. Soc. Haemat., London, 1959, S. Karger, Basel/New York, 2:26, 1960 (156A).

Table 67. Distribution of Radioactivity in Various Organs after Oral Dose of $Co^{60}B_{12}$: Oral Dose 0.56 μg $Co^{60}B_{12}$ (0.5μc)

Subject No.	Age	Diagnosis	Hours between Test and Death	Oral Dose (cpm)	Organ Radioactivity, % of Oral Dose				
					Small Intestine (A)	Extraintest. Organs* (B)	Skeletal Musculature† (C)	Skeleton† (D)	$\dfrac{A}{A+B} \times 100$
1	34	Hodgkin's disease	2	252,902	1.3	0.1‡	0	...	91.6
2	67	myocardial infarction	4	248,853	13.4	0.5‡	5.2‡	1.3‡	95.9
3	70	emphysema, pneumonia	7	235,194	15.2	0.5‡	0.7‡	0.4‡	96.9
4	63	myocardial infarction	24	237,114	1.5	3.4	2.0‡	2.3‡	30.2
5	27	stomach cancer	42	252,221	3.6	9.6	4.3	3.4	27.5
6	64	ASHD§	85	248,833	0.7	10.3	0	1.2‡	6.4
7	70	lung cancer	115	237,497	2.5	48.1	3.1‡	3.1	4.9
8	85	CVA**	137	253,124	3.0	20.2	6.3	2.2	12.9
9	63	ASHD§	309	235,325	2.5	26.2	7.1	1.7	8.6
10	64	Hodgkin's disease	724	247,736	0.4	29.9	2.8‡	1.2‡	1.4
11	68	CVA**	2,724	253,538	0.5	30.9	11.8	2.4‡	1.5

(Taken, with slight changes, from Doscherholmen, Finley, and Hagen: Distribution of radioactivity in man after the oral ingestion of small test doses of radiolabeled cyanocobalamin. J. Lab. Clin. Med., 56:547, 1960, published by the C. V. Mosby Company, St. Louis.)

* Includes liver, spleen, kidneys, pancreas, lungs, and heart.
† Estimated weights.
‡ Not statistically significant.
§ ASHD = arteriosclerotic heart disease.
** CVA = cerebrovascular accident.

shows that in the 3 patients who died during the first 7 hours after the tests, virtually all of the visceral counts were found in the wall of the small bowel. However, after 24 hours the radioactivity of the small intestine had dropped to 30.2 per cent and after 42 hours to 27.5 per cent of the total visceral counts. A further decline to between 4.9 and 12.9

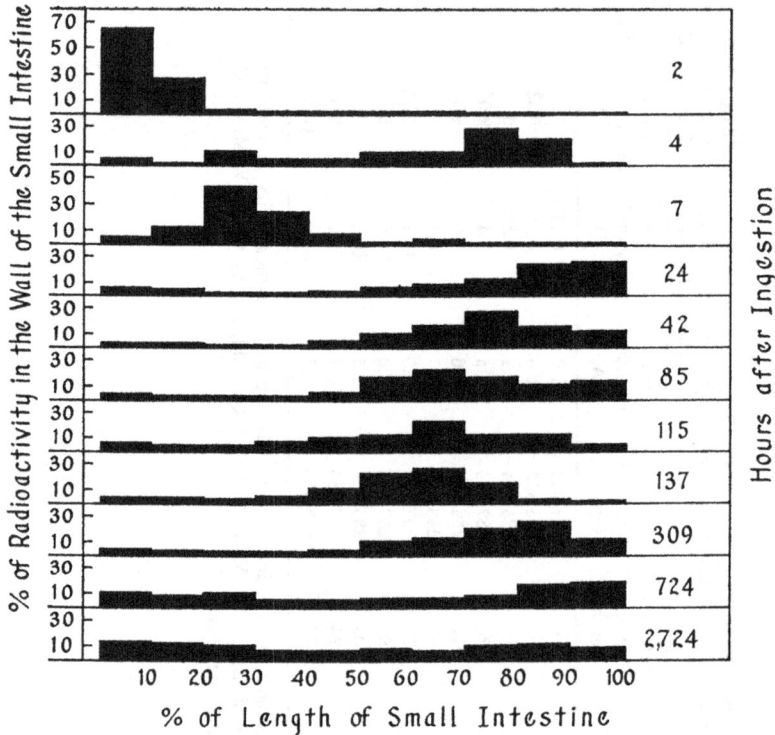

Figure 21. Radioactivity in the wall of the small intestine at various times after oral dose of 0.56 µg B_{12} (0.5 µc Co^{60}). (Taken, with slight changes, from Doscherholmen, Finley, and Hagen: Distribution of radioactivity in man after the oral ingestion of small test doses of radiolabeled cyanocobalamin. J. Lab. Clin. Med., 56:547, 1960, published by the C. V. Mosby Company, St. Louis; and from Doscherholmen, Finley, and Hagen: Organ distribution of radioactivity in man after the oral administration of physiologic test doses of radiolabeled cyanocobalamin. Proc. 7th Congr. Europ. Soc. Haemat., London, 1959, S. Karger, Basel/New York, 2:26, 1960.)

per cent was recorded 85 to 309 hours after the tests, and to between 1 and 2 per cent in the 2 subjects who died 724 and 2,724 hours after ingestion of the vitamin.

In the 6 subjects who died during the first 85 hours after the tests, the total organ radioactivity ranged from 1.4 to 20.9 per cent of the ingested dose, as compared with 31.7 to 56.8 per cent in those who died later. These figures suggested an impaired absorption of the vitamin shortly before death.

Details of the distribution of radioactivity in the small intestine are shown in Fig. 21. For comparison, in each case the organ was divided into ten equal parts and the radioactivities of the corresponding one-foot segments were assigned appropriately. The radioactivity of each tenth was then expressed as a percentage of its respective whole. The radioactivity was usually distributed unevenly: the ileum showed preferential storage of radioactivity in 7 of the subjects, the jejunum in 2, and an even or almost even distribution was recorded in the last 2 patients in the series.

Table 68 summarizes the distribution of radioactivity in the liver, spleen, kidneys, pancreas, lungs, and heart of the last 8 patients. The calculated total organ radioactivity (A) as well as the concentration of radioactivity in each organ (B and C) has been considered. The first 3 subjects in our series are not included because, as indicated in Table 67, the measured radioactivity of their extragastrointestinal organs was too negligible for reliable calculations. Comparison of Columns A shows that the liver contained from 75 to 93 per cent of all the extraintestinal activity and was, therefore, the most important single organ for the permanent storage of cyanocobalamin.

The radioactivity of the extraintestinal organs was also compared on the basis of concentration. Because of the great individual differences in the total amounts of radioactivity observed (Columns B), the comparison was made easier by using the relative concentration figures (Columns C). For the spleen and the kidneys these figures were at their maximum after 24 and 42 hours and they did not differ materially from those of the liver. The values for the spleen and the kidneys subsequently decreased whereas those for the liver increased.

The amounts of radioactivity found in the musculature and the skeleton (Table 67) and in the stomach and colon (Table 69) were rather small and inconsequential.

Because these studies were carried out on seriously ill patients, there may be objections to generalizations from the results. But in these patients the wall of the small intestine served as a temporary storage organ for the radiocyanocobalamin. There was a delayed release and subsequent gradual transfer of the vitamin to other viscera, mainly the liver. These findings confirmed inferences and conclusions drawn from less direct evidence by ourselves and others (160, 232).

The total visceral radioactivity was lower in the subjects who died during the first three and a half days after the tests than in those who died later. In other words, shortly before death the absorption of cyano-

Table 68. Distribution of Radioactivity in Extraintestinal Organs *

Subject	Hours	Liver			Spleen			Kidneys			Pancreas			Lungs			Heart		
		A	B	C	A	B	C	A	B	C	A	B	C	A	B	C	A	B	C
4	24	74.9	837	26.9	6.8	427	84.1	9.1	266	21.2	1.4	129	10.8	5.7	61	4.9	2.1	84	2.7
5	42	78.3	750	82.6	5.1	448	19.5	14.6	888	88.4	0.6	188	5.8	...	...	...	1.3	84	8.7
6	85	90.1	1515	68.0	2.6	369	15.8	2.1	281	9.6	0.4	175	7.8	2.6	45	1.9	1.8	69	2.9
7	115	90.7	7058	68.0	1.4	1116	10.7	2.2	746	7.2	0.9	988	9.5	4.3	270	2.0	0.5	206	2.0
8	187	88.7	4166	65.2	1.7	829	18.0	2.4	816	4.9	0.8	474	7.4	10.8	488	6.8	1.1	172	2.7
9	309	88.7	4291	60.8	0.5	515	7.8	4.4	872	12.4	1.1	870	12.8	8.7	289	4.1	1.4	215	8.0
10	424	89.1	4519	54.6	1.5	435	5.8	6.8	2519	80.4	0.4	471	5.7	1.9	156	1.9	0.8	179	2.2
11	2724	92.6	4841	66.8	0.4	287	8.9	2.4	615	8.4	1.0	988	12.8	1.9	116	1.6	1.8	511	7.0

(Taken, with slight changes, from Doscherholmen, Finley, and Hagen: Distribution of radioactivity in man after the oral ingestion of small test doses of radiolabeled cyanocobalamin. J. Lab. Clin. Med., 56:547, 1960, published by the C. V. Mosby Company, St. Louis.)

* A = Percentage of total extraintestinal radioactivity. B = Observed counts per minute per 100 grams of tissue. C = Percentage of total radioactivity per 100 grams of tissue.

Table 69. Radioactivity of the Stomach and 1-Foot Segments of
Ascending, Transverse, and Sigmoid Colon

Subject	Hours between Test and Death	Oral Dose (cpm)	cpm Regained			
					Colon	
			Stomach	Ascending	Transverse	Sigmoid
2	4	248,853	141			
3	7	235,194	533	46	28	51
4	24	237,114	154	31	44	21
6	85	248,833	65			
7	115	237,497	246	83	54	76
9	309	235,325	346	53	39	42
10	724	247,736	138			
11	2,724	253,538	174			

(Taken, with slight changes, from Doscherholmen, Finley, and Hagen: Distribution
of radioactivity in man after the oral ingestion of small test doses of radiolabeled
cyanocobalamin. J. Lab. Clin. Med., 56:547, 1960, published by the C. V. Mosby
Company, St. Louis.)

cobalamin was diminished even in the presence of adequate amounts of
intrinsic factor. We can only speculate about the cause of the impaired
absorption. Though infections may be responsible for a decreased absorption of vitamin B_{12} (85, 289, 415), this could have been a possible
explanation in only one of these subjects (No. 3, Table 67).

Whereas large doses of IFC can lower the absorption of cyanocobalamin in man (81, 227), significant inhibition was not noted until the optimum of IFC had been exceeded many times (81). Our subjects did
not receive excessive amounts of this substance and, furthermore, they
all received the same dose of IFC. It is therefore unlikely that the addition of this factor caused the lowered absorption.

Since the gastrointestinal assimilation of small amounts of cyanocobalamin is probably an active process of absorption, it is possible that
the impairment of this function shortly before death was related to a
general deterioration of all vital processes in these seriously ill patients.

An uneven distribution of radioactivity was found in the small intestine in most of the subjects. This finding may have an important bear-
ing upon the controversial question as to the site of absorption of cyanocobalamin. Some reports favor absorption from the upper (90, 508),
some from the lower small intestine (39, 61, 124, 202, 352, 392); one report suggests that the whole length of the small bowel is involved (115),
as found in the rat (59, 210, 527). The categorical denial of absorption
from the upper small intestine (39) is contradicted by individual instances with normal absorption from the jejunum (508) or the upper
half of the small intestine (352).

If it is assumed that the vitamin is absorbed from the area of preferential binding, in our subjects the ileum was the most important site for absorption. On the other hand, in each of the two patients who died after 2 and 7 hours, respectively, there was more radioactivity in the jejunum. The significance of these two observations with respect to absorption is open, however, to further interpretation. For example, negligible radioactivity was found in the extraintestinal organs, but this may have been because little absorption of cyanocobalamin normally takes place during the first 4–6 hours (160). The preferential binding of radioactivity in the jejunum in the patient who died after 2 hours may have been due to insufficient time for distribution throughout the intestine. On the other hand, this possibility was less likely in the case of the patient who died after 7 hours, because, for comparison, the subject who died after 4 hours already had increased amounts of radioactivity in the wall of the ileum. Suffice it to say that the finding of preferential binding in the jejunum, especially in the patient who died after 7 hours, suggests that the jejunum cannot be excluded as an area of absorption, at least in some patients.

The even or almost even distribution of radioactivity along the entire length of the small intestine in the last 2 subjects who died after 30 and 113 days, respectively, could possibly mean an even absorption from the small intestine. But since the small bowel contained only 0.4 and 0.5 per cent of the ingested radioactivity at this time, it is more likely that the residual activity represented either permanent storage or utilization of the cyanocobalamin in the bowel wall.

The finding that the liver was the most important organ for the permanent storage of cyanocobalamin is consistent with previous observations of in-vivo radioactivity measurements (131, 220, 221) as well as with the results of bioassays for the cyanocobalamin activity of various organs (269).

Though an almost equal concentration of radioactivity was found in the liver, spleen, and kidneys 24 and 42 hours after the tests, in the 6 subjects who died later the concentration in the liver was two to seventeen times higher than that of the spleen or the kidneys. Although more data are needed to be certain, it appears from these few observations that the spleen and the kidneys may play a more important role in the storage of cyanocobalamin shortly after absorption than later, suggesting that newly absorbed vitamin B$_{12}$ is shifted around among the extraintestinal organs during the first few days after the tests. Observations made after parenteral injections of labeled cyanocobalamin in man (220, 403) and in rats after parenteral (277) and oral (59) administration may be interpreted in a similar manner. In short, the spleen and the kidneys may serve as an extraintestinal temporary storage site for cyanocobalamin.

The wall of the stomach and colon contained inconsequential amounts of radioactivity, a finding in line with previous reports that vitamin B_{12} in physiologic amounts is not absorbed from the colon (115) and that the stomach, if anything, inhibits the absorption of this vitamin (115, 270, 333). The amounts of radioactivity in the skeleton and the skeletal musculature must be taken as only rough estimates because the true weights of these organs were unknown. Furthermore, samples of these structures might not have been representative. Nevertheless, there were small quantities of radioactivity present in both musculature and bones. These findings are consistent with the observations recorded in man after parenteral administration of radiolabeled cyanocobalamin (131).

Kinetics of Ingested Radiocyanocobalamin in Man [*]

The biosynthesis of radiolabeled cyanocobalamin (99) provided investigators with an effective means of studying various aspects of the metabolism of this vitamin. For example, the availability of radio-tagged vitamin B_{12} made it possible to investigate in detail the gastro-intestinal absorption and distribution of the vitamin. Although some attention has been given to the sequential movement of cyanocobalamin after oral ingestion (60), the kinetics have not yet been fully elucidated.

It is the purpose of this section to reflect on the movements of vitamin B_{12} in the body from the time of its ingestion. Aided by the results of studies with isotopically labeled cyanocobalamin we have been able to hypothesize the existence of several different body spaces or compartments for this vitamin. The confines of these compartments to be described may not always correlate well with anatomical boundaries of specific organs. Thus, it is quite likely that some compartments may encompass several organs and that certain organs may participate in more than one of the compartments.

The urinary excretion test (557) under varying conditions, along with plasma (60, 162), fecal (289), and hepatic (221) radioactivity measurements, was employed to gain the knowledge needed. The oral test dose (0.56 μg vitamin B_{12} containing 0.39 μc or 0.50 μc Co^{60}) was

[*] This section is taken with slight changes and additions from Doscherholmen and Hagen, Vitamin B_{12} und Intrinsic Factor, 2. Europäisches Symposion, Hamburg, 1961, Ferdinand Enke Verlag, Stuttgart, 381, 1962 (165A). An abbreviated version appeared in Doscherholmen, Proc. 8th Congr. Europ. Soc. Haemat., Vienna, 1961, S. Karger, Basel/New York, 328, 1962 (153).

Table 70. B$_{12}$ Absorption in Control Subjects to Whom an Oral Dose of
0.56 μg Co^{60}B$_{12}$ (0.5 μc) Was Given

Subject	1 mg. "cold" B$_{12}$, by Hour of Injection		Fecal Radioactivity, % of Oral Dose	24-Hour Urinary Radioactivity*				24-Hour Urinary B$_{12}$*	
				% of Oral Dose, by Collection		% of Absorption, by Collection		% of I.V. Dose, by Collection	
	1st	2nd		1st	2nd	1st	2nd	1st	2nd
G.K.	0	24	26.3	19.6	9.0	26.8	13.3	59.8	71.3
B.D.	6	30	27.0	29.4	6.6	40.2	8.9	82.8	72.0
W.P.	504	528	25.6	0.48	0.37	0.7	0.6	91.1	90.9

(From Doscherholmen and Hagen: Kinetics of ingested radiocyanocobalamin in man. Vitamin B$_{12}$ und Intrinsic Factor, 2. Europäisches Symposium, Hamburg, 1961, Ferdinand Enke Verlag, Stuttgart, 381, 1962.)

* Urine collections started at time of I.V. injections.

administered in the morning after an overnight fast and breakfast was allowed 2 hours later. The parenteral "flushing" injection of 1 mg. "cold" vitamin B$_{12}$ was given at various time intervals after the oral test dose. Twenty-four-hour urine collection was always begun immediately after the loading injection. Vitamin B$_{12}$ activity was determined by bioassay using *Euglena gracilis* var. *bacillaris* according to the method of Ross (548). Valuable information was also obtained from the measurements of radioactivity in the formed elements of the blood and from the autopsy studies (pp. 170–177).

After ingestion of physiologic test doses of radioactive vitamin B$_{12}$, in general, three characteristic urinary excretion responses have been observed, depending upon the time relation of the parenteral injection to the oral test dose. Examples of these typical responses will be given by showing the detailed results from metabolic studies carried out on 3 control subjects. In each instance vitamin B$_{12}$ absorption was determined by the four commonly available absorption methods. In addition, cyanocobalamin concentrations were estimated microbiologically on samples of serum and urine obtained serially. All 3 subjects had normal absorption of labeled vitamin B$_{12}$ and they all handled the large parenteral injections of the vitamin in a normal manner (Table 70, Fig. 22–24).

Subject G.K. was given 1 mg. of non-labeled cyanocobalamin intravenously at the time of the oral test dose and the injection was repeated 24 hours later. Fig. 22 shows that there was a delay in the appearance of radioactivity in the urine after the first parenteral loading dose until the sample collected between the fourth and the sixth hour, by which time a significant level of radioactivity was present in the plasma. On the other hand, there was an immediate increase of urinary radioactivity in the 2-hour sample following the parenteral dose given at 24 hours, when significant plasma radioactivity was still present.

In subject B.D., who received the first intravenous injection 6 hours after the oral dose, there was an immediate excretion of appreciable amounts of radioactivity in the first 2-hour urine sample (Fig. 23). This sample was collected at a time when there was a rapid rise of radioactivity in the plasma. Twenty-four hours later, with the repeated intravenous injection, there was again an immediate increase in radioactivity in the urine coincident with the presence of significant activity in the plasma.

The third subject, W.P., was given the intravenous injections 21 and 22 days following the oral test dose (Fig. 24). In contrast to the other 2 subjects, there were only negligible amounts of radioactivity in all urine samples. Plasma radioactivity was very low during the entire

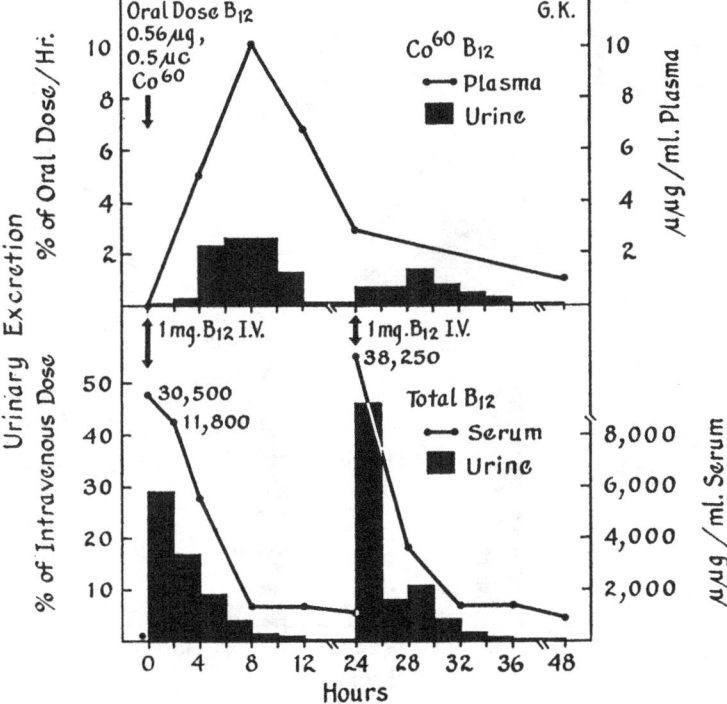

Figure 22. Urinary radioactivity in the Schilling test; comparison with the Co⁶⁰B₁₂ in the plasma and the excretion of non-labeled B₁₂; intravenous "flushing" injections given simultaneously with and 24 hours after oral dose. (From Doscherholmen and Hagen: Kinetics of ingested radiocyanocobalamin in man. Vitamin B₁₂ und Intrinsic Factor, 2. Europäisches Symposion, Hamburg, 1961, Ferdinand Enke Verlag, Stuttgart, 381, 1962.)

time of these urine collections, while the early part of the absorption curve showed that there had been normal absorption of radioactivity. The fecal excretion test (Table 70) and the hepatic radioactivity measurements (Fig. 25) also revealed that normal absorption had occurred.

In summary, the observations in these 3 subjects showed three different urinary excretion responses to the parenteral injection of non-labeled cyanocobalamin. When the parenteral injection was given simultaneously with the oral dose, there was a delay of several hours in the appearance of urinary radioactivity. When the parenteral dose was administered 6, 24, or 30 hours after the oral dose there was immediate excretion of a considerable amount of radioactivity in the urine. But, with late parenteral injection, negligible amounts of urinary radioactivity were present. In each instance the excretion of urinary radioactivity reflected the presence or absence of significant plasma radioactivity.

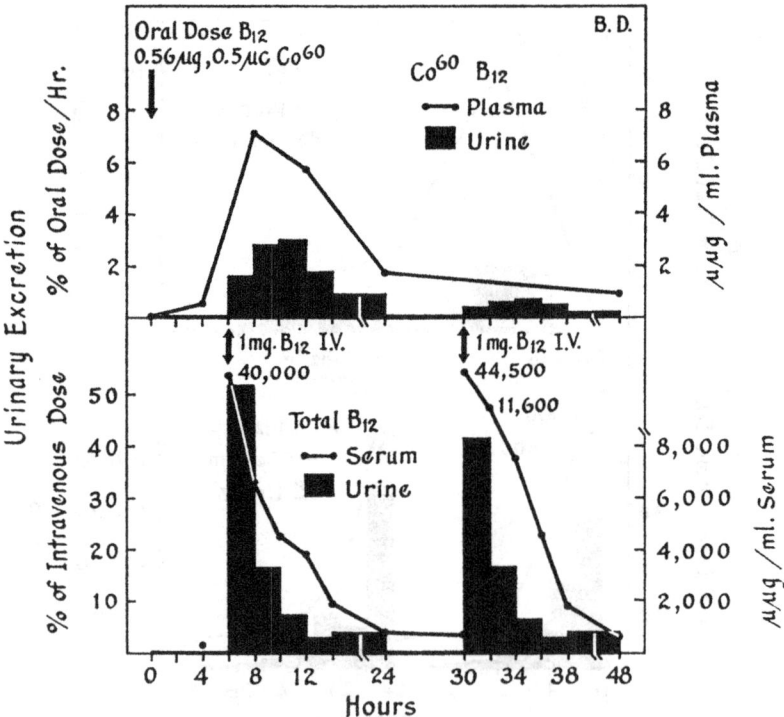

Figure 23. Urinary radioactivity in the Schilling test; comparison with $Co^{60}B_{12}$ in the plasma and the excretion of non-labeled B_{12}; intravenous "flushing" injections given 6 and 30 hours after oral dose. (From Doscherholmen and Hagen: Kinetics of ingested radiocyanocobalamin in man. Vitamin B_{12} und Intrinsic Factor, 2. Europäisches Symposion, Hamburg, 1961, Ferdinand Enke Verlag, Stuttgart, 381, 1962.)

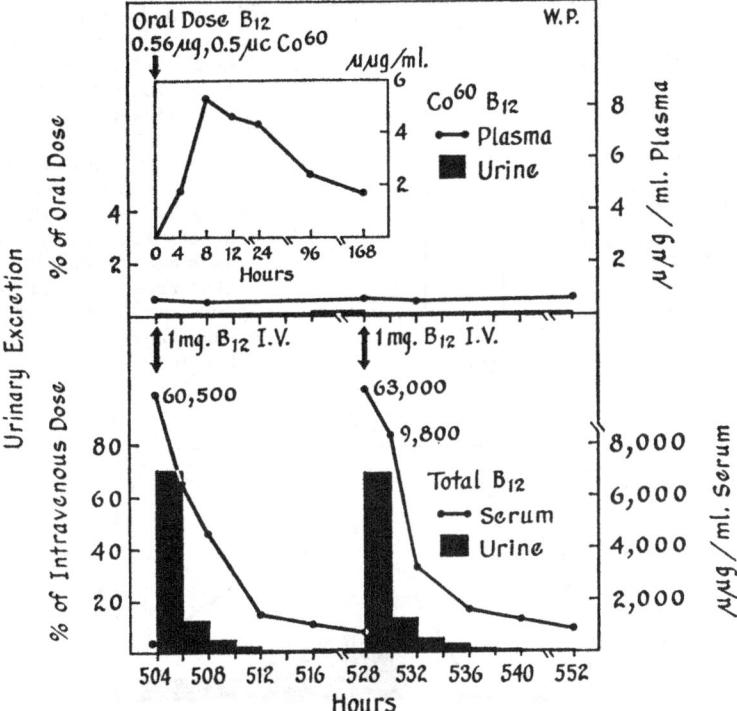

Figure 24. Urinary radioactivity in the Schilling test; comparison with B_{12} in the plasma and the excretion pattern of non-labeled B_{12}; intravenous "flushing" injections given 21 and 22 days after oral dose. (From Doscherholmen and Hagen: Kinetics of ingested radiocyanocobalamin in man. Vitamin B_{12} und Intrinsic Factor, 2. Europäisches Symposion, Hamburg, 1961, Ferdinand Enke Verlag, Stuttgart, 381, 1962.)

After ingestion of physiologic amounts of radiocyanocobalamin it takes about 4 hours before significant quantities of radioactivity appear in the plasma (60, 158, 162) and urine (40, 60, 557). During the interval between the ingestion of the test dose and the appearance of radioactivity in blood and urine, the labeled vitamin must be assumed to be in a body space or compartment from which it is not readily dislodged by the "flushing" procedure of Schilling. Because this interval was relatively short, this body space was labeled a temporary storage compartment.

Approximately 4 to 6 hours after ingestion of the labeled cyanocobalamin, the vitamin apparently begins to move into a second body space and is then readily diverted from its natural course by the parenteral "flushing" procedure and excreted into the urine. Because there has always been a high correlation between the time of appearance of radioactivity in the plasma and urine (Fig. 26) and between the de-

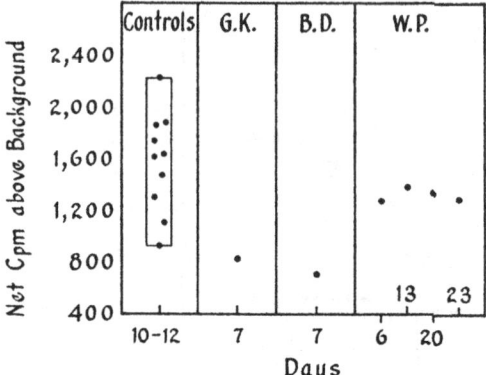

Figure 25. In-vivo hepatic radioactivity 6 to 23 days after oral dose of Co⁶⁰B₁₂; 10 control subjects received no parenteral "flushing" injections; G.K. received injections at 0 and 24 hours, B.D. at 6 and 30 hours, and W.P. 21 and 22 days after oral dose. (From Doscherholmen and Hagen: Kinetics of ingested radiocyanocobalamin in man. Vitamin B₁₂ und Intrinsic Factor, 2. Europäisches Symposion, Hamburg, 1961, Ferdinand Enke Verlag, Stuttgart, 381, 1962.)

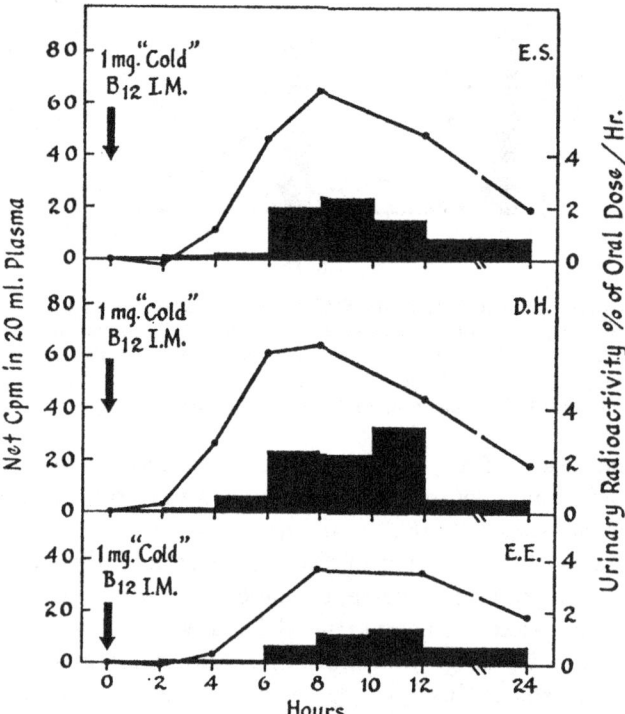

Figure 26. Correlation between delayed appearance of Co⁶⁰B₁₂ in the plasma and urine in 3 control subjects; oral dose 0.56 µg B₁₂ (0.5 µc Co⁶⁰); 1 mg. "cold" B₁₂ given intramuscularly simultaneously with oral dose. (From Doscherholmen and Hagen: Kinetics of ingested radiocyanocobalamin in man. Vitamin B₁₂ und Intrinsic Factor, 2. Europäisches Symposion, Hamburg, 1961, Ferdinand Enke Verlag, Stuttgart, 381, 1962.)

Figure 27. Correlation between the fall-off curve of radioactivity of plasma and the decreasing amount of urinary radioactivity as a function of time; upper part shows the average of 10 plasma Co⁶⁰B₁₂ absorption values with upper and lower ranges obtained in control subjects who did not receive any parenteral B₁₂; lower part shows the average 24-hour urinary excretion values with upper and lower ranges in 9 groups of control subjects containing 10–42 individuals; 1 mg. "cold" B₁₂ was administered intramuscularly at various times after the oral dose and immediately before the urinary collection was begun; oral dose 0.56 μg

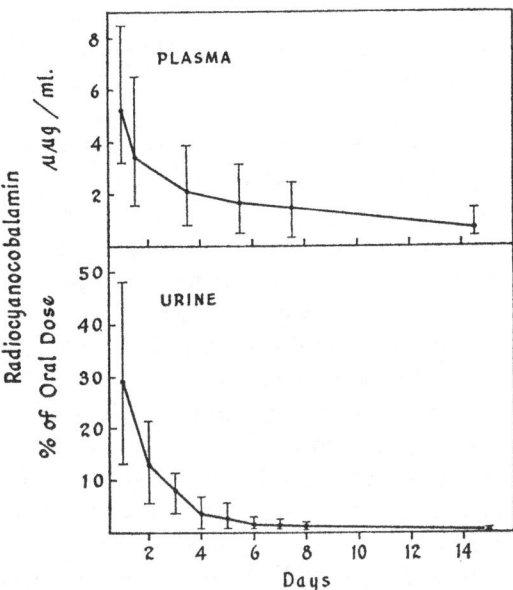

B₁₂ (0.39 or 0.50 μc Co⁶⁰). (From Doscherholmen and Hagen: Kinetics of ingested radiocyanocobalamin in man. Vitamin B₁₂ und Intrinsic Factor, 2. Europäisches Symposion, Hamburg, 1961, Ferdinand Enke Verlag, Stuttgart, 381, 1962.)

cline of plasma radiocyanocobalamin and the urinary radioactivity as a function of time (Fig. 27), the second body space was termed the transport compartment.

The third typical response to the parenteral injection, observed 21 and 22 days after the oral test dose was administered, indicated that by this time the vitamin had moved into a third body space. Because the response did not change with the repeated injection, it was assumed that the stay in this compartment was rather more permanent. This third body space was therefore called a "permanent" storage compartment. It is apparent that the ingested cyanocobalamin was relatively well protected from the "flushing" action of the parenterally injected vitamin B_{12} when in the storage compartments but not when being transported through the second compartment, i.e., the blood stream.

Investigations have been performed to locate the anatomical sites of the temporary and the more permanent storage compartments. Both direct (156) and indirect (160, 232) evidence suggests that the wall of the small intestine serves as a temporary storage space for vitamin B_{12} during its absorption from the gastrointestinal tract in man, and the same holds true for the rat (59), whereas the liver is the most important but not the only organ for the permanent storage of the vitamin.

Fig. 28 summarizes studies on material obtained at autopsy and illustrates the point in question. Up to 7 hours after the ingestion of the labeled test dose virtually all of the visceral radioactivity was found in the wall of the small intestine. After 24 hours the radioactivity of the small bowel had dropped to 30.2 per cent and after 42 hours to 27.5 per cent of the total visceral count. A further decline to between 4.9 and 12.9 per cent was recorded between 85 and 309 hours after the tests, and to between 1 and 2 per cent in the 2 subjects who died 13 and 113 days after ingestion of the vitamin.

The concept of a prolonged transfer of the vitamin from the temporary storage in the intestinal wall to more permanent storage in other organs (60, 156, 160, 232) can explain the slow disappearance rate of plasma radioactivity after oral ingestion of labeled cyanocobalamin (60, 158, 162) in contrast to the rapid falling off after intravenous injections of the vitamin (179, 266, 416, 437, 536, 544). The fact that the ingested vitamin is relatively well protected against the "flushing" action of the parenterally injected vitamin when in the storage compartments, together with a slow transport between the compartments may

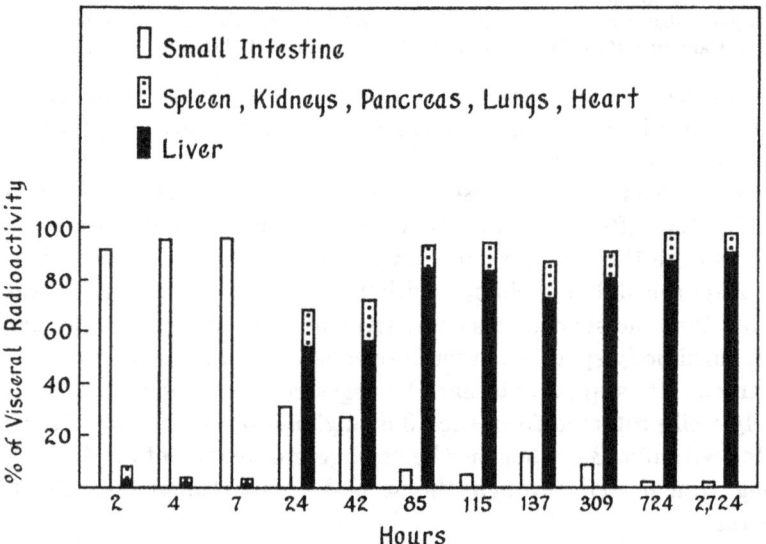

Figure 28. Radioactivity of the small intestine in man compared with that of the major viscera at differing times after oral dose of 0.56 μg B_{12} (0.5 μc Co^{60}). (From Doscherholmen, Finley, and Hagen: Organ distribution of radioactivity in man after the oral administration of physiologic test doses of radiolabeled cyanocobalamin. Proc. 7th Congr. Europ. Soc. Haemat., London, 1959, S. Karger, Basel/New York, 2:26, 1960; and from Doscherholmen and Hagen: Kinetics of ingested radiocyanocobalamin in man. Vitamin B_{12} und Intrinsic Factor, 2. Europäisches Symposion, Hamburg, 1961, Ferdinand Enke Verlag, Stuttgart, 381, 1962.)

be the main reason why only a fraction — on the average approximately a third (82, 380) — of the absorbed radiocyanocobalamin is excreted in the 24-hour urine in the Schilling test, while at the same time a much greater proportion of the injected vitamin is excreted (Table 70) (60, 122, 355, 442). It also explains why "flushing" injections given at intervals during the first day after the oral test (415) are hardly more effective than a single injection despite the fact that similar injections administered on subsequent days will result in additional radioactivity's being excreted (73, 177, 415, 509, 657), and, finally, why an increase in the amount of vitamin B_{12} to 4 or 5 mg. in the "flushing" injection is not much more effective than the conventional 1 mg. dose (177) (Table 28).

Besides the various excretion patterns, the detailed studies in the 3 patients revealed certain other phenomena of great interest. For example, Fig. 25 shows that in subjects G.K. and B.D. the hepatic radioactivity was lower than that usually found in control subjects who did not receive parenteral injections. The comparatively large urinary losses of 40.1 and 49.1 per cent of the absorbed radioactivity, respectively, in the 2 instances may explain this finding. On the other hand, in the third subject, W.P., who received the parenteral injections at a later time, the hepatic radioactivity was in the range found in the control subjects, and, furthermore, there was no significant decrease in hepatic radioactivity with delayed "flushing" injections. The practical lesson to be learned from these experiments is that two early injections will prevent hepatic accumulation of much of the ingested radioactivity whereas two late injections fail in this respect.

Another finding of note was the fact that, although there was immediate excretion of radioactivity in the urine following the 6-, 24-, and 30-hour injections, there was in each instance a delay in the peak amounts excreted. Similar observations have been observed and commented on previously (60). The reason for this phenomenon has been given above (pp. 155–156).

Vitamin B_{12} has a function in the body and we must therefore assume the existence of a compartment of utilization as distinct from the three previously mentioned body spaces. We have used incorporation of radiocyanocobalamin into the formed elements of the blood to demonstrate the existence of such a compartment. The red blood cells contain cyanocobalamin (19, 593) but they are practically impermeable to vitamin B_{12} in vitro, even in the presence of very high concentrations of the vitamin (Table 71), and they have not been found to serve as passive carriers of cyanocobalamin in the blood stream (162). Incorporation of vitamin B_{12} into these cells might for this reason rightfully be an expression of metabolic utilization of the vitamin by these cells. Presumably other body cells also use cyanocobalamin in their metabolism, because they show characteristic changes in vitamin B_{12} deficiency states (50, 51, 52, 191, 192, 241, 389). The formed elements of the blood were chosen to demonstrate the existence of the compartment of utilization because they are so readily available for examination.

Table 71. In-Vitro Uptake of Radiocyanocobalamin from Plasma by Erythrocytes, Plasma Containing 50,000 μμg $Co^{57}B_{12}$ per ml. Incubated with Equal Volumes of Packed Red Blood Cells, Radioactivity of Plasma Determined before and after Incubation with the Erythrocytes

	Radioactivity, cpm/5 ml. Aliquot		
	Plasma		
Experiment Number	Before Incubation with Erythrocytes	After Incubation with Erythrocytes	Erythrocytes Washed Thrice
1	15,156	14,794	...
2	15,188	14,246	72

A 54-year-old man suffering from diverticulosis of the sigmoid colon and gastritis, with normal blood values (hemoglobin 16.3 grams per 100 ml. of blood and hematocrit of 48 per cent) was given an oral test dose of 3.25 μg vitamin B_{12} containing 19.89 μc Co^{57}. The fecal excretion test showed that 30.5 per cent of the oral dose was absorbed, and 70 ml. blood samples were obtained at various times up to 4 weeks after the administration of the test dose. Radioactivity measurements were performed, respectively, on 20 ml. plasma, 20 ml. thrice-washed packed erythrocytes, and the buffy coat of the whole blood sample suspended in 20 ml. water. The results are shown in Fig. 29. The plasma absorption curve revealed a peak concentration of radioactivity after 12 hours, with a gradual decline over the ensuing days—a normal absorption curve. The radioactivity pattern of the erythrocytes was entirely different. There was negligible radioactivity in the red blood cells when the plasma activity was at its peak, and, in contrast to the plasma, the activity of these cells kept rising until a maximum concentration was reached one week after the oral test dose was administered. The radioactivity pattern of the buffy coat was similar to that of the erythrocytes.

This experiment shows that radiocyanocobalamin is incorporated into the red blood cells reminiscent of the manner in which Fe^{59} and N^{15}- or C^{14}-labeled glycine are incorporated into the erythrocytes in vivo (34, 35, 168, 259, 260, 321, 576). It is therefore reasonable to assume

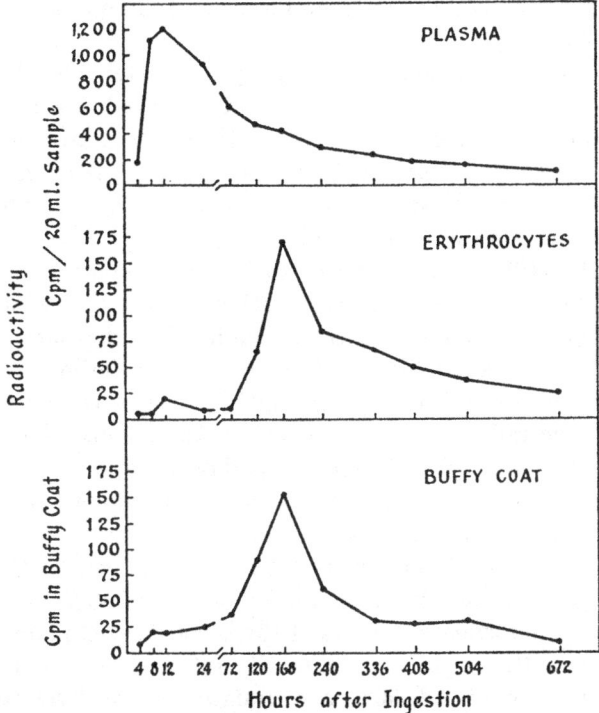

Figure 29. Radioactivity in plasma, thrice-washed erythrocytes, and the buffy coat of 70 ml. blood at various times after oral dose of 3.25 μg B_{12} (19.89 μc Co^{57}); patient a 54-year-old man with gastritis and diverticulosis of the sigmoid colon. (From Doscherholmen and Hagen: Kinetics of ingested radiocyanocobalamin in man. Vitamin B_{12} und Intrinsic Factor, 2. Europäisches Symposion, Hamburg, 1961, Ferdinand Enke Verlag, Stuttgart, 381, 1962.)

that vitamin B_{12} was incorporated into these formed elements of the blood as they were manufactured in the bone marrow. The radioactive vitamin B_{12} disappeared from the erythrocytes much faster than did N^{15} or C^{14} after labeled glycine had been incorporated into these same cells in vivo (34, 35, 370, 576). Thus, when $Co^{57}B_{12}$ was administered, the concentration of radioactivity in the erythrocytes had fallen by 50 per cent 3 days after the peak value was reached. There was no bleeding or hemolysis to account for this rapid change: the most likely explanation is that the radioactivity was lost from the intact cells. Since it is the newly formed red blood cells (reticulocytes) that contain the radio-vitamin, we may infer that the reticulocytes as they mature into erythrocytes lose some, if not all, of their vitamin B_{12}. After the parenteral injection into animals of radioactive cyanocobalamin, findings similar to ours have been observed, with delayed incorporation of activity in the erythrocytes (545) and a rapid decline following the peak activity (545, 650).

The radioactivity pattern of the buffy coat after ingestion of radio-cyanocobalamin was very similar to that observed in man or animals when P^{32}- or S^{35}-labeled L-cystine or tritiated thymidine was incorporated into the white blood cells in vivo (130A, 350, 484, 495, 648). Presumably, then, vitamin B_{12} stayed with the cells in the buffy coat until they left the blood stream or died.

Previously Miller and associates (416) have reported that radioactivity could not be detected in the erythrocytes or white blood cells of normal subjects or patients with leukemia after the parenteral injection of radiocyanocobalamin. In the light of our findings it is possible to suggest that these investigators did not follow their patients long enough for the radioactivity to appear in the formed elements of the blood or that insufficient radioactivity had been given.

From the estimated blood volume and the peripheral venous hematocrit, the maximum amounts of radioactivity in the entire plasma volume and the red cell mass were 3.2 and 0.5 per cent of the absorbed radioactivity, respectively. This small amount of radioactivity incorporated into the formed elements of the blood may explain why radioactive vitamin B_{12} injected parenterally into patients with pernicious anemia in relapse (443B, 503) accumulated in the liver to the same extent as seen in control subjects or patients with pernicious anemia in remission. Apparently a very small amount of the vitamin is needed for the formation of bone marrow and blood, and the in-vivo counters are not sensitive enough to detect the minute differences in hepatic radioactivity which may exist between persons with active blood regeneration and control subjects.

Two laboratory findings have been observed suggesting the existence of an extraintestinal temporary storage compartment for vitamin B_{12} following the oral ingestion of radio-labeled cyanocobalamin. They will be cited briefly.

In the autopsy study (pp. 170–177) it was noted that the spleen and the kidneys contained relatively more radioactivity 24 and 42 hours after the ingestion of the oral test dose than subsequently (Fig. 30), suggesting that these organs played a greater role in the storage of vitamin B_{12} immediately after it was absorbed, and that recently absorbed cyanocobalamin may be shifted around between the organs before it is finally stored more permanently in the liver. In other words, spleen and kidneys apparently partake in an extraintestinal temporary storage of cyanocobalamin.

The second observation in support of extraintestinal temporary stor-

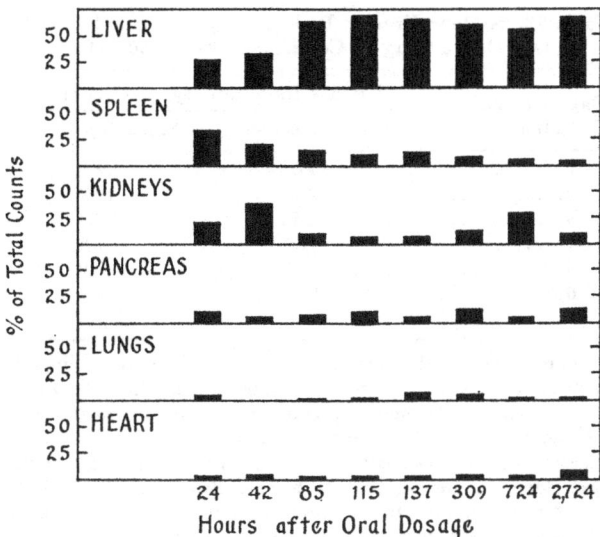

Figure 30. Distribution of radioactivity in extraintestinal organs in man at various times after oral dose of 0.56 μg B₁₂ (0.5 μc Co⁶⁰). (From Doscherholmen and Hagen: Kinetics of ingested radiocyanocobalamin in man. Vitamin B₁₂ und Intrinsic Factor, 2. Europäisches Symposion, Hamburg, 1961, Ferdinand Enke Verlag, Stuttgart, 381, 1962.)

age of vitamin B_{12} was made when the data from the urinary excretion tests were analyzed. A difference in the results was noted when the tests were performed in control subjects with single or multiple injections (Table 72). The subjects in the first column received one injection each morning for a week, with 24-hour urinary radioactivity determined after each injection. The second column contains the results from seven different groups of control subjects. The individuals in the first of these groups received the injection during the morning of the first day, those in the second group on the second day, those in the third group on the third day, and so on. When one compares the urinary excretion figures for the respective days in the two columns it becomes evident that the group receiving daily injections always showed the lowest average excretion figures after the first day. If extraintestinal temporary storage of cyanocobalamin occurs, it will be reduced in subjects receiving daily injections because of the great urinary loss of radioactivity they have sustained. Consequently, less radioactivity will be available for re-entry into the blood stream and excretion into the urine after the first day. These findings support the hypothesis of temporary extraintestinal storage of vitamin B_{12}, followed by redistribution of the vitamin.

Only indirect evidence has been offered for this hypothesis. More

Table 72. 24-Hour Urinary Radioactivity in Control Subjects:
Oral Dose 0.56 μg B_{12} Containing 0.39 or 0.50 μc Co^{60}

Day of Urine Collection	Urinary Radioactivity, % of Oral Dose	
	Daily Injection *	Single Injection †
1....................	24.0	22.4
2....................	9.0	12.8
3....................	2.2	7.8
4....................	1.1	3.6
5....................	0.7	2.9
6....................	0.6	1.6
7....................	0.6	1.5

(From Doscherholmen and Hagen: Kinetics of ingested radiocyanocobalamin in man. Vitamin B_{12} und Intrinsic Factor, 2. Europäisches Symposion, Hamburg, 1961, Ferdinand Enke Verlag, Stuttgart, 381, 1962; and Doscherholmen: Kinetics of ingested radiocyanocobalamin in man. Proc. 8th Congr. Europ. Soc. Haemat., Vienna, 1961, S. Karger, Basel/New York, 1962.)

* Average figures for a group who received one parenteral "flushing" injection every morning for 7 days.

† Average values for 7 groups, each of whom received a single "flushing" injection on the morning of the day on which urine was collected.

direct proof would be desirable, but may be difficult to get. Perusal of the literature, however, reveals findings in support of the hypothesis, findings in man after parenteral administration of radiocyanocobalamin and in the rat after oral as well as after parenteral administration of labeled vitamin B_{12}. Thus virtually all of the radiocyanocobalamin administered intramuscularly in man disappeared from the site of injection in 3 or 4 hours whereas the radioactivity over the liver continued to rise for several days (212, 220, 403). Activity over the spleen and the kidneys seemed to reach its maximum earlier than over the liver and also declined more rapidly (212, 220, 403), suggesting a redistribution of the vitamin from the spleen and the kidneys to more permanent storage in the liver — temporary storage of the vitamin extraintestinally.

After the intravenous injection of radiocyanocobalamin, a rapid disappearance of radioactivity from the blood has invariably been found in control subjects (179, 266, 416, 437, 536, 544). The uptake of radioactivity over the hepatic region under these conditions may be rapid in the beginning (443B) or slow (416), but it invariably continues for many days (266, 416). This continuous rise in hepatic radioactivity seemed greater than could be explained by the amount of radioactivity in the blood (416); the radioactivity must therefore be assumed to have come from somewhere else. These findings again point to redistribution of the vitamin or temporary extraintestinal storage. It is quite likely that organs other than the spleen and the kidneys may take part in this temporary extraintestinal storage, as recently suggested (131). Findings after the parenteral (277) or oral (59) administration of radiocyanocobalamin to rats may likewise be interpreted as supporting the hypothesis of temporary extraintestinal storage. Transfer of radioactive vitamin B_{12} to the liver from extrahepatic sources has in fact recently been described in rats following parenteral injection of the vitamin (606). In the light of these findings in man after parenteral and in the rat after oral and parenteral administration of cyanocobalamin, the indirect evidence given (pp. 188–190, Fig. 30, Table 72) for extraintestinal temporary storage of vitamin B_{12} in man after the oral ingestion of radio-labeled B_{12} takes on much greater importance.

The biological half-life of vitamin B_{12} in the liver has been found to be approximately a year (212, 216, 563). An idea of the half-life of radiocyanocobalamin in the intestinal wall can be got from autopsy material (156) and from the urinary excretion figures (Table 72, A). The fact that 70 per cent of the visceral radioactivity was transferred to storage outside the intestinal tract during the first 24 hours after the test dose was administered (156) suggests a half-life of about 17 hours for the temporary storage of vitamin B_{12} in the intestinal wall. The 24-hour

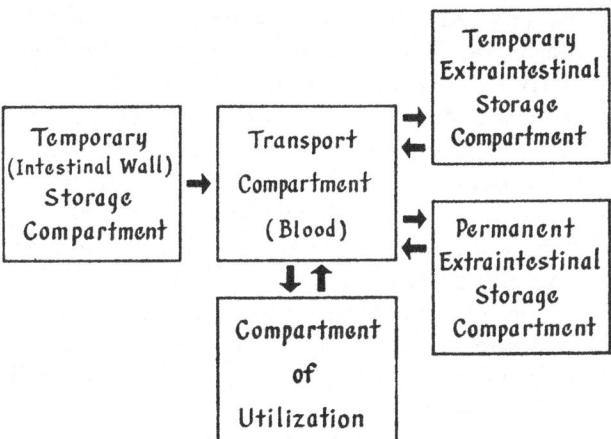

Figure 31. Sequential movement of radioactive B_{12} in man after oral dose; 5-compartmental system deduced from autopsy studies, measurements of radiocyanocobalamin in the formed elements of the blood, and from varying responses to the parenteral "flushing" procedures. (From Doscherholmen: Kinetics of ingested radiocyanocobalamin in man. Proc. 8th Congr. Europ. Soc. Haemat., Vienna, 1961, S. Karger, Basel/New York, 1962; and from Doscherholmen and Hagen: Kinetics of ingested radiocyanocobalamin in man. Vitamin B_{12} und Intrinsic Factor, 2. Europäisches Symposion, Hamburg, 1961, Ferdinand Enke Verlag, Stuttgart, 381, 1962.)

urinary excretion figures represent relative absorption of vitamin B_{12} from the gut or, if we may, discharge from the intestinal storage compartment. Assuming that the absorption is completed in 4–7 days, the daily percentage of transfer from this compartment can be estimated from these figures. Such a calculation shows that approximately two thirds of the radiocyanocobalamin in the intestinal wall is released each 24 hours, corresponding to the half-life for vitamin B_{12} of 18–19 hours for this compartment. Thus there seems to be a good agreement between these two ways of estimating the half-life of vitamin B_{12} in the intestinal wall. The rate of disappearance of radiocyanocobalamin from the transport compartment may be judged by the falling off of the plasma absorption curve. However, because of prolonged influx of radiocyanocobalamin into the blood, this part of the curve is probably even more difficult to evaluate than is the disappearance curve observed after intravenous injection of labeled B_{12} (131). There seem to be three components to this disappearance curve after oral ingestion of radiocyanocobalamin in man, similar to the three-part curve in rabbits (543). The half-life of the vitamin in the compartment of utilization and in the extraintestinal temporary storage compartment is largely unknown.

Understanding the kinetics of orally ingested cyanocobalamin as set forth here may be facilitated by following the vitamin from the time of its ingestion (Fig. 31). After having been absorbed into the intestinal mucosal cells, the molecules are released into the blood gradually and in an orderly manner over a period of time, most of them during the first day after ingestion. From the blood stream the majority of the molecules will move into permanent storage in the liver and possibly also other organs. Some of the molecules will be used in the formation of new blood cells in the bone marrow and in the production of other tissue cells. Some will temporarily move into viscera such as the spleen and the kidneys and probably also other organs, but will soon be rerouted back to the liver for more permanent storage there. When entering the blood stream on its way from the temporary to the more permanent storage compartment, the vitamin seems readily diverted from its normal course to be excreted with the urine by Schilling's "flushing" procedure, whereas it appears practically immune to the same procedure at other times.

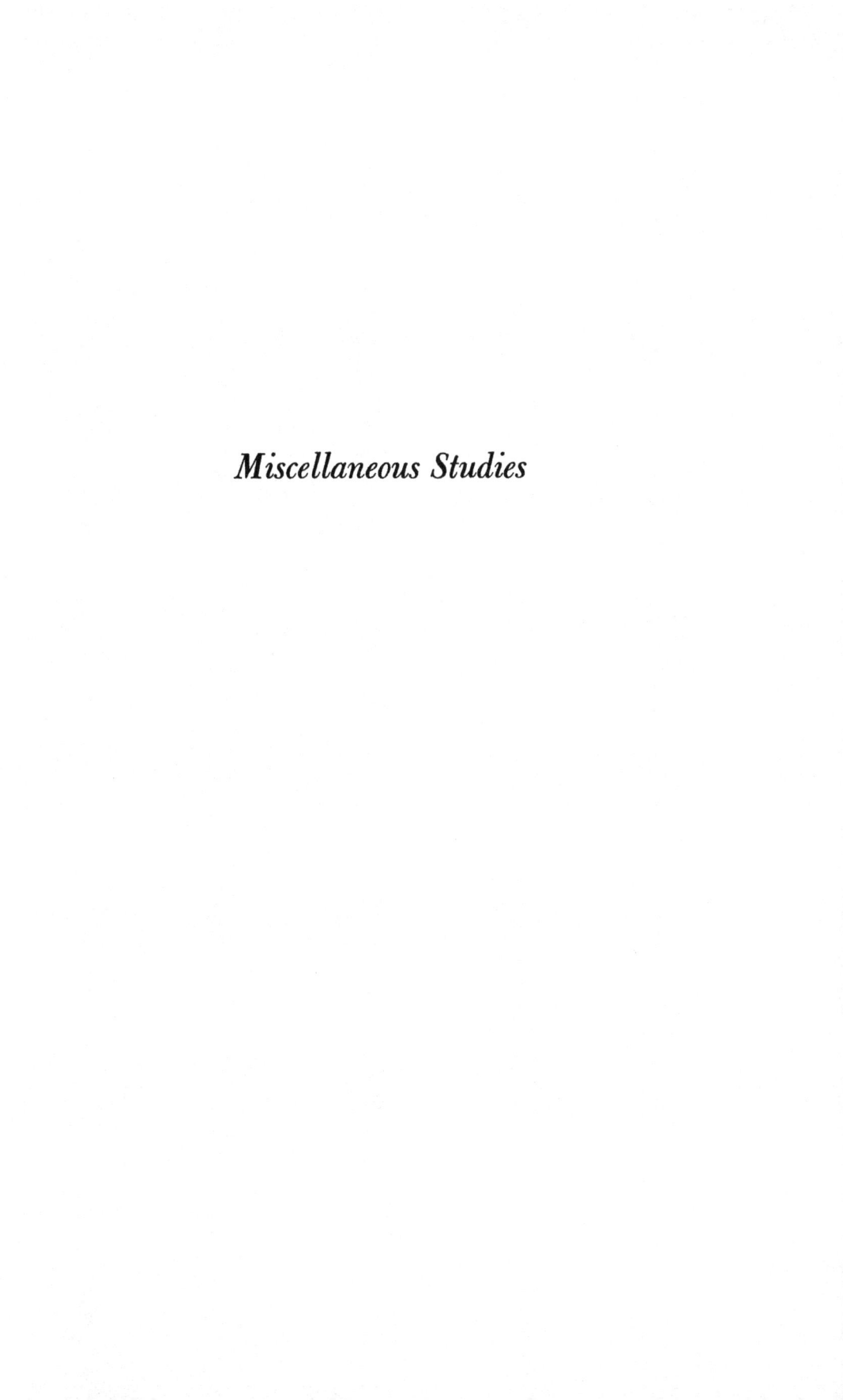

Miscellaneous Studies

5 | ENZYMATIC RELEASE OF VITAMIN B_{12} BOUND EITHER TO THE INTRINSIC FACTOR OR IN THE WALL OF THE SMALL INTESTINE

VITAMIN B_{12} in nature is bound to animal proteins, though proteolytic enzymes can liberate it (522). Cyanocobalamin thus released during the digestive process presumably is bound to the intrinsic factor before being absorbed by the small intestine. Recent investigations have shown that intrinsic factor can remove vitamin B_{12} from proteins in vitro even after the inactivation of the pepsin in gastric juice (126), suggesting that the digestion of protein, in its strictest sense, is not required for the action of intrinsic factor and the absorption of vitamin B_{12}.

When cyanocobalamin is being absorbed from the gastrointestinal tract, it must first enter the intestinal mucosal cells from the intestinal lumen and then be released from these cells into the blood stream. Many investigations have dealt with the problem of the uptake of cyanocobalamin by the small intestine (1, 2, 59, 119, 126, 156, 306, 308, 313, 362, 432, 473, 605, 658, 663A, 664), but nothing is known about the release of the vitamin from the intestinal mucosal cells into the blood stream. Recently it has been found that the IF-B_{12} complex can be split by enzymatic activity (126, 336, 470) and, furthermore, that an enzyme that does this splitting is present in the intestinal wall (126, 301A, 311A, 472A). The physiologic implication of these findings is still debatable.

Release of Vitamin B_{12} from the Intrinsic Factor

Pooled human gastric juice, filtered and neutralized to pH 7.0, rat-stomach homogenate, and commercially available hog-stomach intrin-

NOTE: This chapter appeared in slightly different form in Doscherholmen, Vitamin B_{12} und Intrinsic Factor, 2. Europäisches Symposion, Hamburg, 1961, Ferdinand Enke Verlag, Stuttgart, 472, 1962 (155).

sic factor concentrate were used as sources of IF. The desired amount of $Co^{60}B_{12}$ or $Co^{57}B_{12}$ was added to the solution containing the IF to make up the substrate. These mixtures were incubated for 30 minutes at 37°C. as a standard procedure, although later experiments showed that the binding of vitamin B_{12} to IF occurred instantaneously. Homogenates from the small intestine of rats were used to furnish the B_{12}-releasing activity. These rats, fed an ordinary stock diet, were, after a fast of 18 hours to 3 days, sacrificed with a blow over the head and the small intestines removed. The intestines were rinsed in ice cold phosphate buffer and homogenized with a ground glass homogenizer. A phosphate buffer with a pH of 7.4 was used for the homogenates as well as for making up solutions of radiocyanocobalamin. The desired amount of homogenate of rat intestine and substrate were mixed and incubated in a shaking water bath at 37°C. for 30 minutes to 4 hours. A control mixture consisting of substrate and buffer solution was similarly incubated. Two mixtures similar to the ones incubated at warm temperature were also prepared and kept on ice for identical lengths of time. The liberated cyanocobalamin was measured in the ultrafiltrates of these mixtures radiometrically and by bioassay using the *Euglena gracilis* method (548). Ultrafiltrates were prepared according to the method of Prasad and Flink (506). If the mixture had been warm-incubated, ultrafiltrates were obtained at room temperature whereas ultrafiltrates from the control mixtures kept on ice were prepared in a refrigerated centrifuge at 3–5°C. Measurements of radioactivity (162) were taken on various volumes, but the geometry was kept constant for each experiment so that the figures are comparable. Paper chromatographic studies were carried out on the ultrafiltrable radioactivity according to a previously described technique (380). The solubility characteristic for butanol of the ultrafiltrable radioactivity was also determined and compared with that of radiocyanocobalamin.

Experiments Using Human Gastric Juice as a Source of Intrinsic Factor

The substrate was made up by mixing equal volumes of pooled human gastric juice and a solution containing 1,000 $\mu\mu g$ radio-vitamin B_{12} per ml. This concentration was chosen because it gave a well saturated but not a supersaturated intrinsic factor according to preliminary B_{12}-binding studies of the gastric juice. To 50 ml. of the intestinal homogenate 10 ml. of this substrate were added before the incubation period. Table 73 shows the results of 3 different experiments. The ultrafiltrates obtained from the warm-incubated mixtures of rat intestinal homog-

Table 73. Release of Free $Co^{60}B_{12}$ from the Intrinsic Factor–Vitamin B_{12} Complex by Homogenate from Rat Small Intestine, Human Gastric Juice Used as Source of Intrinsic Factor

Mixture	Incubation Time (hr.)	Counting Volume (ml.)	Radioactivity, cpm		
				Ultrafiltrate	
			Whole Mixture	Incubated	On Ice
Experiment 1					
Substrate + rat intestinal homogenate	4	2	1,444	112	15
Substrate + buffer..	4	2		24	20
Experiment 2					
Substrate + rat intestinal homogenate	4	20	9,342	283	18
Substrate + buffer..	4	20		43	16
Experiment 3					
Substrate + rat intestinal homogenate	1	20	9,348	777	22
Substrate + buffer..	1	20		57	13

(From Doscherholmen: Enzymatic release of vitamin B_{12} bound either to the intrinsic factor or in the wall of the small intestine. Vitamin B_{12} und Intrinsic Factor, 2. Europäisches Symposion, Hamburg, 1961, Ferdinand Enke Verlag, Stuttgart, 472, 1962.)

enates and substrate contained many times more radioactivity than the ultrafiltrates from the control mixtures incubated in the water bath or kept on ice. It is therefore evident that under appropriate conditions the homogenate from rat intestine is able to make radiocyanocobalamin more ultrafiltrable, presumably by releasing it from its binding to intrinsic factor. Incubation of the mixture of substrate and buffer also constantly led to a slight increase in the amount of ultrafiltrable radioactivity, perhaps suggesting that even in the gastric juice some splitting of the B_{12}-IF complex takes place.

The influence of boiling on the activity of the homogenate from the small intestine was investigated in two experiments. In the first, 50 ml. of the homogenate was boiled over an open flame for 5 minutes; in the second it was kept on a boiling water bath for 30 minutes. The evaporated volume of water was replaced before the substrate was added. The results (Table 74) show that most of the activity was destroyed by heat, and that the open flame was more effective in this respect than the boiling water bath. Significant, but not complete, inactivation by heat was also a characteristic for the B_{12}-releasing activity of the extract of the small intestine of rats (126) .

Table 74. Effect of Boiling on the Release of Free Co^{57}B$_{12}$ from the Intrinsic Factor–Vitamin B$_{12}$ Complex, Human Gastric Juice Used as Source of Intrinsic Factor

Mixture	Incubation Time (hr.)	Boiling Time (min.)	Radioactivity, cpm/20 ml. Sample		
				Ultrafiltrates	
			Whole Mixture	Incubated	On Ice
		Experiment 4			
Substrate + rat intestinal homogenate, not boiled	4	...	9,230	1,156	16
Substrate + rat intestinal homogenate, boiled	4	5*		142	...
Substrate + buffer	4	...		75	242
		Experiment 5			
Substrate + rat intestinal homogenate, not boiled	4	...	8,987	4,359	15
Substrate + rat intestinal homogenate, boiled	4	30†		939	...
Substrate + buffer	4	...		188	121

(From Doscherholmen: Enzymatic release of vitamin B$_{12}$ bound either to the intrinsic factor or in the wall of the small intestine. Vitamin B$_{12}$ und Intrinsic Factor, 2. Europäisches Symposion, Hamburg, 1961, Ferdinand Enke Verlag, Stuttgart, 472, 1962.)

* Boiled over open flame.
† Kept in a boiling water bath.

Experiments Using Rat Stomach Homogenate as a Source of Intrinsic Factor

It has been shown that preparations of rat stomach (463, 617, 644) as well as rat gastric juice (463) can serve as sources of intrinsic factor in gastrectomized rats. Rat stomachs, being more readily available, were chosen to furnish this factor in these studies. The substrate consisted of equal volumes of rat stomach homogenate in phosphate buffer and a solution containing 500 $\mu\mu$g Co^{57}B$_{12}$ per ml. Two experiments were performed in which 50 ml. of rat intestinal homogenate was mixed with 15 ml. of the substrate, and a control mixture was made up of substrate and buffer. The two mixtures were incubated for 1 hour at 37°C. in the water bath; two identically prepared mixtures were kept on ice as controls for a similar length of time. Radioactivity measurements were performed on the whole mixtures and the various ultrafiltrates. The results (Table 75) show that the most radioactivity was found in the ultrafiltrates from the warm-incubated mixtures containing substrate and intestinal homogenate, meaning that more ultrafiltrable or free cyanocobalamin was present in these mixtures than in any of the controls. The incubated mixtures containing substrate plus buffer apparently contained more radioactive vitamin B$_{12}$ in a free form than did the corresponding mixtures kept on ice. Some splitting of the B$_{12}$-IF complex or digestion may have taken place in the substrate to account for this phenomenon. It is, however, important to note that much more radiocyanocobalamin was freed from its binding when intestinal homogenate was present in the warm-incubated mixtures. A minute amount of pepsin might conceivably be present in the substrate; it is known that this enzyme can liberate cyanocobalamin from its protein binding (522). Although it is unlikely that pepsin would be very active at the pH used in these experiments, it cannot be ruled out that some peptic activity was present. But since so much more radioactivity was released when intestinal homogenate was added, it becomes evident that the major B$_{12}$-releasing activity came from the intestine.

Table 75. Release of Free Co^{57}B$_{12}$ from the Intrinsic Factor–Vitamin B$_{12}$ Complex by Homogenate from the Small Intestine of Rats, Rat-Stomach Homogenate Used as Source of Intrinsic Factor

Mixture	Radioactivity, cpm/20 ml. Sample		
		Ultrafiltrate	
	Whole Mixture	Incubated	On Ice
Experiment 6			
Substrate + rat intestinal homogenate	7,492	502	12
Substrate + buffer		166	18
Experiment 7			
Substrate + rat intestinal homogenate	6,987	675	31
Substrate + buffer		190	27

(From Doscherholmen: Enzymatic release of vitamin B$_{12}$ bound either to the intrinsic factor or in the wall of the small intestine. Vitamin B$_{12}$ und Intrinsic Factor, 2. Europäisches Symposion, Hamburg, 1961, Ferdinand Enke Verlag, Stuttgart, 472, 1962.)

Experiments Using Hog Stomach IFC as a Source of IF

One capsule containing 1 USP unit of IFC was diluted in 2,000 ml. of phosphate buffer. The substrate consisted of equal volumes of this solution of IFC and a solution containing 1,000 $\mu\mu$g Co^{57}B$_{12}$ per ml. Preliminary vitamin B$_{12}$-binding studies showed that this mixture would give a well saturated but not a supersaturated IFC. Four experiments were carried out wherein 50 ml. homogenate of rat intestine was mixed with 10 ml. of substrate. A control mixture consisted of 10 ml. substrate and 50 ml. of phosphate buffer. Both kinds of mixture were incubated at 37°C. for 1 to 4 hours in the water bath. Two identically prepared mixtures were kept on ice for corresponding lengths of time. Radioactivity was measured in all the mixtures and their corresponding ultrafiltrates. The results (Table 76) show that the highest amount of radioactivity was consistently found in the ultrafiltrates of the warm-in-

Table 76. Release of Free Co^{57}B$_{12}$ from the Intrinsic Factor–Vitamin B$_{12}$ Complex by Homogenate from Small Intestine of Rats, Hog-Stomach Intrinsic Factor Concentrate Used as a Source of Intrinsic Factor

	Time of Incubation (hr.)	Radioactivity, cpm/20 ml. Sample		
			Ultrafiltrate	
Mixture		Whole Mixture	Incubated	On Ice
Experiment 8				
Substrate + rat intestinal homogenate	4	9,285	324	65
Substrate + buffer..	4		20	24
Experiment 9				
Substrate + rat intestinal homogenate	4	8,367	817	5
Substrate + buffer..	4		45	7
Experiment 10				
Substrate + rat intestinal homogenate	1	8,350	314	14
Substrate + buffer..	1		25	17
Experiment 11				
Substrate + rat intestinal homogenate	1	5,524	407	11
Substrate + buffer..	1		52	1

(From Doscherholmen: Enzymatic release of vitamin B$_{12}$ bound either to the intrinsic factor or in the wall of the small intestine. Vitamin B$_{12}$ und Intrinsic Factor, 2. Europäisches Symposion, Hamburg, 1961, Ferdinand Enke Verlag, Stuttgart, 472, 1962.)

cubated mixtures containing substrate and intestinal homogenate, and very little radioactivity was present in ultrafiltrates of the other mixtures.

The B$_{12}$-releasing factor in the homogenate of rat small intestine is thus capable of liberating the vitamin from the IF of its own species as well as from that of hog and man, a result somewhat at variance with that of Cooper and Castle, who did not find any consistent activity of rat intestinal extract when hog-stomach IFC was used (126). The reason for this discrepancy is not entirely clear: it could be variations in methods, or inhibitory substances present in some IFC. We know that too much IFC in the substrate may inhibit the B$_{12}$-releasing activity (Table 77), a phenomenon reminiscent of the finding that the cellular

Table 77. Inhibition of the Release of B$_{12}$ by Excess Intrinsic Factor Concentrate in the Substrate, Substrates and Homogenates Incubated for 2 Hours at 37°C. and Ultrafiltrates Prepared at 2–5°C.

IFC in Substrate (USP unit)	Substrate (ml.)	Rat Intestinal Homogenate (ml.)	Radioactivity, cpm/20 ml.	
			Total Mixture	Ultrafiltrate
1:100	10	50	7,384	5
1:4,000	10	50	7,384	88

uptake of cyanocobalamin is inhibited by an excess of intrinsic factor (81, 227, 306, 308, 311, 610, 614, 616, 617). The receptor protein on the surface of the cells apparently works on the intrinsic factor and not on the B$_{12}$ part of the complex (2, 306, 308, 614). The same may be true of the enzyme responsible for the splitting of the complex. This may explain why the absorption of the IF-B$_{12}$ complex into the cells and the splitting of the complex in vitro by intestinal homogenate are both inhibited by the presence of excess IF.

Release of Co^{57}B$_{12}$ from Its Binding in the Intestinal Wall

The studies so far have shown that homogenates from the small intestine of rats contain some factor which under appropriate conditions can release vitamin B$_{12}$ from the IF-B$_{12}$ complex in vitro. The B$_{12}$-releasing phenomenon must also occur in vivo in order to be of physiologic significance. In other words, the question must be entertained whether bound vitamin B$_{12}$ is released from the mucosal cells of the small intestine. In man (156, 160) as well as in rats (59) the small intestine serves as a temporary storage compartment for cyanocobalamin after the oral ingestion of radiocyanocobalamin, and radioautographs have shown the radioactivity to be in the mucosal cells (59). To answer this important question, in-vitro experiments were performed on small intestinal homogenates from rats. The rats fasted for 18 hours and were then given oral test doses of 0.005–0.01 μg vitamin B_{12} containing 0.01 to 0.04 μc Co^{57} through a stomach tube. The rats were sacrificed 1–2 hours later and the small intestine removed, rinsed in phosphate buffer, and homogenized. The homogenates from two rats were mixed and diluted to 100 ml. with buffer solution. Half of this mixed homogenate was incubated for 4 hours at 37°C. in the water bath while the other half was kept on ice as a control for the same length of time. In this experiment ultrafiltrates were prepared from the warm-incubated homogenate and the control at 2–5°C. and at room temperature. The results (Table 78) show that the ultrafiltrate from the warm-incubated homogenate prepared in the refrigerated centrifuge contained almost as much radioactivity as that prepared at room temperature. The ultrafiltrate of the cold homogenate prepared in the refrigerated centrifuge contained no radioactivity. Some activity, however, appeared in the ultrafiltrate prepared at room temperature from the same control homogenate. It is apparent, therefore, that some release of free vitamin B_{12} took place even at room temperature. But it should be noted that much more radioactivity was released with incubation at 37°C.

It is evident from this study that under appropriate conditions vitamin B_{12} can be released from its binding in the intestinal wall. We assume that this reaction is the same as that witnessed when vitamin B_{12} was released from the IF-B_{12} complex in vitro in previous experiments.

Table 78. Release of $Co^{57}B_{12}$ from the Homogenate of the Small Intestine of Rats Given 0.005 μg $Co^{57}B_{12}$ (0.01 μc) Orally 1 Hour before Sacrifice

Experiment 12	Radioactivity, cpm/2 ml. Aliquot
Homogenate, incubated at 37°C.	327
Corresponding ultrafiltrate, prepared at room temperature	93
Corresponding ultrafiltrate, prepared at 2–5°C.	83
Homogenate, kept on ice	324
Corresponding ultrafiltrate, prepared at 2–5°C.	0
Corresponding ultrafiltrate, prepared at room temperature	17

(From Doscherholmen: Enzymatic release of vitamin B_{12} bound either to the intrinsic factor or in the wall of the small intestine. Vitamin B_{12} und Intrinsic Factor, 2. Europäisches Symposion, Hamburg, 1961, Ferdinand Enke Verlag, Stuttgart, 472, 1962.)

Since there is good reason to believe that the IF-B$_{12}$ complex is absorbed into the mucosal cells of the small intestine (1, 2, 306, 308, 663A, 664), this assumption seems tenable.

The next experiment aimed at learning the effect of heat on the release of radiocyanocobalamin from its binding in the intestinal wall. For this purpose rats were given radiocyanocobalamin orally in a manner similar to that of the previous experiment. The homogenates of small intestines from three rats were mixed and diluted to 300 ml. with buffer solution; 100 ml. of this mixed homogenate was kept in the boiling water bath for 5 or 15 minutes, and the homogenates then divided into equal parts. Half was incubated for an hour at 37°C. in the shaking water bath while the other half was kept on ice as a control for the same length of time. Another 100 ml. of the mixed homogenate was not boiled, but was divided into two equal parts. One was kept on ice for an hour, the other incubated in the water bath at 37°C. as a control for the boiled samples. Radioactivities of the various portions of the mixed homogenates and their respective ultrafiltrates are seen in Table 79. The non-boiled mixture which was kept on ice showed no ultrafiltrable radioactivity. The corresponding warm-incubated homogenate showed about 10 per cent ultrafiltrable or free radiocyanocobalamin. The boiled homogenates that had been kept on ice showed 20–30 per cent ultrafiltra-

Table 79. Effect of Boiling on the Release of Free Co^{57}B$_{12}$ from the Homogenate of the Small Intestine of Rats, Oral Dose 0.005 μg Co^{57}B$_{12}$ (0.01 μc)

Experiment 13	Radioactivity, cpm/4 ml. Aliquot	
	Homogenate	Ultrafiltrate
Boiled Homogenate		
Boiled for 5 minutes, then incubated at 37°C.	260	95
Boiled for 5 minutes, then kept on ice for 1 hour.	266	89
Boiled for 15 minutes, then incubated at 37°C.	232	58
Boiled for 15 minutes, then kept on ice for 1 hour.	242	51
Non-Boiled Homogenate		
Incubated at 37°C.	321	31
Kept on ice for 1 hour.	342	1

(From Doscherholmen: Enzymatic release of vitamin B$_{12}$ bound either to the intrinsic factor or in the wall of the small intestine. Vitamin B$_{12}$ und Intrinsic Factor, 2. Europäisches Symposion, Hamburg, 1961, Ferdinand Enke Verlag, Stuttgart, 472, 1962.)

ble radioactivity. When portions of the same homogenates were incubated at warm temperatures they showed only insignificantly greater ultrafiltrable radioactivity.

This experiment shows that heating in itself results in the release of some of the bound cyanocobalamin from the intestinal wall. Furthermore, it also shows that the B_{12}-releasing activity in the intestinal homogenate is heat-labile and almost completely destroyed after being in a boiling water bath for 5–15 minutes.

The effect of time on the release of radioactivity from the intestinal homogenate was also investigated. Mixed homogenate from rat small intestine was incubated for 0, 30, 60, 90, and 120 minutes in the shaking water bath at 37°C. The 0-minute homogenate served as a control for the other samples and was removed from the water bath as soon as its temperature was the same as that of the water bath. A good correlation was found between the length of incubation and the amount of free or ultrafiltrable radioactivity present in the homogenates (Table 80). Thus, after 30, 60, 90, and 120 minutes of incubation there was, respectively, 1.2, 2.8, 4.8, and 8.1 per cent ultrafiltrable radioactivity in the homogenates over and above the control value.

A study was designed to discover the optimum pH for the B_{12}-releasing activity in the intestinal wall. For this purpose, rat small intestines were homogenized in normal saline solution and diluted in various phosphate buffer solutions with pH ranging from 5 to 9. Two drops of a 10 per cent solution of NaOH had to be added to bring the pH of the homogenate above 8.4. The final pH values, ranging from 5 to 9.2, were determined on the homogenates immediately before they were incubated in the water bath. All the ultrafiltrates in this experiment were prepared in the refrigerated centrifuge. Table 81 shows that there was

Table 80. Influence of Time on the Release of Radiocyanocobalamin from the Homogenate of Small Intestines of Rats

Minutes of Incubation	Radioactivity, cpm/10 ml. Sample	
	Whole Homogenate	Ultrafiltrate
0............................	5,128	52
30...........................		113
60...........................		194
90...........................		300
120..........................		469

(From Doscherholmen: Enzymatic release of vitamin B_{12} bound either to the intrinsic factor or in the wall of the small intestine. Vitamin B_{12} und Intrinsic Factor, 2. Europäisches Symposion, Hamburg, 1961, Ferdinand Enke Verlag, Stuttgart, 472, 1962.)

Table 81. Influence of pH on the Release of Radiocyanocobalamin from the Homogenates of Small Intestines of Rats

pH	Radioactivity, cpm/10 ml. Aliquot	
	Homogenate	Ultrafiltrate
5.0	7,104	218
6.0		401
7.0		1,005
7.8		1,791
9.2		1,435

(From Doscherholmen: Enzymatic release of vitamin B$_{12}$
bound either to the intrinsic factor or in the wall of the small
intestine. Vitamin B$_{12}$ und Intrinsic Factor, 2. Europäisches Symposion, Hamburg, 1961, Ferdinand Enke Verlag, Stuttgart, 472,
1962.)

little release of radioactivity at pH 5 and that the maximum release
occurred on the alkaline side at pH 7.8.

The influence of these various factors — heat, time, and pH — on the
B$_{12}$-releasing factor in the intestinal wall suggests that we are dealing
here with an enzymatic reaction.

Characterization of the Ultrafiltrable Radioactivity

It was necessary to prove that the radioactivity found in the various
ultrafiltrates in our experiments was due to radiocyanocobalamin and
not to degradation products of the vitamin. This was accomplished in
three different ways: by paper chromatography, by solubility studies
of the ultrafiltrable radioactivity, and by determination of the vitamin
B$_{12}$ activity in the various ultrafiltrates.

The Rf value of Co^{57}B$_{12}$ and of the unknown radioactivity was determined radiometrically and the pink color was used to estimate the corresponding value for the "cold" concentrated vitamin B$_{12}$. Table 82
shows that the Rf values of the unknown radioactivities were similar
to those of pink vitamin B$_{12}$ applied to the same paper strips. When
pink B$_{12}$ and control Co^{57}B$_{12}$ were applied to separate paper strips, their
Rf values were different. Apparently something in the concentrated butanol extracts of the ultrafiltrates of the intestinal homogenate or the
mixture of the intestinal homogenate with the substrate speeded up
the migration of the cyanocobalamin in this system. The recently described complexing tendency of vitamin B$_{12}$ (282) may explain this
phenomenon.

The partition coefficient for Co^{57}B$_{12}$ in butanol over water was determined and found to be 0.839 when the vitamin solution was supersaturated with ammonium sulfate (Table 82). The corresponding fig-

Table 82. Solubility and Chromatography Characteristics of $Co^{57}B_{12}$, Non-Radioactive B_{12}, and the Ultrafiltrable Radioactivity of Various Experiments

Source of Ultrafiltrate	Partition Coefficient	Rf Value
Experiment 3. Human Intrinsic Factor		
Substrate + rat intestinal homogenate, incubated	0.833	0.67–0.75*
Experiment 6. Rat Intrinsic Factor		
Substrate + rat intestinal homogenate, incubated	0.853	0.67–0.75*
Experiment 10. Hog Intrinsic Factor		
Substrate + rat intestinal homogenate, incubated	0.857	0.67–0.75*
Experiment 12 (Table 78)		
Homogenate of rat small intestine, incubated	0.823	0.49–0.78*
Control Experiments		
$Co^{57}B_{12}$ in buffer solution	0.839	0.50–0.58*
Non-radioactive B_{12}	...	0.48–0.57†
Non-radioactive B_{12} added to Exp. 3, 6, and 10.............	...	0.66–0.77†

(From Doscherholmen: Enzymatic release of vitamin B_{12} bound either to the intrinsic factor or in the wall of the small intestine. Vitamin B_{12} und Intrinsic Factor, 2. Europäisches Symposion, Hamburg, 1961, Ferdinand Enke Verlag, Stuttgart, 472, 1962.)

* Rf values determined radiometrically.

† Rf values determined from migration of the pink color.

Table 83. B_{12} Activity (μμg/ml. ultrafiltrate) in Ultrafiltrates of Mixtures of Rat Intestinal Homogenates and Solutions Containing the Intrinsic Factor–Vitamin B_{12} Complex

	Source of Intrinsic Factor					
	Rat Stomach (Exp. 7)		Human Gastric Juice (Exp. 3)		Hog-Stomach IFC (Exp. 8)	
Mixture	Total	Free	Total	Free	Total	Free
Substrate + homogenate, incubated at 37°C..........	808	945	260	268	730	958
Substrate + homogenate, kept on ice.................	29	31	18	17	4	4
Substrate + buffer, incubated at 37°C..........	48	50	26	26	0	..
Substrate + buffer, kept on ice.................	8	11	5	4	0	..

(From Doscherholmen: Enzymatic release of vitamin B_{12} bound either to the intrinsic factor or in the wall of the small intestine. Vitamin B_{12} und Intrinsic Factor, 2. Europäisches Symposion, Hamburg, 1961, Ferdinand Enke Verlag, Stuttgart, 472, 1962.)

Table 84. B_{12} Activity in Ultrafiltrate from Homogenate of Rat Small Intestine as Measured by the *Euglena gracilis* Method; Rats Given 0.005 μg $Co^{67}B_{12}$ (0.01 μc) Orally 1 Hour before Sacrifice

	B_{12} Activity in Ultrafiltrate, μμg/ml.	
	Total	Free
Homogenate, incubated at 37°C. in a water bath for 4 hours.............	548	715
Homogenate, kept on ice for 4 hours	0	..

(From Doscherholmen: Enzymatic release of vitamin B_{12} bound either to the intrinsic factor or in the wall of the small intestine. Vitamin B_{12} und Intrinsic Factor, 2. Europäisches Symposion, Hamburg, 1961, Ferdinand Enke Verlag, Stuttgart, 472, 1962.)

ures for the unknown radioactivities in experiments 3, 6, 10, and 12 ranged from 0.823 to 0.857. These figures are for all practical purposes identical with that of control radiocyanocobalamin.

The vitamin B_{12} activity in the various ultrafiltrates was determined by the *Euglena gracilis* method. The results show that the highest vitamin B_{12} activity was always found in the ultrafiltrates of the warm-incubated mixtures containing substrate plus intestinal homogenate (Table 83), or the warm-incubated intestinal homogenate (Table 84), whereas little or no activity was detected in any of the other ultrafiltrates. These findings support the contention that the radioactivity measured in the ultrafiltrates is due to radiocyanocobalamin and not to some metabolite of the vitamin.

It was noted that the ultrafiltrates contained more vitamin B_{12} activity than was foreseen from their respective contents of radioactivity. The most likely explanation for this is that the intestinal mucosa also contained a large amount of non-radioactive vitamin B_{12} which also was released from its bound form by the enzymatic activity of the intestinal homogenate. It is known that the transport of vitamin B_{12} from the intestinal wall to the organs of storage and utilization is a slow process (59, 119, 156, 160) and that the wall of the small bowel in the rat (59, 119) as well as in man (156, 160) serves as a temporary storage organ for cyanocobalamin. The finding of a relatively high content of vitamin B_{12} activity in the ultrafiltrates of the warm-incubated mixtures was therefore not surprising.

The reproducibility of the results in the *Euglena gracilis* method is most often within ±15 per cent. The differences between the free and the total vitamin B_{12} concentrations in the ultrafiltrates may all fall within the range of reproducibility of this bioassay method.

These three methods for identifying vitamin B_{12} give reasonable assurance that the radioactivities measured in the ultrafiltrates represent free radio-labeled vitamin B_{12}. Cooper and Castle also concluded that the radioactivities in their dialysates were free cyanocobalamin (126). These authors used the partition coefficient of the radioactivity for benzyl alcohol over water for the characterization of the dialysable radioactivity.

Table 85. B_{12}-Binding Capacity of Hog-Stomach Intrinsic Factor Concentrate: Reduction of Binding Power after Incubation with Homogenate of Small Intestines from Rats

$Co^{57}B_{12}$ ($\mu\mu g$/ml.)	% of Ultrafiltrable Radioactivity	
	IFC + Homogenate	IFC + Buffer
500	31.8	0.3
1,000	36.4	0.1

(From Doscherholmen: Enzymatic release of vitamin B_{12} bound either to the intrinsic factor or in the wall of the small intestine. Vitamin B_{12} und Intrinsic Factor, 2. Europäisches Symposion, Hamburg, 1961, Ferdinand Enke Verlag, Stuttgart, 472, 1962.)

The existence of an intestinal enzyme capable of releasing vitamin B_{12} bound to intrinsic factor in vitro may or may not in itself be of physiologic significance. It should be remembered that the fish tapeworm has also been found to possess an enzyme capable of releasing cyanocobalamin from the IF-B_{12} complex (336, 470). The fact that the intestinal enzyme can release B_{12} after it has been bound in the intestinal wall in vivo seems, however, to give the observed phenomenon of in-vitro B_{12}IF-splitting much greater importance The release by the intestinal homogenate of vitamin B_{12} bound to IF in vitro and the release of cyanocobalamin bound in the intestinal wall in vivo are two phenomena probably caused by one and the same enzyme. It is most likely that we are dealing with an intracellular enzyme whose main function is to degrade or digest the intrinsic factor after the IF-B_{12} complex has been brought into the mucosal cells by pinocytosis, as recently suggested by Abels (1, 2). Vitamin B_{12} would thus be released in a free form and could move into the extracellular fluid space and blood according to the physical laws of diffusion. It is not known whether this intestinal enzyme is identical with previously described enzymes, but this possibility has been discussed (126). The phenomenon of intracellular digestion in the mucosal cells of the small intestine as part of the absorptive process has recently been described in regard to the absorption of carbohydrates (420). It is quite likely that in the absorption of vitamin B$_{12}$ under physiologic conditions we are also dealing with an intracellular digestive process, which will destroy the intrinsic factor or at least its binding site for vitamin B$_{12}$. In favor of this hypothesis is the fact that a reduction of the IFC's B$_{12}$-binding power has been observed after the incubation with homogenate of rat small intestine (Table 85).

The fate of the IF after its absorption into the mucosal cells of the small intestine is not known. If it is discharged into the blood stream we should be able to detect its presence in the plasma by appropriate tests. Schilling and Schloesser, using radioactive technique, were unable to find intrinsic factor activity in 200–400 ml. of human plasma (561). This and other experiments (254, 641) may be cited as evidence against the absorption of the gastric intrinsic factor. No definite proof exists today for the contention that the gastric IF is absorbed from the gastrointestinal tract, although certain experiments do not rule out this possibility (10, 83, 166, 307, 313, 334, 361, 422–426, 477, 493, 515). Apparently an extragastric IF is present in the plasma (10, 83, 313), but the relation of this plasma factor to the gastric IF is still not clear. More information is needed to elucidate the fate of the gastric IF after its absorption into the intestinal mucosal cells, its relation to the plasma factor, and the manner in which vitamin B$_{12}$ is discharged from these cells into the blood stream.

6 | TRANSPORT OF B_{12} IN THE BLOOD

Determination of Vitamin B_{12} Serum Binding Capacity by Ultrafiltration

VITAMIN B_{12} is present in the serum in a free and in a bound form, as first pointed out by Ross (547). The amount of free cyanocobalamin in the serum is just a small fraction of the total serum vitamin B_{12} (22, 421, 441). A specific B_{12}-binding protein exists in the blood (394, 414, 418, 419, 498, 647). Some evidence indicates non-specific binding of cyanocobalamin to serum proteins as well (36, 38, 404, 546A). Furthermore, when added to it in vitro, serum also has the ability to bind additional vitamin B_{12} (22, 26, 38, 363, 419, 443A, 498).

Several methods have been used for the determination of B_{12}-binding power. In Ternberg and Eakin's method (619) the inhibition of the growth response of microorganisms to vitamin B_{12} is utilized as a measure of B_{12}-binding capacity, since bound vitamin B_{12} is unavailable as a growth factor for bacteria. The method of Hutner and associates using *Euglena gracilis* as an assay for the determination of vitamin B_{12} (325) was adapted for human serum by Ross (548) and Mollin and Ross (441), and has been used to detect both free and total vitamin B_{12} in the serum. Several authors have used this bioassay method for the study of the B_{12}-binding power of serum (22, 26, 363, 442, 498). Dialysis experiments have been used to detect the binding power of various substances for vitamin B_{12} such as lysozyme (45, 108), gastric juice (108, 245, 619), cerebrospinal fluid (406), tear fluid (255), saliva (37), heparin (108), and serum (36, 38, 404). Absorption of free vitamin B_{12} by a resting strain of *Lactobacillus leichmannii* was used by Davis and associates in the study of the B_{12}-binding power of human serum (108, 138–140) and absorption onto activated charcoal was used by O. Neal Miller (421).

It is the purpose of this chapter to describe still another method for the study of the binding power of serum for cyanocobalamin, a method based upon the use of radiocyanocobalamin and ultrafiltration.

Ultrafiltration was carried out after the method of Clegg (117) as modified by Prasad and by Prasad and Flink (505, 506). The ultrafiltrate obtained contained no protein as confirmed by chemical determination, by precipitation with trichloracetic acid and alcohol, and by paper electrophoresis (505, 506). Five to ten milliliters of whole serum or serum dilutions were mixed with equal volumes of solutions containing various amounts of radio-labeled cyanocobalamin ranging from 250 $\mu\mu$g/ml. to 25,000 $\mu\mu$g/ml. Two milliliters of the mixture were transferred to a counting vial and the rest of the mixture transferred to a cellophane bag and immediately centrifuged for 75 minutes at 2,500 rpm. Two milliliters of the ultrafiltrate were transferred to a counting vial. The radioactivity was determined in the 20 ml. scintillation counter using the automatic sample changer and a preset count of 12,800. The results may be expressed in two ways. One can either use the radioactivity in the ultrafiltrate, expressed as a percentage of the activity in the whole mixture, or he can use the reciprocal of this value, which gives an expression of the percentage of vitamin B$_{12}$ bound in the mixture. This latter value was chosen for this chapter. No attempt was made to correct for the volume occupied by the serum proteins, since it represents a small, constant, and insignificant error (505). Saline control solutions were subjected to ultrafiltration procedures in the same manner as serum or dilutions of serum.

The B$_{12}$-binding capacity was determined in this manner on two lots of undiluted pooled serum and on serum dilutions of 1:4 and 1:10 on one of these lots. The results are shown graphically in Fig. 32. The two curves representing the undiluted pooled sera have a similar appearance, showing, in general, three distinct parts: The first, almost horizontal, part, showed a high binding capacity of around 90 per cent of the added dose up to the level of 3,000 $\mu\mu$g/ml. The second part was characterized by a gradual decline in the percentage of vitamin B$_{12}$ bound and this again was followed by a third, almost horizontal, part starting at the level of 10,000 $\mu\mu$g/ml. When the studies were performed on serum dilutions of 1:4 and 1:10 the binding curves seemed to consist of only two distinct parts, the first very steep, and the second almost horizontal. Ultrafiltration of various saline control solutions of Co^{60}-labeled cyanocobalamin showed that between 32.1 and 35.3 per cent of the radioactivity was retained inside the cellophane bags in a control experiment (Table 58). These figures then should be considered as "blanks" for this method, since there was no known B$_{12}$-binding substance present in the control saline solutions.

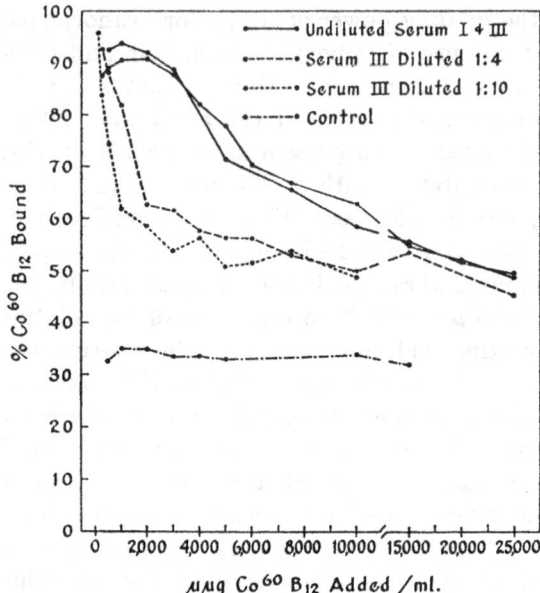

Figure 32. B$_{12}$-binding power of undiluted serum and serum diluted 1:4 and 1:10; control mixture contained normal saline instead of serum.

These binding curves fit the idea of the existence of specific as well as non-specific binding of vitamin B$_{12}$ in the serum. The first parts of the curves are believed to represent the binding by the specific binding protein, whereas the later, more horizontal parts of the curves represent non-specific binding. The difference in the curves between undiluted and diluted serum is owing to the presence of a smaller amount of the specific binding protein in diluted serum. These findings are in agreement with those produced by the dialysis technique (36, 404). That technique shows that the absolute binding capacity of serum increases as the amount of vitamin B$_{12}$ added is raised (36), because of the non-specific binding of vitamin B$_{12}$ in the serum. With the bioassay method it has been found that the B$_{12}$-binding power of serum is limited (363, 498). The reason for the discrepancy is believed to lie in the different techniques used: apparently the bioassay method cannot detect non-specific binding by serum proteins.

The reproducibility of the results in this ultrafiltration procedure was tested on three sera on different days and found to be good, as seen in Table 86. The greatest difference between two corresponding values was 1.4 per cent. The influence of time and temperature on the binding was also investigated (Table 87). The binding capacity was found to be the same at 37°C. as at room temperature, and, furthermore, the binding in vitro seemed to take place instantaneously, so that incubation was deemed unnecessary. The influence of pH was investigated by adding hydrochloric acid to the mixture of plasma and radioactive vitamin B$_{12}$ (Table 88). When the pH was varied between 4.0 and 8.5, no significant difference in the binding power could be detected. The question arose as to whether the results would be changed if the residue from one filtration was put into another cellophane bag and the same procedure reproduced. The amount of B$_{12}$ added to the pooled serum was 5,000 $\mu\mu$g/ml. The results of the first ultrafiltration showed a binding capacity of 73.2 per cent, and when the residue was subjected to ultrafiltration, the binding capacity was found to be 71.8 per cent, two

Table 86. Reproducibility of Repeated Tests

Serum	Test Dose, B$_{12}$ ($\mu\mu$g/ml.)	% of Added B$_{12}$ Bound	
		1st Test	2nd Test
Pooled serum I	5,000	71.5	70.8
Pooled serum II	5,000	75.2	76.6
Dr. W.*	5,000	93.5	93.6

* Diagnosis: chronic myeloid leukemia.

Table 87. The Influence of Time and Temperature on the Binding Capacity of Pooled Serum II When 5,000 $\mu\mu$g/ml. Labeled B$_{12}$ Was Added

Temperature	Time (hr.)	% of B$_{12}$ Bound
37°C.	½	76.5
37°C.	1	75.2
37°C.	2	75.5
37°C.	3	75.3
37°C.	4	76.5
37°C.	17	76.5
19°C.	0	74.7
19°C.	1	75.0

Table 88. Influence of pH on B$_{12}$ Serum-Binding Capacity: 5,000 $\mu\mu$g/ml. B$_{12}$ Added to Pooled Serum III Prior to the Addition of HCl

pH	B$_{12}$ Bound
4.0	74.4%
5.0	72.5
6.0	78.7
7.0	74.7
8.5	75.2

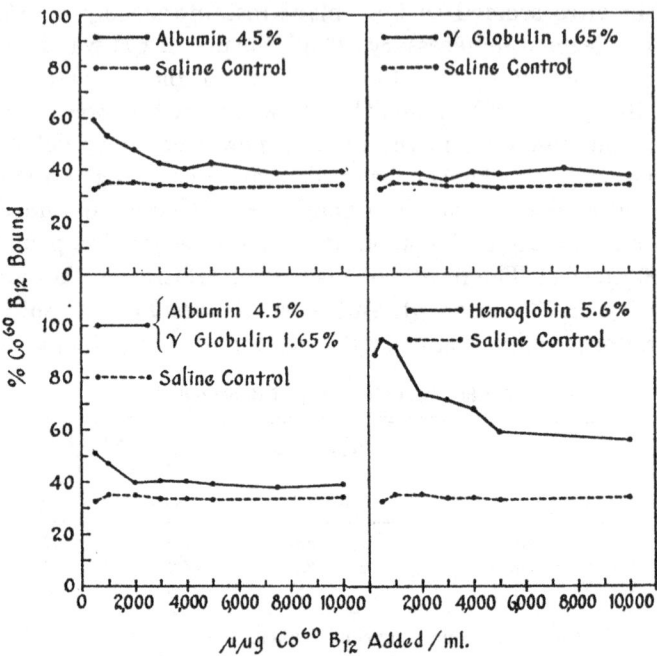

Figure 33. B_{12}-binding power of a 4.5 per cent solution of human albumin, 1.65 per cent solution of gamma globulin, a mixture of these two, and a 5.6 per cent solution of human hemoglobin; control contained normal saline instead of these solutions.

values within the reproducibility of the test. There was no difference in the results whether saline solution, distilled water, or an ultrafiltrate of serum was used as a diluent in these experiments.

Since the above described experiments suggested non-specific binding of B_{12} in serum, we decided to test the binding power of commercially available human albumin and gamma globulin. Fig. 33 shows the binding curves obtained with a 4.5 per cent solution of human albumin and 1.65 per cent solution of human gamma globulin as well as with a solution containing both of these proteins. The results make it clear that both of these proteins bound small amounts of cyanocobalamin in vitro. The binding curves were quite flat except for the initial part of the albumin curve, and they resembled the later part of the curves in Fig. 32. These almost horizontal curves suggest non-specific binding of vitamin B_{12}.

The electrophoretic pattern of the human albumin and gamma globulin solutions was compared with that of human serum (Fig. 34). The two proteins appear to have a fairly uniform pattern, although some trailing was noted for the albumin solution. Since the specific B_{12}-binding protein is believed to belong to the alpha globulins, it is quite pos-

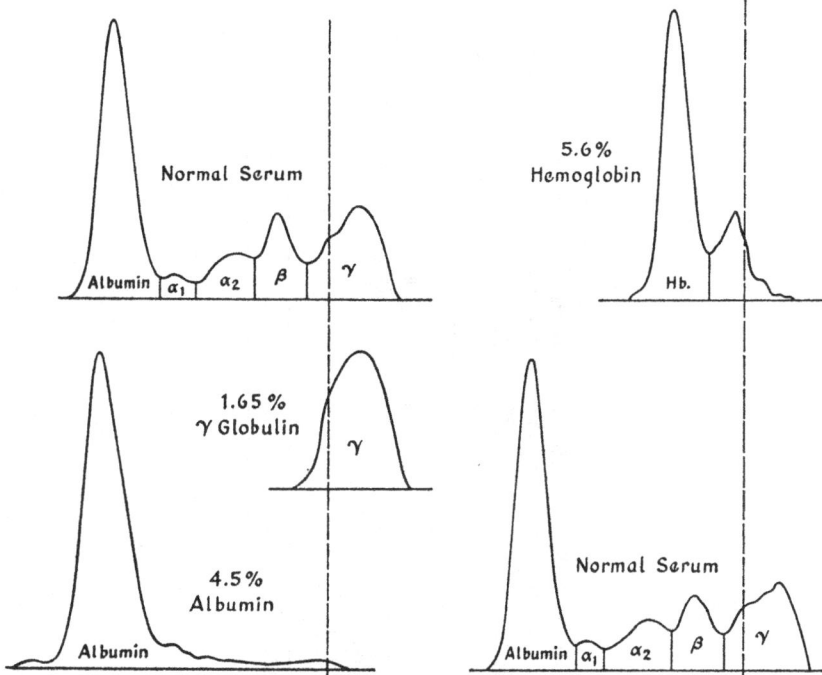

Figure 34. Electrophoretic pattern of normal human serum compared with a 4.5 per cent solution of serum albumin, 1.65 per cent solution of gamma globulin, and a 5.6 per cent solution of human hemoglobin.

sible that a slight amount of this binding protein was present in the albumin fraction. The configuration of the first part of the binding curve obtained with the albumin solution also suggests the presence of a very small amount of the specific binding protein in this solution.

The B$_{12}$-binding curve was also determined for a 5.6 per cent solution of hemoglobin prepared according to a previously described method (455) which was identical with that of whole serum. The electrophoretic pattern of this hemoglobin was compared with that of serum (Fig. 34). Since this binding study was not performed on crystalline hemoglobin and our solution might conceivably contain more than one protein, it is difficult to claim that the binding curve in question was definitely caused by hemoglobin. Kato has, however, previously found that crystalline human oxyhemoglobin will bind vitamin B$_{12}$ in vitro (340). The origin of the specific B$_{12}$-binding protein in the blood is not known. The finding in this study may lead to a working hypothesis that it originates from the formed elements of the blood. Mollin and Ross (443A) think that breakdown of granulocytes may lead to the

Table 89. B$_{12}$-Binding Capacity of Serum Diluted 1:4 from 5 Control Subjects and 1 Sample of Pooled Serum

Source of Serum	B$_{12}$ Bound, as % of Various Amounts (in ml.) of Added Co^{60}B$_{12}$								
	250	500	1,000	2,000	3,000	4,000	5,000	10,000	15,000
J.A.	91.9	84.9	80.3	68.5	62.3	54.4	52.8	49.7	47.3
D.J.	89.6	92.4	76.7	68.6	63.5	62.3	56.9	53.3	
A.D.	90.7	87.7	83.1	76.8	64.0	68.1	54.9	52.0	
H.H.	94.6	90.7	84.4	72.8	66.1	...	60.6	54.3	
L.G.	90.7	80.1	66.4	64.4	58.5	...	53.3	46.5	
Pool III	92.8	88.2	82.0	63.1	61.8	57.8	56.6	50.3	53.7
Average	91.7	87.3	78.8	67.5	62.7	59.4	55.9	51.0	50.5

Table 90. B₁₂-Binding Capacity of Serum from Patients with Chronic Myeloid and Chronic Lymphatic Leukemia: Serum in Dilutions of 1:4 Was Mixed with Equal Volumes of Co⁵⁷B₁₂ Solutions and Subjected to Ultrafiltration; Radioactivity Measurements Were Performed on the Mixtures and Their Corresponding Ultrafiltrates

Patient	WBC	B_{12} Bound, as % of Various Amounts (in ml.) of Added $Co^{57}B_{12}$							
		500	1,000	2,000	3,000	4,000	5,000	10,000	15,000
Chronic Myeloid Leukemia									
V.O.	19,150	100.0	78.1	58.1	50.2	49.3	47.1	28.1	42.8
P.H.	92,000	100.0	99.8	75.2	64.5	59.8	53.0	51.4	49.7
N.F.	59,000	99.7	99.5	99.7	91.2	77.6	69.4	52.7	45.0
D.V.	134,000	98.1	96.1	84.5	66.5	57.1	49.3	40.3	35.7
Average	...	99.5	93.4	79.4	68.1	61.0	54.7	43.1	43.3
Chronic Lymphatic Leukemia									
J.S.	36,000	80.7	62.0	51.8	50.1	48.7	49.4	46.9	47.4
G.R.	180,000	88.2	63.9	51.9	45.4	43.6	43.5	37.0	40.4
C.L.	19,400	86.7	62.1	49.7	43.7	42.6	39.4	38.1	36.1
J.L.	29,200	87.7	64.4	52.9	49.8	48.3	47.6	46.7	47.2
J.D.	164,000	92.3	66.7	54.9	48.6	46.5	44.5	48.2	44.1
Average		87.9	64.4	52.4	47.9	45.9	44.8	42.6	43.2

liberation of B_{12}-binding material in the blood. Besides this theoretical consideration, a practical implication resulted: the exclusion of all sera for binding studies if even the slightest hemolysis was present.

Abnormalities of vitamin B_{12} binding have been observed in sera from patients with acute and chronic myeloid leukemia. We decided to investigate whether the present method could verify the hypothesis that myeloid leukemia is associated with increased binding of vitamin B_{12} in vitro. In preparation for such a study, we had to decide whether to use whole or diluted serum. The amount of serum needed to make a complete binding curve with undiluted serum is 40–50 ml. (approximately 80 ml. of blood). Because it seems impractical to remove so much blood from leukemic subjects, we decided to perform the binding studies with diluted serum. Preliminary binding studies on six sera (Table 89) (one pooled lot and five from normal subjects) showed that a serum dilution of 1:4 would be satisfactory. With such a dilution, only 10 ml. of serum would be needed for a complete binding curve. This amount of serum did not seem objectionable from a clinical standpoint, and consequently the binding studies in leukemic subjects were performed on dilutions of 1:4. Five patients with chronic lymphatic leukemia, four with chronic myelogenous leukemia are included (Table 90).

Comparing the average values for the binding capacities, we can see that the patients with chronic myeloid leukemia had higher values than those with chronic lymphatic leukemia (Table 90) and the control subjects (Table 89) in concentrations of up to 4,000 $\mu\mu$g vitamin B_{12} per ml. of serum. When more than 5,000 $\mu\mu$g $Co^{60}B_{12}$ were added per ml. of serum the binding capacity of sera from patients with chronic myeloid leukemia and chronic lymphatic leukemia seemed to be of the same magnitude and slightly below that of control subjects. Patients with chronic lymphatic leukemia had average binding capacities below the normal control values at all levels tested except the 500 $\mu\mu$g.

The most likely interpretation of these findings is that in chronic myeloid leukemia there is an increase in the specific binding of vitamin B_{12}, while the non-specific binding may be normal or even slightly decreased. In chronic lymphatic leukemia, on the other hand, there may be a decrease in both the specific and the non-specific binding of cyanocobalamin. In chronic lymphatic leukemia a decrease in the B_{12}-binding capacity of serum proteins has also been found by other investigators (178, 296, 510), whereas in myelogenous leukemia the binding power is increased (see pp. 122–132). The abnormalities in the binding of vitamin B_{12} may explain the disturbances found in the plasma absorption of cyanocobalamin and in the serum vitamin B_{12} in myelogenous and lymphatic leukemia.

7 | ALTERATION OF HEPATIC STORAGE OF RADIOCYANOCOBALAMIN

THE liver is the most important storage organ for vitamin B_{12}. After oral or parenteral administration of radio-labeled cyanocobalamin, surface counting over various sites has shown that the liver accumulates most of the radioactivity (220, 221, 403). It also retains the radioactivity with great avidity. Indeed, from 86 to 94 per cent of the maximal activity was found after three months (221) and about 50 per cent after a year (216, 563). The biological half-life of vitamin B_{12} in the body has recently been calculated to be approximately a year (242, 521). The liver radioactivity seems unaffected by a single intramuscular injection of 1 mg. "cold" vitamin B_{12} given a week after the administration of the radio-vitamin (402).

The purpose of the present investigation was to observe the effect of a large series of 1 mg. parenteral doses of "cold" vitamin B_{12} on hepatic storage of radioactivity after orally administered radio-labeled cyanocobalamin.

A test dose of 0.46 μg vitamin B_{12} containing 0.5 μc Co^{60} was administered in approximately 100 ml. of water to two healthy female volunteers after an overnight fast and two hours before breakfast. Plasma radioactivity as well as a 24-hour urinary excretion study started after 24 hours showed that they both absorbed the vitamin normally. External monitoring over the organ areas was carried out according to the method of Glass with a probe scintillation counter. Uptake of radioactivity over the liver, spleen, and precordium was determined 9–13 days after administration of the tests. The radioactivities recorded between one and two weeks after the tests were taken as the 100 per cent values. One of the subjects was given a series of one hundred 1 mg.

NOTE: This chapter appeared in slightly different form in Doscherholmen and Hagen Proc. Soc. Exp. Biol. Med., 95:667, 1957, Society of Experimental Biology and Medicine (165).

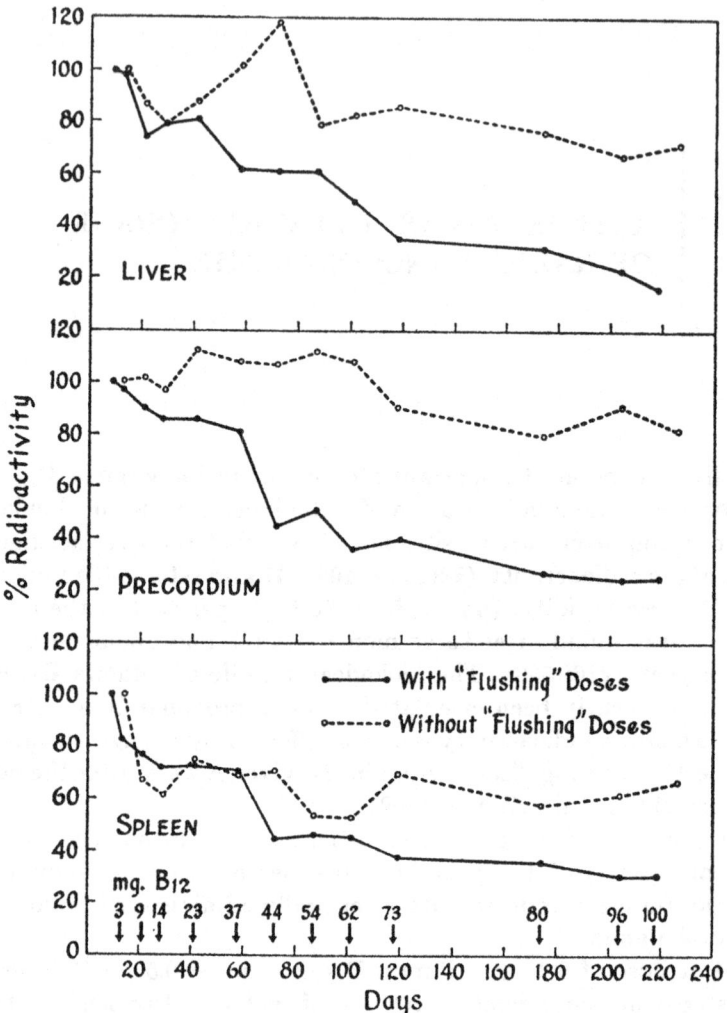

Figure 35. Effect of parenteral injections of B₁₂ on body stores of radioactive B₁₂; net cpm for 100 per cent values were 905, 599, and 421 for the liver, precordium, and spleen, respectively, in the experimental subject; comparable figures for control subject were 507, 382, and 295; cumulative amounts of parenteral "cold" B₁₂ are shown at bottom of graph. (From Doscherholmen and Hagen: Alteration of hepatic storage of radiolabeled vit. B₁₂. Proc. Soc. Exp. Biol. Med., 95:667, 1957.)

parenteral injections of non-radioactive cyanocobalamin during the ensuing 7 months, while the other subject served as a control. Twenty-four-hour urine collections were made at intervals and the amounts of radioactivity excreted were determined.

Fig. 35 shows that repeated 1 mg. parenteral doses of "cold" vitamin B_{12} caused a marked increase in the rate of disappearance of radioactivity over the liver as well as over the precordium and spleen. The radioactivity over the liver declined to 49.5 per cent 101 days after administration of the test when 62 mg. cyanocobalamin had been administered, and to 15.8 per cent 218 days after the test when 100 mg. had been given. In the control subject, liver radioactivity amounted to 82.6 per cent and 71.4 per cent on the 101st day and the 226th day, respectively, after the test.

Table 91 summarizes the amounts of urinary radioactivity in each subject. The control subject did not excrete measurable radioactivity 10 days after the single flushing injection of cyanocobalamin she had received. After the parenteral vitamin B_{12} injections, the experimental subject had definite radioactivity in urine each time it was examined. The amount excreted was 0.7 per cent of the administered dose at the start of the injections and decreased to 0.3 per cent toward the end.

The results of this study show that the radioactivity stored in the liver can be reduced by a series of parenteral injections of vitamin B_{12}. Because of simultaneous decline in the radioactivity over the spleen and the precordium, we thought it unlikely that the loss of hepatic radioactivity resulted from an accumulation of radioactivity in other or-

Table 91. Effect of Repeated Intramuscular Injections of 1 mg. "Cold" B_{12} on Urinary Excretion of Radioactivity

Time at Which Urinary Collection Was Started	24-Hour Urinary Radioactivity, % of Oral Dose	
	Experimental Subject	Control Subject
24 hours	17.7*	4.9*
8 days	0†	
9 days	0.7*	
10 days		0†
21 days	0.5*	
30 days	0.4*	
186 days	0.3*	

(From Doscherholmen and Hagen: Alteration of hepatic storage of radiolabeled vitamin B_{12}. Proc. Soc. Exp. Biol. Med., 95:667, 1957.)

* B_{12} parenterally immediately before start of urinary collection.

† No B_{12} parenterally.

gans. The finding of radioactivity in the urine showed that the kidneys were at least one route of loss from the body. A rough estimate suggested that about 40 per cent of the test dose was excreted in the urine during the series of injections started the ninth day after administration of the oral test. No attempts were made to prove that the radioactivity was lost in the form of cyanocobalamin, although this has been contended for the usual Schilling test (380). The findings in this study are in agreement with the report of Schloesser, Deshpande, and Schilling, who found an increased disappearance rate of hepatic radioactivity when a subject received 1 mg. "cold" vitamin B_{12} intramuscularly twice a day for 7 days (563). It has recently been shown that there is an enterohepatic circulation of cyanocobalamin (250, 251, 253, 475, 523–525), and most likely some radioactivity was also lost with the feces. No attempts, however, were made to measure this loss.

Although the hepatic radioactivity in the control subject declined slower than in the experimental subject, the rate was still faster than expected from the physical decay of Co^{60} alone. This is in agreement with previous observations (216, 221, 563), and indicates a release of stored radioactivity. Assuming that the stored radioactivity represents radioactive cyanocobalamin (403), and with a normal intake and absorption of vitamin B_{12}, this finding suggests an exchange between stored cyanocobalamin in the liver and that of the rest of the body. Such a turnover can, apparently, be enhanced by parenteral injections of large amounts of vitamin B_{12}.

8 SUMMARY

BECAUSE of the great importance of vitamin B_{12} studies in the investigation of patients with pernicious anemia an evaluation was made of the value of the most commonly used B_{12}-absorption test, the urinary excretion method. In general, there was a good separation between subjects with pernicious anemia and control patients. Thus, in 29 tests performed on 21 patients with a clinical diagnosis of Addison's pernicious anemia, a very low urinary excretion value was observed. In 80 tests on 69 control patients, 2 revealed urinary excretion values in the range found in pernicious anemia; 1 of these showed normal, the other very high fecal excretion values. Though an undefined error can possibly account for the findings in the first patient, it is likely that low absorption existed in the second patient. The test was discriminatory whether the test dose contained 0.1, 0.5, or 1.0 μg of radiocyanocobalamin. Since an inverse relation was observed between the size of the oral test dose and the percentage of the test material excreted in the urine, subsequent absorption studies were carried out with test doses of the order of magnitude of 0.5 μg.

The reproducibility of the results of the urinary excretion test was found to be satisfactory and superior to that of the fecal excretion test performed simultaneously.

Patients with Addison's pernicious anemia generally showed absorption values in the normal range when IFC was administered with the radiocyanocobalamin, meaning that the Schilling test can be used to evaluate the intrinsic factor activity. For maximum absorption an optimum relation seems to exist between the amount of IFC and the amount of radiocyanocobalamin ingested. By increasing the dose of IFC above this optimum no further absorption is observed, and some decrease in the absorption value may even be seen when this optimum is exceeded.

223

Patients with total gastrectomy behaved as did those with Addison's pernicious anemia. Patients with partial gastrectomy, on the other hand, showed normal, borderline, or low absorption values. Thus, 12 of 35 patients with subtotal gastrectomy had excretion values below 10 per cent and 3 below 5 per cent. Macrocytic anemia was present in 6 patients and megaloblastic bone marrow in 3. There was satisfactory response to parenteral vitamin B_{12} therapy in 2.

Patients with histamine-fast achlorhydria were generally found to have absorption values within the normal range, but 1 had 0 per cent excretion on one occasion and 9.3 per cent on another. The average figure in the group of histamine-fast achlorhydria patients was slightly below that in the corresponding control group.

A group of 11 patients with posterolateral column disease was studied. Anemia was, however, not a problem in any of them. Of these, 3 showed absorption values in the pernicious anemia range; their absorption figures improved greatly with the addition of IFC, leading to the belief that they suffered from Addison's pernicious anemia. The absorption tests were normal in the other 8 patients.

The 5 patients suffering from intestinal pernicious anemia and showing an abnormally low urinary excretion test, in contrast to patients with Addison's pernicious anemia and gastrectomy, showed no improvement in the absorption values with the addition of IFC. After pretreatment with tetracycline, however, 1 patient with small bowel diverticula showed normal absorption of radiocyanocobalamin. Folic acid therapy failed in 2 of these patients because one developed a fulminating subacute combined degeneration of the spinal cord and the other a megaloblastic anemia after a temporary remission. Parenteral vitamin B_{12} therapy has kept their anemias in remission.

No consistent pattern in the absorption of cyanocobalamin was found in patients with regional ileitis, non-tropical sprue, and secondary steatorrhea.

Three patients with megaloblastic anemias showed normal absorption of Vitamin B_{12}. One of these patients was in the puerperium, one had a presumed folic acid deficiency and one was a vegetarian. Seven patients with leukemia and six with cirrhosis of the liver also had normal absorption. One patient with myelofibrosis revealed normal while another with the same disease had impaired absorption. Seven of eight patients with neuritis of various types showed absorption values within the normal range. One patient with diabetic neuropathy and nocturnal diarrhea showed a low absorption value. Another patient also with nocturnal diarrhea and diabetes showed impaired absorption of radiocyanocobalamin.

False positive urinary excretion tests were observed in uremia, after vomiting and after parenteral "loading" doses of non-labeled cyanocobalamin. In contrast to normal subjects a single parenteral injection given to patients with uremia resulted in a considerable amount of radioactivity excreted in the urine after the first day.

The optimum time for the "flushing" injection was investigated and found to be 6 hours after the administration of the oral test dose of radiocyanocobalamin. When daily "flushing" injections were administered additional amounts of radioactivity were excreted with the urine.

The influence of the size of the parenteral dose on the urinary radioactivity was investigated. A five-fold increase in the average excretion value was observed when the dose was increased from 0.1 to 1 mg. However, a further five-fold increase in the parenteral dose resulted in only a 20 per cent additional increment in the average excretion value.

The influence of multiple "flushing" injections was also investigated. There was little improvement in the average excretion figures with this procedure unless a small "preloading" injection was administered 24 hours before the Schilling test was performed.

A new method for the determination of the absorption of radiocyanocobalamin was described, using measurement of radioactivity in the blood or plasma after the ingestion of physiologic test doses of Co^{60}-labeled vitamin B_{12}. With this method it was possible to differentiate between the 9 patients with pernicious anemia and the 36 control subjects. In the control subjects and also in the pernicious anemia patients given intrinsic factor there was a relative delay of 3–4 hours before measurable amounts of radioactivity appeared in the plasma. The peak was reached in the 8–12-hour interval after the ingestion of the test dose. Following the peak blood concentration the radioactivity gradually declined with small amounts usually persisting for more than one week. The reproducibility of the plasma absorption test was found to be a little better than that of the urinary excretion test performed simultaneously. A good correlation was found between the plasma absorption and the urinary excretion tests.

This latter finding was confirmed in a subsequent study of 42 control subjects and 14 patients with Addison's pernicious anemia. (Oral dose 0.56 μg B_{12} 0.5 μc Co^{60}.) In this investigation the parenteral injection was given at 6 hours. The plasma absorption values were determined at 6 and 8 hours. The 24-hour urinary radioactivity was determined as well as the amount of activity excreted between the two blood samplings. The 8-hour plasma values were just as discriminatory as the 24-hour urinary excretion figures. The 6-hour plasma values were just as discriminatory as the 2-hour urine values, but both of these latter values were less discriminatory than the 8-hour plasma and the 24-hour urinary excretion values. Carbamylcholine chloride increased the absorption values in some control subjects with low absorption values. It also improved the absorption figures in two patients with Addison's pernicious anemia to such an extent that the results would have been difficult to evaluate or the diagnosis of malabsorption of vitamin B_{12} would have been missed entirely if this drug had been used routinely. Incidentally, it was discovered that in control subjects the average 8-hour plasma value with "flushing" at 6 hours was 8.0 ± 2.8 $\mu\mu$g/ml. as compared to 4.7 ± 1.5 $\mu\mu$g/ml. without such treatment.

In a third plasma absorption study an attempt was made to measure the radioactivity of the plasma with half the amount of radioactivity used in the oral dose of the previous study. The 8-hour plasma value was determined in 37 control patients and 10 subjects with Addison's pernicious anemia. A "flushing" dose of non-labeled cyanocobalamin was injected at 6 hours. Again a good separation was obtained between the patients with pernicious anemia and the control subjects.

In the previously mentioned plasma absorption studies 20 ml. plasma volumes were used for counting purposes. An attempt was made to reduce the volume of plasma needed without sacrificing the accuracy of the test. Scintillation spectrometry of $Co^{57}B_{12}$ was chosen for this purpose, using a plasma volume of 4 ml. (Oral test dose 0.56 μg B_{12} 0.5 μc Co^{57}.) In 10 control patients and 4 subjects with malabsorption of cyanocobalamin there was no overlap in the 8-hour absorption values. The augmented plasma absorption test gave higher counts in the control group as would be expected, but it also required a parenteral "flushing" injection. Therefore, with this modification of the test, only 4 ml. of plasma is needed for successful separation of patients with pernicious anemia from control patients.

In a group of 10 patients with various types of gastrectomy a comparison was made between the 8-hour plasma absorption values and the 24-hour urinary excretion figures. The results showed a good correlation between these two parameters of vitamin B_{12} absorption.

Plasma absorption of radiocyanocobalamin was studied in 6 patients with chronic myeloid leukemia, 14 with chronic lymphatic leukemia, 9 with acute or subacute myeloid leukemia, and 3 with non-leukemic neutrophilic leukocytosis. Patients with chronic myeloid leukemia had higher plasma absorption values, later peaks, and more sustained curves than control subjects. Patients with chronic lymphatic leukemia had lower absorption values than control subjects, but the configuration of their absorption curves was normal. The absorption curves in patients with acute and subacute myeloid leukemia did not show a uniform pattern. The plasma absorption curves in the three patients with non-leukemic neutrophilic leukocytosis had a normal configuration. When three successive doses of radio-labeled cyanocobalamin were administered with 3- and 4-day intervals, there was a gradual accumulation of radioactivity in the plasma of a patient with chronic myeloid leukemia whereas a patient with chronic lymphatic leukemia and one control subject showed no similar build-up of radioactivity in the plasma.

Food had no apparent influence on the late appearance of radioactivity in the plasma. A relatively good absorption was found throughout the day even when the test material was administered shortly before or after meals. In fact, only one control subject out of 50 given the test doses immediately before or after meals showed an impaired absorption value.

The plasma absorption of radiocyanocobalamin under the influence of parenteral "loading" with non-labeled vitamin B_{12} was studied more closely in 31 control subjects. A distortion in the configuration of the absorption curves was seen after the parenteral "loading." The changes were more marked with 100 μg and 1,000 μg than with 30 μg "loading" doses. The alteration in the appearance of the curves was more pronounced when the "loading" injections were given 4 to 7 hours after rather than simultaneously with the oral doses. The changes consisted of a rapid increase in radioactivity in the plasma after the 4-, the 5-, the 6-, and the 7-hour injections and, following the peak concentrations, a faster than normal decline of the absorption curves.

The plasma absorption of radiocyanocobalamin was studied both with physiologic and massive oral doses in control subjects and patients with pernicious anemia. Because the absorption curves with small oral test doses were completely different from those observed after massive doses, the inference was made that a dual mechanism exists for the absorption of vitamin B_{12} from the gastrointestinal tract.

The plasma absorption curves obtained from portal venous blood and peripheral venous blood from patients with portacaval shunts showed delay in the appearance of radioactivity similar to that in the peripheral blood of normal subjects. The delay in the appearance of radioactivity in the blood was therefore felt to lie in the intestine. Intestinal transit time was excluded as the causative factor, however, and it was concluded that the delayed plasma absorption with physiologic oral test doses was due to temporary storage of cyanocobalamin in the intestinal wall and a slow release into the blood stream.

The basic mechanism of the Schilling test was investigated. It was discovered that the parenterally injected vitamin B_{12} caused some of the radiocyanocobalamin in the plasma to appear in an ultrafiltrable form. Furthermore, the urinary radioactivity reflected the ultrafiltrable radioactivity in the plasma rather than the plasma radioactivity. In contrast to normal subjects, a patient with uremia had a considerable amount of ultrafiltrable radioactivity in the plasma after the first day. This phenomenon explains the continuing excretion of urinary radioactivity beyond the first day of the test in this type of patient. An excellent correlation was found between the amount of radioactivity excreted with the urine and the filtered load of radioactivity in the kidneys. The true kidney clearance for the ultrafiltrable radiocyanocobalamin was somewhat less than the simultaneously performed endogenous creatinine clearance. The parenteral "flushing" injection saturated the vitamin B_{12} binding capacity of the blood. Furthermore, it also afforded a mechanism for the release of the bound radiocyanocobalamin absorbed into the blood from the gut. Studies of the ultrafiltrable radioactivity in the plasma before, and 5 and 10 minutes after the intravenous injection of "cold" vitamin B_{12} showed that the major portion of the increment in plasma radioactivity above the preinjection level was present in a non-ultrafiltrable form and a smaller amount was ultrafiltrable. This finding raises a question as to the possibility that vitamin B_{12} may be absorbed in a bound as well as a free form.

Organ distribution of radioactivity was studied in man after the oral ingestion of small test doses of radiocyanocobalamin. The liver was the main permanent storage organ for the vitamin. In most patients the ileum was the most important site for the temporary storage of vitamin B_{12} in the small intestine and presumably for the absorption of this vitamin.

The kinetics of ingested radiocyanocobalamin in man was also investigated. From the various responses to the "flushing" procedure of Schilling, measurements of radioactivity in the erythrocytes and from the autopsy studies it was concluded that a five-compartmental system exists for cyanocobalamin in the body.

Homogenates from the small intestines of rats were found capable of releasing cyanocobalamin from the IF-vitamin B_{12} complex in vitro. Radiocyanocobalamin bound in the intestinal wall was also found to be released in a free form under appropriate conditions, presumably by an enzyme.

The B_{12}-binding capacity of serum was studied in vitro using radiocyanocobalamin and an ultrafiltration technique. The binding curves of sera from normal subjects and patients with chronic myeloid leukemia and chronic lymphatic leukemia were characterized. Increased binding capacity in the lower concentrations was typical of chronic myeloid leukemia.

The purpose of one study was to observe the effect of a large series of 1 mg. parenteral doses of "cold" vitamin B_{12} on hepatic storage of radioactivity after orally administered radiocyanocobalamin. The rate of disappearance of the radioactivity was much faster with than without the repeated parenteral injections. Massive parenteral doses of non-labeled vitamin B_{12}, therefore, were exchanged with radiocyanocobalamin stored in the liver.

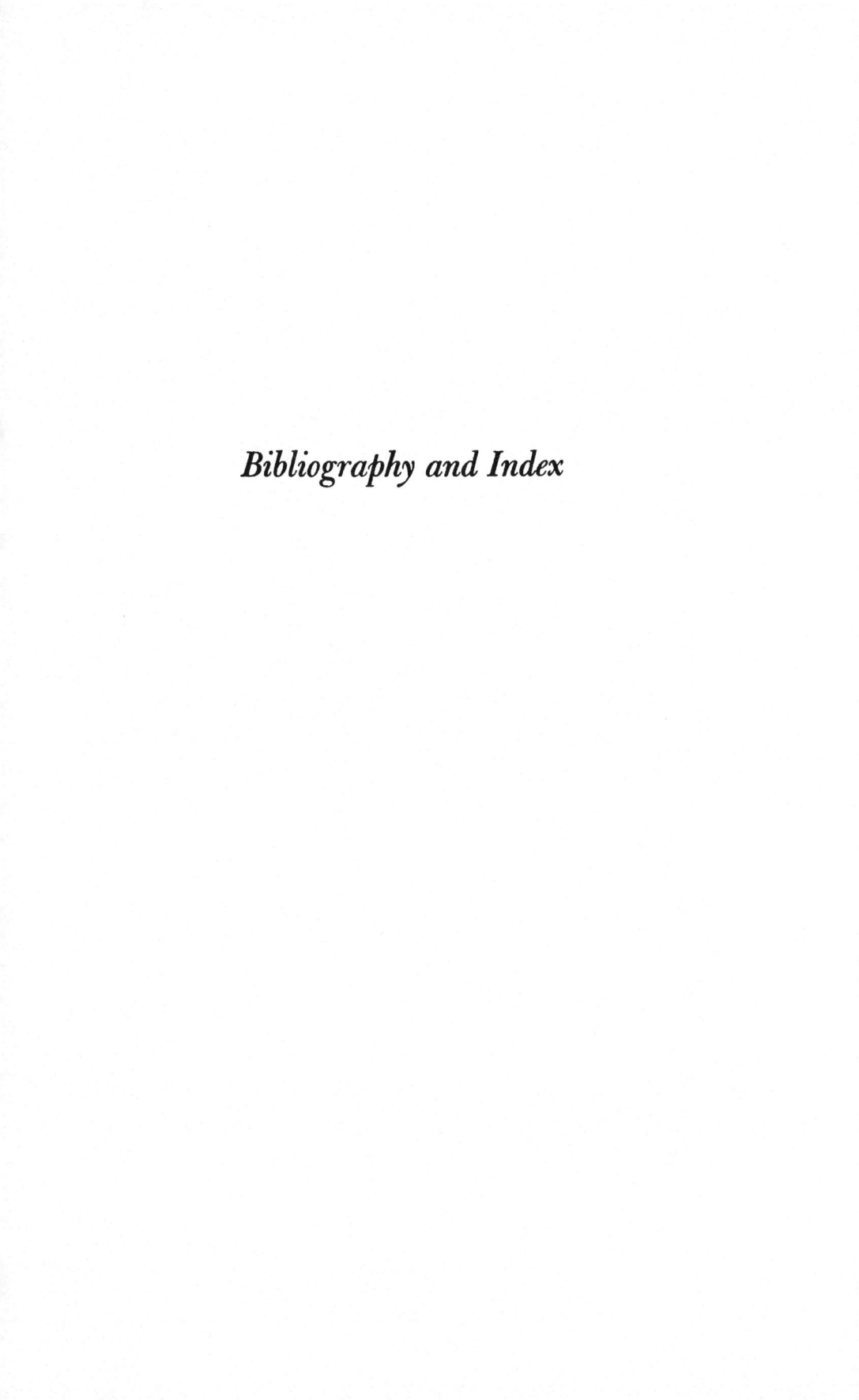

Bibliography and Index

BIBLIOGRAPHY

1. Abels, J.: Intrinsic Factor van Castle en Resorptie van Vitamine B₁₂. Doctoral Thesis, University of Groningen, Netherlands, March 11, 1959.
2. ———, J. J. M. Vegter, M. G. Woldring, J. H. Jans, and H. O. Nieweg: The physiologic mechanism of vitamin B_{12} absorption. Acta Med. Scand., 165:105, 1959.
3. Abels, J., M. G. Woldring, H. O. Nieweg, J. G. Faber, and J. A. deVries: Ethylenediamine tetraacetate and the intestinal absorption of vitamin B_{12}. Nature, 183:1395, 1959.
4. Adams, J. F.: Intrinsic factor. Brit. Med. J., 1:644, 1958.
5. ———, and D. A. Seaton: Reproducibility and reliability of the Schilling test. J. Lab. Clin. Med., 58:67, 1961.
6. Allcock, E.: Absorption of vitamin B_{12} in man following extensive resection of the jejunum, ileum, and colon. Gastroenterology, 40:81, 1961.
7. Allen, G., and C. F. Critchley: Macrocytic anaemia. Brit. Med. J., 1:667, 1951.
8. Alsted, G.: Pernicious anaemia after nitric acid corrosion of the stomach. Lancet, 1:76, 1937.
9. Arias, I. M., L. Apt, and M. Pollycove: Absorption of radioactive vitamin B_{12} in nonanemic patients with combined-system disease. New Engl. J. Med., 253: 1005, 1955.
10. Astaldi, G., and G. Cardinali: Cytology of B_{12} deficiency in vitro. Vitamin B_{12} und Intrinsic Factor, 1. Europäisches Symposion, Hamburg, 1956, Ferdinand Enke Verlag, Stuttgart, 341, 1957.
11. Badenoch, J.: The blind loop syndrome. Modern Trends in Gastroenterology, 2:231, 1958.
12. ———: The use of labelled vitamin B_{12} and gastric biopsy in the investigation of anaemia. Proc. Roy. Soc. Med., 47:426, 1954.
13. ———, and P. D. Bedford: Massive diverticulosis of the upper intestine presenting with steatorrhoea and megaloblastic anaemia. Quart. J. Med., 23:462, 1954.
14. ———, and J. R. Evans: Massive diverticulosis of the small intestine with steatorrhoea and megaloblastic anaemia. Quart. J. Med., 24:321, 1955.
15. Badenoch, J., S. T. Callender, J. R. Evans, A. L. Turnbull, and L. J. Witts: Megaloblastic anaemia of pregnancy and the puerperium. Brit. Med. J., 1:1245, 1955.
16. Badenoch, J., J. R. Evans, and W. C. D. Richards: The stomach in hypochromic anaemia. Brit. J. Haemat., 3:175, 1957.
17. ———, and L. J. Witts: Megaloblastic anaemia following partial gastrectomy and gastro-enterostomy. Brit. J. Haemat., 1:339, 1955.
18. Badenoch, J., and W. C. D. Richards: The gastric lesion in anaemia with particular reference to biopsy. Gastroenterologia, 79:329, 1953.

19. Baker, H., I. Pasher, and H. Sobotka: Vitamin B$_{12}$ distribution between plasma and cells. Nature, 180:1043, 1957.
20. Baker, S. J., and D. L. Mollin: The relationship between intrinsic factor and the intestinal absorption of vitamin B$_{12}$. Brit. J. Haemat., 1:46, 1955.
21. Banerjee, D. K., and J. B. Chatterjea: Serum vitamin B$_{12}$ in vegetarians. Brit. Med. J., 2:992, 1960.
22. Banerjee, D. K., S. Chose, S. K. Ghosh, and J. B. Chatterjea: Free serum vitamin B$_{12}$ level in certain hematologic disorders. Blood, 15:630, 1960.
22A. Barker, H. A.: Chemistry and biology of the vitamin-B$_{12}$-coenzymes. Vitamin B$_{12}$ und Intrinsic Factor, 2. Europäisches Symposion, Hamburg, 1961, Ferdinand Enke Verlag, Stuttgart, 82, 1962.
23. Barker, W. H., and L. E. Hummel: Macrocytic anemia in association with intestinal strictures and anastomoses. Review of the literature and report of two new cases. Bull. Johns Hopkins Hosp., 64:215, 1939.
24. Baskin, R., H. L. Demorest, and S. Sandhaus: Gamma counting efficiency of two well-type NaI crystals. Nucleonics, 12:46, August, 1954.
25. Bastrup-Madsen, P.: Non-anaemic neuropathy due to deficiency of anti-pernicious-anaemia principle. Acta Psychiat. Scand., Suppl., 108:35, 1956.
26. Beard, M. F., W. R. Pitney, and E. H. Sanneman: Serum concentrations of vitamin B$_{12}$ in patients suffering from leukemia. Blood, 9:789, 1954.
27. ———, M. J. Sakol, and H. H. Moorhead: Serum concentrations of vitamin B$_{12}$ in acute leukemia. Ann. Intern. Med., 41:323, 1954.
27A. Beck, W. S.: The metabolic functions of vitamin B$_{12}$. New Engl. J. Med., 266:708, 1962.
28. Berk, L., W. B. Castle, A. D. Welch, R. W. Heinle, R. Anker, and M. Epstein: Observations on the etiologic relationship of achylia gastrica to pernicious anemia. X. Activity of vitamin B$_{12}$ as food (extrinsic) factor. New Engl. J. Med., 239:911, 1948.
29. Berlin, H., R. Berlin, G. Brante, J. G. Andresen, and S.-G. Sjöberg: Studies on intrinsic factor and pernicious anemia. II. Correlation of intrinsic factor activity to B$_{12}$-binding power in different hog pylorus preparations. Scand. J. Clin. Lab. Invest., 11:154, 1959.
30. Berlin, H., R. Berlin, G. Brante, and S.-G. Sjöberg: Studies on intrinsic factor and pernicious anemia. I. Oral uptake of vitamin B$_{12}$ in pernicious anemia with increasing doses of an intrinsic factor concentrate. Scand. J. Clin. Lab. Invest., 10:278, 1958.
30A. ———: Studies on intrinsic factor and pernicious anemia. Scand. J. Clin. Lab. Invest., 13:245, 1961.
31. Berlin, R., H. Berlin, G. Brante, and S.-G. Sjöberg: Failures in long-term oral treatment of pernicious anemia with B$_{12}$-intrinsic factor preparations. Acta Med. Scand., 161:143, 1958.
33. ———: Refractoriness to intrinsic factor-B$_{12}$ preparations abolished by massive doses of intrinsic factor. Acta Med. Scand., 162:317, 1958.
34. Berlin, N. I., J. H. Lawrence, and H. C. Lee: The life span of the red blood cell in chronic leukemia and polycythemia. Science, 114:385, 1951.
35. ———: The pathogenesis of the anemia of chronic leukemia: Measurement of the life span of the red blood cell with glycine-2-C^{14}. J. Lab. Clin. Med., 44:860, 1954.
35A. Bernstein, L., and M. Weatherall: Statistics for Medical and Other Biological Students. E. & S. Livingston Ltd., Edinburgh and London, 1952.
36. Bertcher, R. W., and L. M. Meyer: Co^{60} vitamin B$_{12}$ binding capacity of normal human serum. Proc. Soc. Exp. Biol. Med., 94:169, 1957.
37. ———, and I. F. Miller: Co^{60} vitamin B$_{12}$ binding capacity of normal human saliva. Proc. Soc. Exp. Biol. Med., 99:513, 1958.
38. Bertcher, R. W., L. M. Meyer, H. Varmus, and C. Mulzac: Some characteristics of binding of vitamin B$_{12}$ by normal human serum. Acta Haemat., 23:287, 1960.

39. Best, W. R., J. H. Frenster, and M. M. Zolot: Observations on intrinsic factor and the intestinal absorption of vitamin B₁₂. J. Lab. Clin. Med., 50:793, 1957.
40. Best, W. R., W. A. Landmann, and L. R. Limarzi: Time pattern of vitamin B₁₂ Co⁶⁰ urinary excretion in man after oral administration and parenteral "flushing." Blood, 11:352, 1956.
41. Best, W. R., W. F. White, J. Louis, and L. R. Limarzi: Experiences with the Schilling test using Co⁶⁰ labeled vitamin B₁₂ in pernicious anemia, sprue, and other conditions. J. Lab. Clin. Med., 44:767, 1954.
42. Best, W. R., W. F. White, K. C. Robbins, W. A. Landmann, and S. L. Steelman: Studies on urinary excretion of vitamin B₁₂ Co⁶⁰ in pernicious anemia for determining effective dosage of intrinsic factor concentrate. Blood, 11:338, 1956.
43. Bethell, F. H., M. C. Meyers, and R. B. Neligh: Vitamin B₁₂ in pernicious anemia and puerperal macrocytic anemia. J. Lab. Clin. Med., 33:1477, 1948.
44. Bierring, E., and I. Ebbesen: Schilling-prövernes teoretiske baggrund og kliniske betydning. Ugeskr. Laeg., 122:277, 1960.
45. Bird, O. D., and B. Hoevet: The vitamin B₁₂-binding power of proteins. J. Biol. Chem., 190:181, 1951.
46. Bishop, R. C., M. Toporek, N. A. Nelson, and F. H. Bethell: The relationship of binding power to intrinsic factor activity. J. Lab. Clin. Med., 46:796, 1955.
47. Blachford, R. D., and D. W. Dawson: Association of jejunal diverticulosis with macrocytic anaemia. Brit. Med. J., 1:1407, 1956.
48. Blackburn, E. K., G. H. Spray, H. T. Swan, G. R. Tudhope, and G. M. Wilson: Oral treatment of pernicious anaemia with vitamin B₁₂ and desiccated hog duodenal extract. Brit. Med. J., 2:535, 1959.
49. Bockus, H. L.: Gastroenterology. W. B. Saunders Co., Philadelphia and London, 468, 1949.
50. Boen, S. T.: Changes in epithelial cells in vitamin B₁₂ deficiency. Vitamin B₁₂ und Intrinsic Factor, 1. Europäisches Symposion, Hamburg, 1956, Ferdinand Enke Verlag, Stuttgart, 386, 1957.
51. ———: Changes in the nuclei of squamous epithelial cells in pernicious anaemia. Acta Med. Scand., 159:425, 1957.
52. ———, J. A. Molhuysen, and J. Steenbergen: Nuclear changes in oral epithelial cells in subacute combined degeneration of the spinal cord due to vitamin B₁₂ deficiency. Lancet, 2:294, 1958.
53. Boger, W. P., D. S. Brashear, and J. J. Gavin: Enhancement of serum vitamin B₁₂ by D-sorbitol. Amer. J. Clin. Nutr., 7:318, 1959.
54. Boger, W. P., and E. T. Parmelee: Influence of D-sorbitol on plasma concentrations of vitamin B₁₂. Metabolism, 8:126, 1959.
55. von Bonsdorff, B.: Pathogenesis of vitamin B₁₂ deficiency, with special reference to tapeworm pernicious anaemia. Vitamin B₁₂ und Intrinsic Factor, 1. Europäisches Symposion, Hamburg, 1956, Ferdinand Enke Verlag, Stuttgart, 311, 1957.
56. ———: Vitamin B₁₂ deficiency in carriers of Diphyllobothrium latum. Proc. 6th Internat. Congr. Trop. Med. Malaria, 2:541, 1958.
57. ———: Bred bandmask som orsak till B₁₂-vitaminbrist. Farmaceutisk Notisblad, 68:185, 1959.
58. ———, W. Nyberg, and R. Gräsbeck: Vitamin B₁₂ deficiency in carriers of the fish tapeworm Diphyllobothrium latum. Proc. 7th Congr. Europ. Soc. Haemat., London, 1959; Acta Haemat., 24:15, 1960.
59. Booth, C. C., I. Chanarin, B. B. Anderson, and D. L. Mollin: The site of absorption and tissue distribution of orally administered ⁵⁶Co-labelled vitamin B₁₂ in the rat. Brit. J. Haemat., 3:253, 1957.
60. Booth, C. C., and D. L. Mollin: Plasma, tissue and urinary radioactivity after oral administration of ⁵⁶Co-labelled vitamin B₁₂. Brit. J. Haemat., 2:223, 1956.
61. ———: The site of absorption of vitamin B₁₂ in man. Lancet, 1:18, 1959.
62. Bounett, R., J. R. Cannon, A. W. Johnson, I. Sutherland, A. R. Todd, and

E. Lester Smith: The structure of vitamin B_{12} and its hexacarboxylic acid degradation product. Nature, 176: 328, 1955.

63. Bourne, M. S., and S. Oleesky: Dietary deficiency of vitamin B_{12}. Brit. Med. J., 2: 511, 1960.

64. Bradley, J. E., E. L. Smith, S. J. Baker, and D. L. Mollin: The use of the radioactive isotope of cobalt Co^{58} for the preparation of labelled vitamin B_{12}. Lancet, 2: 476, 1954.

65. Brante, G., and T. Ernberg: The in vitro uptake of vitamin B_{12} by Diphyllobothrium latum and its blockage by intrinsic factor. Scand. J. Clin. Lab. Invest., 9: 313, 1957.

66. ———: The mechanism of pernicious tapeworm anemia studied with ^{60}Co-labelled vitamin B_{12}. Acta Med. Scand., 160: 91, 1958.

67. Brock, J. F.: Intestinal stricture and megalocytic anaemia. Lancet, 1: 72, 1939.

68. Brodine, C., B. I. Friedman, E. L. Saenger, and J. J. Will: The absorption of vitamin B_{12} labeled with radioactive cobalt^{60} following subtotal gastrectomy. J. Lab. Clin. Med., 53: 220, 1959.

69. Brody, E. A., S. Estren, and L. R. Wasserman: The kinetics of intravenously injected radioactive vitamin B_{12}: Studies on normal subjects and patients with chronic myelocytic leukemia and pernicious anemia. Blood, 15: 646, 1960.

70. ———: Treatment of pernicious anemia by oral administration of vitamin B_{12} without added intrinsic factor. New Engl. J. Med., 260: 361, 1959.

71. Brown, M. R.: The pathology of the gastro-intestinal tract in pernicious anemia and subacute combined degeneration of the spinal cord. New Engl. J. Med., 210: 473, 1934.

72. Buchholz, C. H.: Concentration of vitamin B_{12} from urine by absorption on carbon. J. Lab. Clin. Med., 52: 653, 1958.

73. Bull, F. E.: Radioactive vitamin B_{12} absorption in the evaluation of intrinsic factor. M.S. Thesis, University of Minnesota, 1960.

74. ———, D. C. Campbell, and C. A. Owen, Jr.: The diagnosis and treatment of pernicious anemia. Med. Clin. N. Amer., 40: 1005, 1956.

75. Bunge, M. B., L. L. Schloesser, and R. F. Schilling: Intrinsic factor studies IV. Selective absorption and binding of cyanocobalamin by gastric juice in the presence of excess pseudovitamin B_{12} or 5,6-dimethylbenzimidazole. J. Lab. Clin. Med., 48: 735, 1956.

76. Burkholder, P. R.: Microbiological studies on materials which potentiate oral vitamin B_{12} therapy in Addisonian anemia. Arch. Biochem., 39: 322, 1952.

77. Burnet, MacF.: Auto-immune disease. I. Modern immunological concepts. Brit. Med. J., 2: 645, 1959.

78. ———: Auto-immune disease. II. Pathology of the immune response. Brit. Med. J., 2: 720, 1959.

79. Butt, H. R., and C. H. Watkins: Occurrence of macrocytic anemia in association with lesions of the bowel. Ann. Intern. Med., 10: 222, 1936.

80. Callender, S. T., and M. A. Denborough: A family study of pernicious anaemia. Brit. J. Haemat., 3: 88, 1957.

81. Callender, S. T., and J. R. Evans: Observations on the relationship of intrinsic factor to the absorption of labelled vitamin B_{12} from the intestine. Clin. Sci., 14: 387, 1955.

82. ———: The urinary excretion of labelled vitamin B_{12}. Clin. Sci., 14: 295, 1955.

83. Callender, S. T., and L. G. Lajtha: On the nature of Castle's hemopoietic factor. Blood, 6: 1234, 1951.

84. Callender, S. T., and G. H. Spray: Preparation of haemopoietically active extracts from faeces. Lancet, 1: 1391, 1951.

85. Callender, S. T., A. Turnbull, and G. Wakisaka: Estimation of intrinsic factor of Castle by use of radioactive vitamin B_{12}. Brit. Med. J., 1: 10, 1954.

86. ———: Intrinsic factor after total gastrectomy. Clin. Sci., 13: 221, 1954.

87. Calvert, R. J., E. Hurworth, and A. L. MacBean: Megaloblastic anemia from methophenobarbital. Blood, 13: 894, 1958.
88. Cameron, D. G., G. M. Watson, and L. J. Witts: The clinical association of macrocytic anemia with intestinal stricture and anastomosis. Blood, 4: 793, 1949.
89. ———: The experimental production of macrocytic anemia by operations on the intestinal tract. Blood, 4: 803, 1949.
90. Castle, W. B.: Development of knowledge concerning the gastric intrinsic factor and its relation to pernicious anemia. New Engl. J. Med., 249: 603, 1953.
91. ———: Observations on the etiologic relationship of achylia gastrica to pernicious anemia. I. The effect of the administration to patients with pernicious anemia of the contents of the normal human stomach recovered after the ingestion of beef muscle. Amer. J. Med. Sci., 178: 748, 1929.
92. ———: Factors involved in the absorption of vitamin B₁₂. Gastroenterology, 37: 377, 1959.
93. ———: Oral treatment of pernicious anemia. Lancet, 2: 270, 1958.
94. ———, C. W. Heath, and M. B. Strauss: Observations on the etiologic relationship of achylia gastrica to pernicious anemia. IV. A biologic assay of the gastric secretion of patients with pernicious anemia having free hydrochloric acid and that of patients without anemia or with hypochromic anemia having no free hydrochloric acid, and of the role of intestinal impermeability to hematopoietic substances in pernicious anemia. Amer. J. Med. Sci., 182: 741, 1931.
95. ———, and R. W. Heinle: Observations on the etiologic relationship of achylia gastrica to pernicious anemia. VI. Site of interaction of food and gastric factors: failure of in vitro incubation to produce thermostable hematopoietic principle. Amer. J. Med. Sci., 194: 618, 1937.
96. Castle, W. B., C. W. Heath, M. B. Strauss, and W. C. Townsend: The relationship of disorders of the digestive tract to anemia. J.A.M.A., 97: 904, 1931.
97. Castle, W. B., and W. C. Townsend: Observations on the etiologic relationship of achylia gastrica to pernicious anemia. II. The effect of the administration to patients with pernicious anemia of beef muscle after incubation with normal human gastric juice. Amer. J. Med. Sci., 178: 764, 1929.
98. ———, and C. W. Heath: Observations on the etiologic relationship of achylia gastrica to pernicious anemia. III. The nature of the reaction between normal human gastric juice and beef muscle leading to clinical improvement and increased blood formation similar to the effect of liver feeding. Amer. J. Med. Sci., 180: 305, 1930.
99. Chaiet, L., C. Rosenblum, and D. T. Woodbury: Biosynthesis of radioactive vitamin B₁₂ containing cobalt⁶⁰. Science, 111: 601, 1950.
100. Chalmers, J. N. M., and K. Boheimer: Megaloblastic anaemia and anticonvulsant therapy. Lancet, 2: 920, 1954.
101. Chalmers, J. N. M., and Z. M. Hall: Treatment of pernicious anaemia with oral vitamin B₁₂ without known source of intrinsic factor. Brit. Med. J., 1: 1179, 1954.
102. Chalmers, J. N. M., and N. K. Shinton: Absorption of orally administered vitamin B₁₂ in pernicious anaemia. Lancet, 2: 1298, 1958.
103. ———: Effect of D-sorbitol on the absorption of orally administered vitamin B₁₂. Nature, 183: 120, 1959.
104. Chanarin, I., P. C. Elmes, and D. L. Mollin: Folic-acid studies in megaloblastic anaemia due to primidone. Brit. Med. J., 2: 80, 1958.
105. Chanarin, I., J. Laidlaw, L. W. Loughridge, and D. L. Mollin: Megaloblastic anaemia due to phenobarbitone. The convulsant action of therapeutic doses of folic acid. Brit. Med. J., 1: 1099, 1960.
105A. Chaudhuri, S.: Vitamin B₁₂ in megaloblastic anaemia of pregnancy and tropical nutritional macrocytic anaemia. Brit. Med. J., 2: 825, 1951.
106. Chernish, S. M., O. M. Helmer, P. J. Fouts, and K. G. Kohlstaedt: The effect of intrinsic factor on the absorption of vitamin B₁₂ in older people. Amer. J. Clin. Nutr., 5: 651, 1957.

107. Chesterman, D. C., W. F. J. Cuthbertson, and H. F. Pegler: Vitamin B_{12} excretion studies. Biochem. J., 48: LI, 1951.

108. Chow, B. F., and R. L. Davis: Some observations on substances combining with vitamin B_{12}. Recent Advances in Nutrition Research. Nutrition Symposium Series, 5: 17, 1952.

109. Chow, B. F., J. P. Gilbert, K. Okuda, and C. Rosenblum: The urinary excretion test for absorption of vitamin B_{12}. I. Reproducibility of results and agewise variation. Amer. J. Clin. Nutr., 4: 142, 1956.

110. Chow, B. F., P. Meier, and S. M. Free, Jr.: Absorption of vitamin B_{12} enhanced by D-sorbitol. Amer. J. Clin. Nutr., 6: 30, 1958.

111. Chow, B. F., H. Prystowsky, A. E. Hellegers, and V. Wong: Studies on the absorption of vitamin B_{12} in human pregnancy with especial reference to the effect of D-sorbitol. Amer. J. Obstet. Gynec., 76: 91, 1958.

112. Chow, B. F., S. Tauber, I. Woldow, S. Yeh, and B. Ranke: Influence of D-sorbitol on absorption of vitamin B_{12} by patients with pernicious anemia and achlorhydria. Amer. J. Clin. Nutr., 7: 328, 1959.

113. Chow, B. F., W. L. Williams, K. Okuda, and R. Gräsbeck: The urinary excretion test for absorption of vitamin B_{12}. II. Effect of crude and purified intrinsic factor preparation. Amer. J. Clin. Nutr., 4: 147, 1956.

114. Christenson, W. N., J. E. Ultmann, and D. M. Roseman: Megaloblastic anemia during primidone (mysoline) therapy. J.A.M.A., 163: 940, 1957.

115. Citrin, Y., C. DeRosa, and J. A. Halsted: Sites of absorption of vitamin B_{12}. J. Lab. Clin. Med., 50: 667, 1957.

116. Clark, A. C. L., and C. C. Booth: Deficiency of vitamin B_{12} after extensive resection of the distal small intestine in an infant. Arch. Dis. Child., 35: 595, 1960.

117. Clegg, R. E.: A simple method of preparing an ultrafiltrate. Chemist Analyst, 38: 87, December, 1949.

118. Clement, D. H., C. A. Nichol, and A. D. Welch: A case of juvenile pernicious anemia: study of the effects of folic acid and vitamin B_{12}. Blood, 17: 618, 1961.

119. Coates, M. E., and E. S. Holdsworth: The mechanism of vitamin B_{12} absorption in animals, in Proc. 7th Congr. Internat. Soc. Hemat., Grune & Stratton, New York, 3: 96, 1960.

120. Colle, E., L. Greenberg, and W. Krivit: Studies of a patient with selective deficiency in absorption of vitamin B_{12}. Blood, 18: 48, 1961.

121. Conley, C. L., and J. R. Krevans: Development of neurologic manifestations of pernicious anemia during multivitamin therapy. New Engl. J. Med., 245: 529, 1951.

122. Conley, C. L., J. R. Krevans, B. F. Chow, C. Barrows, and C. A. Lang: Observations on the absorption, utilization and excretion of vitamin B_{12}. J. Lab. Clin. Med., 38: 84, 1951.

123. Cooke, W. T.: Anaemia and the alimentary tract. Lancet, 2: 255, 1958.

124. ———, E. V. Cox, M. J. Meynell, and R. Gaddie: Importance of the ileum in the absorption of vitamin B_{12}. Lancet, 2: 1231, 1957.

125. Cooper, B. A.: Failure of sorbitol to replace intrinsic factor in the gastrectomized rat. Nature, 182: 647, 1958.

126. ———, and W. B. Castle: Sequential mechanisms in the enhanced absorption of vitamin B_{12} by intrinsic factor in the rat. J. Clin. Invest., 39: 199, 1960.

127. Cornell, G. N., H. Gilder, F. Moody, C. Frey, and J. M. Beal: The pattern of absorption following surgical shortening of the bowel. Bull. N.Y. Acad. Med., 37: 675, 1961.

129. Cox, A. J.: The stomach in pernicious anemia. Amer. J. Path., 19: 491, 1943.

130. Cox, E. V., M. J. Meynell, R. Gaddie, and W. T. Cooke: Interrelation of vitamin B_{12} and iron. Lancet, 2: 998, 1959.

130A. Craddock, C. G., S. Perry, and J. S. Lawrence: The dynamics of leukopenia and leukocytosis. Ann. Intern. Med., 52: 281, 1960.

131. Cronkite, E. P., E. Henley, D. L. Driscoll, L. M. Meyer, F. C. Dohan, J. R.

Rubini, and W. Wollins: Studies on the kinetics of intravenously injected ^{60}cobalt labeled vitamin B$_{12}$ in man, in Proc. 7th Congr. Internat. Soc. Hemat., Grune & Stratton, New York, 3:158, 1960.

132. Crowder, R. V., Jr., W. T. Thompson, Jr., and H. G. Kupfer: Acquired agammaglobulinemia with multiple allergies and pernicious anemia. A.M.A. Arch. Intern. Med., 103:445, 1959.

133. Dallman, P. R., and L. K. Diamond: Vitamin B$_{12}$ deficiency associated with disease of the small intestine. J. Pediat., 57:689, 1960.

134. Das Gupta, C. R., and J. B. Chatterjea: Folic acid in the treatment of macrocytic anaemia in pregnancy. Indian J. Med. Res., 37:455, 1949.

135. Davidson, L. S. P.: The gastro-intestinal flora in pernicious anaemia. J. Path. Bact., 312:557, 1928.

136. ———: Megaloblastic anaemia and subacute combined degeneration from tuberculous disease of the small intestine. Gastroenterologia, 79:342, 1953.

137. Davidson, W. M. B., and J. L. Markson: The gastric mucosa in iron deficiency anaemia. Lancet, 2:639, 1955.

137A. Davis, B. D., and E. S. Mingioli: Mutants of Escherichia coli requiring methionine or vitamin B$_{12}$. J. Bact., 60:17, 1950.

138. Davis, R. L., and B. F. Chow: Vitamin B$_{12}$ binding substances in human serum. Fed. Proc., 13:33, 1954.

139. ———: Some applications of the rapid uptake of vitamin B$_{12}$ by resting Lactobacillus leichmannii organisms. Science, 115:351, 1952.

140. Davis, R. L., R. C. Duvall, and B. F. Chow: Serum vitamin B$_{12}$ level and binding substance of tuberculous patients with and without liver disease. J. Lab. Clin. Med., 49:422, 1957.

142. Davis, R. L., L. L. Layton, and B. F. Chow: Uptake of radioactive vitamin B$_{12}$ by various microorganisms. Proc. Soc. Exp. Biol. Med., 79:273, 1952.

143. Day, L. A., B. E. Hall, and G. L. Pease: Macrocytic anemia of pregnancy refractory to vitamin B$_{12}$ therapy: response to treatment with folic acid: report of case. Proc. Staff Meet., Mayo Clinic, 24:149, 1949.

144. Deller, D. J., H. Germar, and L. J. Witts: Effect of food on absorption of radioactive vitamin B$_{12}$. Lancet, 1:574, 1961.

145. Demorest, H. L., and J. H. Erickson: Automatic sample changer for well-type scintillation counter. Nucleonics, 12:68, July, 1954.

146. Dick, A. P.: Association of jejunal diverticulosis and steatorrhoea. Brit. Med. J., 1:145, 1955.

147. Dixon, C. F., J. G. Burns, and H. Z. Griffin: Pernicious anemia following ileostomy. J.A.M.A., 85:17, 1925.

147A. Doig, A., and R. H. Girdwood: The absorption of folic acid and labelled cyanocobalamin in intestinal malabsorption, with observations on the faecal excretion of fat and nitrogen and the absorption of glucose and xylose. Quart. J. Med., 29:333, 1960.

147B. ———, J. J. R. Duthie, and J. D. E. Knox: Response of megaloblastic anaemia to prednisolone. Lancet, 2:966, 1957.

148. Doig, R. K.: Gastric biopsy and the investigation of the megaloblastic anaemias. Proc. Roy. Soc. Med., 47:423, 1954.

151. Doig, R. K., and I. J. Wood: Gastric biopsy in pernicious anaemia. Med. J. Aust., 2:565, 1950.

152. ———: Gastritis. Modern Trends in Gastroenterology, 2:208, 1958.

152A. Doscherholmen, Alfred: Basic mechanisms of the Schilling test. J. Lab. Clin. Med., 58:813, 1961.

153. ———: Kinetics of ingested radiocyanocobalamin in man. Proc. 8th Congr. Europ. Soc. Haemat., Vienna, 1961, S. Karger, Basel/New York, 1962.

154. ———: Scintillation spectrometry of Co^{57}-vitamin B$_{12}$ in the diagnosis of pernicious anemia. Vitamin B$_{12}$ und Intrinsic Factor, 2. Europäisches Symposion, Hamburg, 1961, Ferdinand Enke Verlag, Stuttgart, 345, 1962.

155. ———: Enzymatic release of vitamin B$_{12}$ bound either to the intrinsic factor or in the wall of the small intestine. Vitamin B$_{12}$ und Intrinsic Factor, 2. Europäisches Symposion, Hamburg, 1961, Ferdinand Enke Verlag, Stuttgart, 472, 1962.

155A. ———: Studies on the basic mechanisms of the Schilling test. Fed. Proc., 21: 472, 1962.

155B. ———: The basic mechanism of the Schilling test. Proc. 9th Congr. Internat. Soc. Hemat., Mexico City, 1962, to be published by Grune & Stratton, New York, in press.

156. ———, P. R. Finley, and P. S. Hagen: Distribution of radioactivity in man after the oral ingestion of small test doses of radiolabeled cyanocobalamin. J. Lab. Clin. Med., 56:547, 1960.

156A. ———: Organ distribution of radioactivity in man after the oral administration of physiologic test doses of radiolabelled cyanocobalamin. Proc. 7th Congr. Europ. Soc. Haemat., London, 1959, S. Karger, Basel/New York, 2:26, 1960.

157. Doscherholmen, A., and P. S. Hagen: Absorption of Co^{60} labeled vitamin B$_{12}$ in intestinal blind loop megaloblastic anemia. J. Lab. Clin. Med., 44:790, 1954.

157A. ———: Vitamin B$_{12}$ absorption: clinical evaluation of the Schilling test. Clin. Res., 4:83, 1956.

157B. ———: A dual vitamin B$_{12}$ plasma absorption mechanism. J. Clin. Invest., 36: 884, 1957.

158. ———: A dual mechanism of vitamin B$_{12}$ plasma absorption. J. Clin. Invest., 36:1551, 1957.

159. ———: Comparison of the plasma absorption and the urinary excretion tests as measures of absorption of cyanocobalamin. J. Lab. Clin. Med., 52:809, 1958.

159A. ———: Delay of absorption of radiolabeled cyanocobalamin in the intestinal wall in the presence of intrinsic factor. J. Clin. Invest., 37:888, 1958.

159B. ———: Clinical evaluation of the Schilling test. Proc. 6th Congr. Internat. Soc. Hemat., Boston, 1956, Grune & Stratton, New York, 328, 1958.

160. ———: Delay of absorption of radiolabeled cyanocobalamin in the intestinal wall in the presence of intrinsic factor. J. Lab. Clin. Med., 54:434, 1959.

160A. ———: Delay of absorption of radiolabeled cyanocobalamin in the intestinal wall in the presence of intrinsic factor. Proc. 7th Congr. Internat. Soc. Hemat., Rome, 1958, Grune & Stratton, New York, 2:1419, 1960.

161. ———: New observations on vitamin B$_{12}$ absorption. Editorial, Univ. Minn. Med. Bull., 27:204, 1956.

162. ———: Radioactive vitamin B$_{12}$ absorption studies: Results of direct measurement of radioactivity in the blood. Blood, 12:336, 1957.

163. ———: Radioactive vitamin B$_{12}$ absorption studies: Results of direct measurement of radioactivity in the blood. Proc. 6th Internat. Congr. of the Internat. Soc. Hemat., Grune & Stratton, New York, 347, 1958.

164. ———: Radioactive vitamin B$_{12}$ absorption studies: Results of direct measurement of radioactivity in the blood. J. Clin. Invest., 35:699, 1956.

165. ———: Alteration of hepatic storage of radiolabeled vitamin B$_{12}$. Proc. Soc. Exp. Biol. Med., 95:667, 1957.

165A. ———: Kinetics of ingested radiocyanocobalamin in man. Vitamin B$_{12}$ und Intrinsic Factor, 2. Europäisches Symposion, Hamburg, 1961, Ferdinand Enke Verlag, Stuttgart, 381, 1962.

166. Driscoll, T., J. Faulkner, B. Carroll, and P. C. Johnson: Effects of gastric juice fractions on uptake of labeled vitamin B$_{12}$ by rat liver slices. Proc. Soc. Exp. Biol. Med., 101:336, 1959.

167. Drouet, P.-L., K. Wolff, and M. G. Rauber: Etude de la vitamine B$_{12}$ hépatique par la ponction-biopsie. Premiers résultats dans la maladie de Biermer. Bull. Soc. Med. Hôp. Paris, 67:281, 1951.

168. Dubach, R., C. V. Moore, and V. Minnich: Studies in iron transportation and metabolism. J. Lab. Clin. Med., 31:1201, 1946.

169. Dunn, A. L., J. R. Walsh, and J. M. Holthaus: Radioactive cyanocobalamin (vitamin B_{12}) in renal disease. Arch. Intern. Med., 101:927, 1958.

170. Eberle, B. T., and G. I. Gleason: Cobalt[57] labeled vitamin B_{12} and its advantages in regard to radiation absorbed dose to the liver and counting efficiency. Clin. Research, 8:208, 1960.

171. Editorial: Vitamin B_{12} neuropathy after gastrectomy. Brit. Med. J., 2:1507, 1960.

172. Editorial: Anaemia in pregnancy. Lancet, 2:1360, 1958.

173. Ellenbogen, L., B. F. Chow, and W. L. Williams: Effect of intrinsic factor on absorption of vitamin B_{12} in healthy individuals. Amer. J. Clin. Nutr., 6:26, 1958.

174. Ellenbogen, L., V. Herbert, and W. L. Williams: Effect of D-sorbitol on absorption of vitamin B_{12} by pernicious anemia patients. Proc. Soc. Exp. Biol. Med., 99:257, 1958.

175. Ellenbogen, L., and W. L. Williams: Quantitative assay of intrinsic factor activity by urinary excretion of radioactive vitamin B_{12}. Blood, 13:582, 1958.

176. ———, and H. C. Lichtman: Successful maintenance of pernicious anaemia patients with vitamin B_{12} and intrinsic factor for long periods. Brit. Med. J., 2:1066, 1960.

177. Ellenbogen, L., W. L. Williams, S. F. Rabiner, and H. C. Lichtman: An improved urinary excretion test as an assay for intrinsic factor. Proc. Soc. Exp. Biol. Med., 89:357, 1955.

178. Erdmann-Oehlecker, S.: Der Vitamin B_{12}-Stoffwechsel bei Hämoblastosen, Vitamin B_{12} und Intrinsic Factor, 1. Europäisches Symposion, Hamburg, 1956, Ferdinand Enke Verlag, Stuttgart, 456, 1957.

179. Estren, S., E. A. Brody, and L. R. Wasserman: The disappearance of intravenously administered vitamin B_{12}. Studies in normal subject and in patients with pernicious anemia. Amer. J. Clin. Nutr., 8:259, 1960.

180. ———: The metabolism of vitamin B_{12} in pernicious and other megaloblastic anemias. Advances Intern. Med., 9:11, 1958.

181. Estren, S., and L. R. Wasserman: Pernicious anemia. I. Remission by small oral doses of purified vitamin B_{12}. Proc. Soc. Exp. Biol. Med., 91:499, 1956.

182. Evans, J. R.: The absorption of vitamin B_{12} in the megaloblastic anaemias. Proc. Nutr. Soc., 15:126, 1956.

182A. Faber, K.: Perniciös anaemi som fölge af tarmlidelse. Hospitalstidende, 3:601, 1895.

182B. ———: Perniciöse Anämie bei Dünndarmstricturen. Berl. Klin. Wschr., 34:643, 1897.

183. ———: Anämische Zustände bei der chronischen Achylia gastrica. Berl. Klin. Wschr., 50:958, 1913.

185. ———: Chronic gastritis: Its relation to achylia and ulcer. Lancet, 2:901, 1927.

186. ———: Gastritis and Its Consequences. Oxford University Press, London, 16, 1935.

189. ———, and C. E. Bloch: Ueber die pathologischen Veränderungen am Digestionstractus bei der perniciösen Anämie und über die sogenannte Darmatrophie. Z. Klin. Med., 40:98, 1900.

189A. Faber, K., and G. Lange: Die Pathogenese und Aetiologie der chronischen Achylia gastrica. Z. Klin. Med., 66:53, 1908.

190. Fantes, K. H., J. E. Page, L. F. J. Parker, and E. L. Smith. Crystallin antipernicious anaemia factor from liver. Proc. Roy. Soc. Biol., 137:592, 1949.

191. Farrant, P. C.: Nuclear changes in oral epithelium in pernicious anaemia. Lancet, 1:830, 1958.

192. ———: Nuclear changes in squamous cells from buccal mucosa in pernicious anaemia. Brit. Med. J., 1:1694, 1960.

193. Faulkner, J., B. Carroll, T. Driscoll, and P. C. Johnson: Co[60]-vitamin B_{12} binding by chromatographic fractions of human gastric contents. Amer. J. Clin. Nutr., 8:512, 1960.

194. Fenwick, S.: On Atrophy of the Stomach and on the Nervous Affections of the Digestive Organs. J. and A. Churchill, London, 1880.

195. ———: On atrophy of the stomach. Lancet, 2:78, 1870.

195A. Fisher, R. A. L.: Statistical Methods for Research Workers. Oliver & Boyd, Edinburgh, 1948.

196. Fone, D. J., W. T. Cooke, M. J. Meynell, and E. L. Harris: Co^{58} B_{12} absorption (hepatic surface count) after gastrectomy, ileal resection, and in coeliac disorders. Gut, 2:218, 1961.

197. Fouts, P. J., O. M. Helmer, and S. M. Chernish: Absorption of radioactive B_{12} in patients with pernicious anemia after long-term oral and parenteral therapy. Ann. Intern. Med., 52:29, 1960.

198. Friedlander, P. H., and V. Gorvy: Steatorrhoea. Brit. Med. J., 2:809, 1955.

199. Frost, J. W., and M. I. Goldwein: Observations on vitamin B_{12} absorption in primary pernicious anemia during administration of adrenocortical steroids. New Engl. J. Med., 258:1096, 1958.

200. ———, and B. D. Kaufman: Studies of B_{12} Co^{60} absorption in malabsorption syndrome: Results before and during specific therapy. Ann. Intern. Med., 47:293, 1957.

201. Gaffney, G. W., D. M. Watkin, and B. F. Chow: Vitamin B_{12} absorption: Relationship between oral administration and urinary excretion of cobalt^{60}-labeled cyanocobalamin following a parenteral dose. J. Lab. Clin. Med., 53:525, 1959.

202. Gardner, F. H.: Gastrointestinal flora and the red cells. Amer. J. Dig. Dis., 2:175, 1957.

203. ———, J. W. Harris, R. F. Schilling, and W. B. Castle: Observations on the etiologic relationship of achylia gastrica to pernicious anemia. XI. Hematopoietic activity in pernicious anemia of a beef muscle extract containing food (extrinsic) factor upon intravenous injection without contact with gastric (intrinsic) factor. J. Lab. Clin. Med., 34:1502, 1949.

204. Gatenby, P. B. B.: The anaemias of pregnancy in Dublin. Proc. Nutr. Soc., 15:115, 1956.

205. Gellman, D. D.: Diverticulosis of the small intestine with steatorrhoea and megaloblastic anaemia. Lancet, 2:873, 1956.

206. Girdwood, R. H.: Rapid estimation of the serum vitamin B_{12} level by a microbiological method. Brit. Med. J., 2:954, 1954.

207. ———: The intestinal content in pernicious anemia of factors for the growth of Streptococcus faecalis and Lactobacillus leichmannii. Blood, 5:1009, 1950.

208. ———: The occurrence of growth factors for Lactobacillus leichmannii, Streptococcus faecalis, and Leuconostoc citrovorum in the tissues of pernicious anaemia patients and controls. Biochem. J., 52:58, 1952.

209. ———: The possible effects of gastro-intestinal bacteria on the absorption of vitamin B_{12}. Rev. Hemat. (Paris), 10:187, 1955.

210. ———, and A. Doig: Importance of the ileum in the absorption of vitamin B_{12}. Lancet, 2:1064, 1957.

212. Glass, G. B. J.: Deposition and storage of vitamin B_{12} in the normal and diseased liver. Gastroenterology, 36:180, 1959.

213. ———: Biochemistry and physiology of Castle's intrinsic factor and its relationship to the metabolism of vitamin B_{12}. Rev. Hemat. (Paris), 10:137, 1955.

214. ———: Intestinal absorption and hepatic uptake of vitamin B_{12} in diseases of the gastrointestinal tract. Gastroenterology, 30:37, 1956.

215. ———: Oral treatment of pernicious anaemia. Lancet, 2:747, 1958.

216. ———: Radioactive vitamin B_{12} in the liver. III. Hepatic storage and discharge of Co^{60} B_{12} in pernicious anemia. J. Lab. Clin. Med., 52:875, 1958.

217. ———: Scintillation measurements of the uptake of radioactive vitamin B_{12} by the liver in normal humans and patients with pernicious and other macrocytic anemias. Bull. N.Y. Acad. Med., 30:717, 1954.

217A. ———: Gastric intrinsic factor and its function in the metabolism of vitamin B_{12}. Physiol. Rev., 43:529, 1963.

218. ———, and L. J. Boyd: Differentiation of macrocytic anemias and diagnosis of pernicious anemia and sprue in remission by accelerated measurement of hepatic uptake of radioactive Co^{60} B_{12}. Ann. Intern. Med., 47:274, 1957.

219. ———, and L. Ebin: Radioactive vitamin B_{12} in the liver. I. Hepatic uptake of Co^{60} B_{12} in liver disease. J. Lab. Clin. Med., 52:849, 1958.

220. Glass, G. B. J., L. J. Boyd, and G. A. Gellin: Surface scintillation measurements in humans of the uptake of parenterally administered radioactive vitamin B_{12}. Blood, 10:95, 1955.

221. ———, and L. Stephanson: Uptake of radioactive vitamin B_{12} by the liver in humans: Test for measurement of intestinal absorption of vitamin B_{12} and intrinsic factor activity. Arch. Biochem., 51:251, 1954.

222. Glass. G. B. J., L. J. Boyd, A. L. Luhby, and L. Stephanson: Assay of intrinsic factor preparations: Comparison of the hepatic uptake of radioactive Co^{60} B_{12} with the hematopoietic response in pernicious anemia. J. Lab. Clin. Med., 46:60, 1955.

223. Glass, G. B. J., L. J. Boyd, M. A. Rubinstein, and C. S. Svigals: Relationship of glandular mucoprotein from human gastric juice to Castle's intrinsic antianemic factor. Science, 115:101, 1952.

224. Glass, G. B. J., L. J. Boyd, and L. Stephanson: Intestinal absorption of vitamin B_{12} in humans as studied by isotope technic. Proc. Soc. Exp. Biol. Med., 86:522, 1954.

225. ———: Intestinal absorption of vitamin B_{12} in man. Science, 120:74, 1954.

226. ———: Inverse relationship between intake and utilization of vitamin B_{12} in the intestine. Fed. Proc., 13:54, 1954.

227. ———, and E. L. Jones: Metabolic interrelations between intrinsic factor and vit. B_{12}. III. B_{12} absorption at varied intrinsic factor doses. Proc. Soc. Exp. Biol. Med., 88:1, 1954.

228. Glass, G. B. J., A. A. Goldbloom, L. J. Boyd, R. Laughton, S. Rosen, and M. Rich: Intestinal absorption and hepatic uptake of radioactive vitamin B_{12} in various age groups and the effect of intrinsic factor preparations. Amer. J. Clin. Nutr., 4:124, 1956.

229. Glass, G. B. J., and R. W. Laughton: Efficiency of intestinal absorption of vitamin B_{12} measured by hepatic uptake of $Co^{60}B_{12}$. Proc. Soc. Exp. Biol. Med., 95:325, 1957.

230. Glass, G. B. J., and W. L. Mersheimer: Metabolic turnover of vitamin B_{12} in the normal and diseased liver. Amer. J. Clin. Nutr., 8:285, 1960.

231. Glass, G. B. J., G. T. Pack, and W. L. Mersheimer: Uptake of radioactive vitamin B_{12} by the liver in patients with total and subtotal gastrectomy. Gastroenterology, 29:666, 1955.

232. Glass, G. B. J., and H. Schaffer: Further observations on the intestinal absorption of vitamin B_{12} as measured by hepatic uptake of $Co^{60}B_{12}$. Bull. N.Y. Med. Coll., 19:74, 1956.

233. Glass, G. B. J., F. D. Speer, H. E. Nieburgs, A. Ishimori, E. L. Jones, H. Baker, S. A. Schwartz, and R. Smith: Gastric atrophy, atrophic gastritis, and gastric secretory failure. Correlative study by suction biopsy and exfoliative cytology of gastric mucosa, paper electrophoretic and secretory assays of gastric secretion, and measurements of intestinal absorption and blood levels of vitamin B_{12}. Gastroenterology, 39:429, 1960.

234. Goldberg, S. R., B. K. Trivedi, and L. Oliner: Radioactive vitamin B_{12} studies. Experience with the urinary excretion test and the measurement of absorbed plasma radioactivity. J. Lab. Clin. Med., 49:583, 1957.

235. Goldhamer, S. M.: Macrocytic anemia in cancer of the stomach, apparently due to lack of intrinsic factor. Amer. J. Med. Sci., 195:17, 1938.

236. ———: The gastric juice in patients with pernicious anemia in induced remission. Amer. J. Med. Sci., 193:23, 1937.

237. ———: The presence of the intrinsic factor of Castle in the gastric juice of patients with pernicious anemia. Amer. J. Med. Sci., 191:405, 1936.

238. Gordin, R.: Megaloblastic anaemia during anticonvulsant therapy. Acta Med. Scand., 162:401, 1958.

239. ———: Vitamin B$_{12}$ absorption in corticosteroid-treated pernicious anaemia. Acta Med. Scand., 164:159, 1959.

241. Graham, R. M., and M. H. Rheault: Characteristic cellular changes in epithelial cells in pernicious anemia. J. Lab. Clin. Med., 43:235, 1954.

242. Gräsbeck, R.: Calculations on vitamin B$_{12}$ turnover in man. With a note on the maintenance treatment in pernicious anemia and the radiation dose received by patients ingesting radiovitamin B$_{12}$. Scand. J. Clin. Lab. Invest., 11:250, 1959.

243. ———: Familjar selektiv B$_{12}$-malabsorption med proteinuri. Ett perniciosaliknande syndrom. Nord. Med., 63:322, 1960.

244. ———: Physiology and pathology of vitamin B$_{12}$ absorption, distribution, and excretion. Advances Clin. Chem., 3:299, 1960.

245. ———: Studies on the vitamin B$_{12}$-binding principle and other biocolloids of human gastric juice. Acta Med. Scand., Suppl. 314, 1956.

246. ———, R. Gordin, I. Kantero, and B. Kuhlbäck: Selective vitamin B$_{12}$ malabsorption and proteinuria in young people, a syndrome. Acta Med. Scand., 167:289, 1960.

247. Gräsbeck, R., and I. Kantero: A case of juvenile vitamin B$_{12}$ deficiency. Acta Paediat. (Upps.), Suppl. 118, 48:140, 1959.

248. ———, and M. Siurala: Influence of calcium ions on vitamin B$_{12}$ absorption in steatorrhoea and pernicious anaemia. Lancet, 1:234, 1959.

249. Gräsbeck, R., and W. Nyberg: Inhibition of radiovitamin B$_{12}$ absorption by ethylenediaminetetraacetate (EDTA) and its reversal by calcium ions. Scand. J. Clin. Lab. Invest., 10:448, 1958.

250. ———, G. Perman, and P. Reizenstein: Excretion of endogenous vitamin B$_{12}$. Acta Physiol. Scand., Suppl. 145, 42:52, 1957.

251. Gräsbeck, R., W. Nyberg, and P. Reizenstein: Biliary and fecal vitamin B$_{12}$ excretion in man. An isotope study. Proc. Soc. Exp. Biol. Med., 97:780, 1958.

252. Gräsbeck, R., W. Nyberg, and M. Siurala: Urinexkretion av radioaktivt B$_{12}$-vitamin (Schilling test). Nord. Med., 56:1656, 1956.

253. Gräsbeck, R., and K. Okuda: The biliary and faecal excretion of vitamin B$_{12}$. Scand. J. Clin. Lab. Invest., Suppl. 31:274, 1957.

254. Gräsbeck, R., L. Runeberg, and K. Simons: Intrinsic factor and radio-vitamin B$_{12}$ excretion in rats. Acta Physiol. Scand., 47:370, 1959.

255. Gräsbeck, R., and I.-T. Takki-Luukkainen: Vitamin B$_{12}$ binding substance in human tear fluid. Acta Ophthal., 36:860, 1958.

256. Green, C., and A. L. Latner: Intestinal absorption of vitamin B$_{12}$. Lancet, 2:156, 1958.

257. Greenberg, S. M., J. F. Herndon, E. G. Rice, E. T. Parmelee, J. J. Gulesich, and E. J. Van Loon: Enhancement of vitamin B$_{12}$ absorption by substances other than intrinsic factor. Nature, 180:1401, 1957.

258. Gregory, M. E., and E. S. Holdsworth: Unpublished observations cited by S. K. Kon in Biochemistry of Vitamin B$_{12}$. Biochemical Society Symposia No. 13, Cambridge University Press, London, 30, 1955.

259. Grinstein, M., M. D. Kamen, and C. V. Moore: Observation on the utilization of glycine in the biosynthesis of hemoglobin. J. Biol. Chem., 174:767, 1948.

260. ———: The utilization of glycine in the biosynthesis of hemoglobin. J. Biol. Chem., 179:359, 1949.

261. Grossowicz, N., J. Aronovitch, and M. Rachmilewitz: Determination of vitamin B$_{12}$ in human serum by a mutant of Escherichia coli. Proc. Soc. Exp. Biol. Med., 87:513, 1954.

262. Haenel, U.: Über einen Fall von alimentärer Megalocytärer Anämie während der Schwangerschaft (alimentäre Schwangerschaftsperniciosa). Klin. Wschr., 28: 471, 1950.

263. Hall, B. E.: Studies on the nature of the intrinsic factor of Castle. Brit. Med. J., 2:585, 1950.

264. Hall, C. A.: The plasma disappearance of radioactive vitamin B_{12} in myeloproliferative diseases and other blood disorders. Blood, 18:717, 1961.

265. ———: Plasma vitamin B_{12} removal in myeloproliferative disorders. Clin. Res., 8:210, 1960.

266. ———: The plasma disappearance of intravenously administered cobalt[58] vitamin B_{12}. J. Clin. Invest., 39:1312, 1960.

267. Halsted, J. A: A matter of nomenclature. New Engl. J. Med., 255:719, 1956.

268. ———, J. Carroll, A. Dehghani, M. Loghmani, and A. S. Prasad: Serum vitamin B_{12} concentration in dietary deficiency. Amer. J. Clin. Nutr., 8:374, 1960.

269. Halsted, J. A., J. Carroll, and S. Rubert: Serum and tissue concentration of vitamin B_{12} in certain pathologic states. New Engl. J. Med., 260:575, 1959.

270. Halsted, J. A., M. Gasster, and E. J. Drenick: Absorption of radioactive vitamin B_{12} after total gastrectomy. New Engl. J. Med., 251:161, 1954.

271. Halsted, J. A., P. M. Lewis, and M. Gasster: Absorption of radioactive vitamin B_{12} in the syndrome of megaloblastic anemia associated with intestinal stricture or anastomosis. Amer. J. Med., 20:42, 1956.

272. Halsted, J. A., P. M. Lewis, E. E. Hvolboll, M. Gasster, and M. E. Swendseid: An evaluation of the fecal recovery method for determining intestinal absorption of cobalt[60]-labeled vitamin B_{12}. J. Lab. Clin. Med., 48:92, 1956.

273. Halsted, J. A., M. E. Swendseid, P. M. Lewis, and M. Gasster: Mechanisms involved in the development of vitamin B_{12} deficiency. Gastroenterology, 30:21, 1956.

274. Hare, R. S., and K. Hare: Determination of creatinine in blood and urine. Fed. Proc., 8:68, 1949.

275. Harris-Jones, J. N., H. T. Swan, and G. R. Tudhope: Pernicious anemia without gastric atrophy and in the presence of free hydrochloric acid: report of a case. Blood, 12:461, 1957.

276. Harrison, R. J., C. C. Booth, and D. L. Mollin: Vitamin-B_{12} deficiency due to defective diet. Lancet, 1:727, 1956.

277. Harte, R. A., B. F. Chow, and L. Barrows: Storage and elimination of vitamin B_{12} in the rat. J. Nutr., 49:669, 1953.

277A. Hartfall, S. J., and L. J. Witts: The intrinsic factor of Castle in simple achlorhydric anaemia. Guy's Hosp. Rep., 83:24, 1953.

278. Harvey, J. C.: The vitamin B_{12} deficiency state engendered by total gastrectomy. Surgery, 40:977, 1956.

279. Haugen, H. N., and E. M. Blegen: The true endogenous creatinine clearance. Scand. J. Clin. Lab. Invest., 5:67, 1953.

280. Hausmann, K.: Über den Gehalt von Lebern Perniciosakranker an antiperniciös wirksamer Substanz nach verschiedenartiger Therapie und über die Beziehungen der bei Perniciosakranken blutbildenden Stoffe zueinander. Vitamin-Hormon-Fermentforschung, 4:162, 1951.

281. ———, and K. Milli: Haemopoietic effect of vitamin-B_{12}-peptide conjugate of low molecular weight. Lancet, 1:889, 1959.

282. Havemeyer, R. N., and T. Higuchi: The complexing tendencies of cyanocobalamin with inorganic compounds. J. Amer. Pharm. Ass. (Sci.), 49:356, 1960.

283. Hawkins, C. F., and M. J. Meynell: Macrocytosis and macrocytic anaemia caused by anticonvulsant drugs. Quart. J. Med., 27:45, 1958.

284. Hawksley, J. C., and E. Meulengracht: Intestinal strictures and its association with pernicious anaemia. Lancet, 2:124, 1936.

285. Heathcote, J. G., and F. S. Mooney: The oral treatment of pernicious anaemia, a new approach. Lancet, 1:982, 1958.

286. ———: Oral treatment of pernicious anaemia. Lancet, 1:1177, 1958.
287. Heinle, R. W., F. H. Bethell, W. B. Castle, I. M. London, and W. T. Salter: Control of U.S.P. anti-anemia preparations. Special report of the United States Pharmacopeia anti-anemia preparations advisory board. J.A.M.A., 151:40, 1951.
288. Heinle, R. W., and A. D. Welch: Folic acid in pernicious anemia. J.A.M.A., 133:739, 1947.
289. ———, V. Scharf, G. C. Meacham, and W. H. Prusoff: Studies of excretion (and absorption) of Co^{60} labeled vitamin B$_{12}$ in pernicious anemia. Trans. Ass. Amer. Physicians, 65:214, 1952.
290. Heinrich, H. C.: Die biochemischen Grundlagen der Diagnostik und Therapie der Vitamin B$_{12}$ Mangelzustände (B$_{12}$-Hypo-und-Avitaminosen) des Menschen und der Haustiere. IV. Mitteilung. Resorption. Verteilung und Exkretion der B$_{12}$ Vitamine bei der oralen Therapie der perniziösen Anämie mit kristallisiertem Vitamin B$_{12}$ + "intrinsic factor." Klin. Wschr., 32:867, 1954.
291. ———: Zur Frage der Beeinflussung des Vitamin-Stoffwechsels durch Sorbose und Sorbit. Klin. Wschr., 37:526, 1959.
292. ———: Die biochemischen Grundlagen der Diagnostik und Therapie der Vitamin B$_{12}$-Mangelzustände (B$_{12}$-Hypo-und-Avitaminosen) des Menschen und der Haustiere. Untersuchungen zum Vitamin B$_{12}$ Stoffwechsel des Menschen während der Gravidität und Lactation. Klin. Wschr., 32:205, 1954.
293. ———: Radio-Vitamin B$_{12}$ in der klinischen Diagnostik, in Schwiegk, H., und Turba, F., Künstliche Radioaktive Isotope in Physiologie, Diagnostik und Therapie, Springer-Verlag, Berlin, 1029, 1961.
294. ———: Radiometrische Intrinsic Factor — Studien am Menschen und am Schwein, Vitamin B$_{12}$ und Intrinsic Factor, 1. Europäisches Symposion, Hamburg, 1956, Ferdinand Enke Verlag, Stuttgart, 213, 1957.
295. ———, and S. Erdmann-Oehlecker: Der Vitamin B$_{12}$ Stoffwechsel bei Hämoblastosen. II. Die intravitale Bindung (transport) der B$_{12}$ Vitamine an die Serumproteinfraktionen bei Hämoblastosen. Clin. Chim. Acta, 1:311, 1956.
296. ———: Der Vitamin B$_{12}$-Stoffwechsel bei Hämoblastosen. III. Resorption, Blutverteilung, Serumproteinbindung, Retention und Exkretion der B$_{12}$-Vitamine bei Hämoblastosen nach oraler und parenteraler B$_{12}$ Applikation. Clin. Chim. Acta, 1:326, 1956.
298. Heinrich, H. C., and H. Lahann: Der orale Vitamin-B$_{12}$-Resorptions-Exkretionstest. Deutsch. Med. Wschr., 78:1475, 1953.
299. Heinrich, H. C., and M. Staak: Sorbitol, an inhibitor of intestinal absorption of vitamin B$_{12}$. Amer. J. Clin. Nutr., 8:247, 1960.
300. Hemsted, E. H., and J. Mills: Vitamin B$_{12}$ in pernicious anemia. Lancet, 2:1302, 1958.
301. Herbert, V.: The Megaloblastic Anemias. Grune & Stratton, New York and London, 1959.
301A. ———: Mechanism of absorption of vitamin B$_{12}$. Fed. Proc., 19:884, 1960.
302. ———: A procedure for the study of the uptake of Co^{60}-B$_{12}$ by rat liver slices in the presence of hog intrinsic factor concentrates. Clin. Res. Proc., 6:12, 1958.
303. ———: Sorbitol and vitamin B$_{12}$ absorption. Amer. J. Clin. Nutr., 6:547, 1958.
304. ———: Development of a possible in vitro assay for intrinsic factor. Proc. Soc. Exp. Biol. Med., 97:668, 1958.
305. ———: Mechanism of intrinsic factor action in the isolated rat small intestine. J. Clin. Invest., 37:901, 1958.
306. ———: Mechanism of intrinsic factor action in everted sacs of rat small intestine. J. Clin. Invest., 38:102, 1959.
307. ———: Studies of the mechanism of the effect of hog intrinsic factor concentrate on the uptake of vitamin B$_{12}$ by rat liver slices. J. Clin. Invest., 37:646, 1958.
308. ———: Studies on the role of intrinsic factor in vitamin B$_{12}$ absorption, transport, and storage. Amer. J. Clin. Nutr., 7:433, 1959.

309. ———, M. Bierfass, L. R. Wasserman, S. Estren, and E. Brody: Effect of D-sorbitol on absorption of vitamin B_{12} by human subjects able to produce intrinsic factor. Amer. J. Clin. Nutr., 7:325, 1959.

311. Herbert, V., Z. Castro, and L. R. Wasserman: Stoichiometric relation between liver-receptor, intrinsic factor and vitamin B_{12}. Proc. Soc. Exp. Biol. Med., 104:160, 1960.

311A. Herbert, V., B. A. Cooper, and W. B. Castle: The site of vitamin B_{12}-intrinsic factor complex "releasing factor" activity in the rat small intestine. Proc. Soc. Exp. Biol. Med., 110:315, 1962.

311B. Herbert, V., S. Estren, E. Brody, and L. R. Wasserman: Oral treatment of pernicious anaemia. Lancet, 2:801, 1958.

312. Herbert, V., and I. M. London: Enhancement of vitamin B_{12} uptake by rat liver slices in the presence of hog intrinsic factor concentrate. Clin. Res. Proc., 5:289, 1957.

313. Herbert, V., and T. H. Spaet: Distribution of "intrinsic factor" activity. Amer. J. Physiol., 195:194, 1958.

314. Hernberg, C. A.: Concerning the anti-anaemic influence of the gastric juice in pernicious botriocephalus anaemia. Acta Med. Scand., Suppl. 78:582, 1936.

315. ———: On the occurrence of the intrinsic factor in the gastric juice in pernicious botriocephalus anaemia. Acta Med. Scand., Suppl. 123:255, 1941.

316. Hobson, Q. J. G., J. G. Selwyn, and D. L. Mollin: Megaloblastic anaemia due to barbiturates. Lancet, 2:1079, 1956.

317. Hodgkin, D. C., J. Pickworth, J. H. Robertson, K. N. Trueblood, R. J. Prosen, and J. G. White: The crystal structure of the hexacarboxylic acid derived from B_{12} and the molecular structure of the vitamin. Nature, 176:325, 1955.

317A. Horrigan, D. L., and R. W. Heinle: Refractory macrocytic anemia with defect in vitamin B_{12} binding and with response to normal plasma. J. Lab. Clin. Med., 40:811, 1952.

318. Horster, H.: Experimentelle Therapie bei intestinaler Autointoxikation. Z. Ges. Exp. Med., 95:514, 1934/35.

319. ———: II. Über abnorme Dünndarmflora und ihre pathogenetische Bedeutung bei experimenteller intestinaler Intoxikation. Z. Ges. Exp. Med., 84:740, 1932.

320. ———, and W. Tönnis: V. Versuche zur Beeinflussung der experimentellen intestinalen Autointoxikation. Z. Ges. Exp. Med., 84:775, 1932.

321. Huff, R. L., P. J. Elmlinger, J. F. Garcia, J. M. Oda, M. C. Cockrell, and J. H. Lawrence: Ferrokinetics in normal persons and in patients having various erythropoietic disorders. J. Clin. Invest., 30:1512, 1951.

322. Hunter, W.: A discussion on pernicious anaemia and allied conditions. Brit. Med. J., 2:1299, 1907.

323. Hurst, A. F.: Precursors of carcinoma of the stomach. Lancet, 217:1023, 1929.

324. ———: The unity of gastric disorders. I. The hypersthenic and hyposthenic gastric constitutions. Brit. Med. J., 2:89, 1933.

325. Hutner, S. H., L. Provasoli, E. L. R. Stokstad, C. E. Hoffmann, M. Belt, A. L. Franklin, and T. H. Jukes: Assay of anti-pernicious anemia factor with Euglena. Proc. Soc. Exp. Biol. Med., 70:118, 1949.

326. Ivy, A. C., M. I. Grossman, and W. H. Bachrach: Peptic Ulcer. The Blakiston Company, Philadelphia, 515, 1950.

327. Izak, G., M. Rachmilewitz, Y. Stein, B. Berkovici, A. Sadovsky, Y. Aronovitch, and N. Grossowicz: Vitamin B_{12} and iron deficiencies in anemia of pregnancy and puerperium. Arch. Intern. Med., 99:346, 1957.

328. Jacobson, E. D., R. B. Chodos, and W. W. Faloon: An experimental malabsorption syndrome induced by neomycin. Amer. J. Med., 28:524, 1960.

329. Jacobson, E. D., and W. W. Faloon: Malabsorptive effects of neomycin in commonly used doses. J.A.M.A., 175:187, 1961.

330. Jännes, J.: Observations concerning the absorption of vitamin B_{12} by cells of Escherichia coli. Acta Physiol. Scand., 31:183, 1954.

331. Jensenius, H.: Results of Experimental Resections of the Small Intestine on Dogs (Experimental Enteroprival Sprue). Nyt Nordisk Forlag, Copenhagen, 1945.

332. Jewesbury, E. C. O.: Subacute combined degeneration of the cord and achlorhydric peripheral neuropathies without anaemia. Lancet, 2:307, 1954.

333. Johnson, P. C., and E. S. Berger: Enhanced urinary excretion of Co^{60} vitamin B$_{12}$ produced by delayed release capsules. Blood, 13:457, 1958.

334. Johnson, P. C., and T. B. Driscoll: Effect of different intrinsic factor preparations on Co^{60} vitamin B$_{12}$ uptake in rat liver slices. Proc. Soc. Exp. Biol. Med., 98:731, 1958.

335. Joske, R. A., E. S. Finckh, and I. J. Wood: Gastric biopsy: a study of 1,000 consecutive successful gastric biopsies. Quart. J. Med., 24:269, 1955.

336. Kaipainen, W. J., and K. Ohela: Effect of tapeworm extract on vitamin B$_{12}$ bound to gastric juice. Ann. Med. Intern. Fenn., 48:77, 1959.

337. ———: Urinary excretion of radiovitamin B-12 in pernicious tapeworm anaemia. Ann. Med. Intern. Fenn., 46:49, 1957.

338. Kaipainen, W. J., and G. Tötterman: The effect of intrinsic factor in pernicious tape-worm anemia. Scand. J. Clin. Lab. Invest., 9:391, 1957.

339. Kampen, E. J. van, and C. A. Graafland: Studies in refractory pernicious anaemia. An investigation with radioactive vitamin B$_{12}$-^{58}Co. Clin. Chim. Acta, 4:175, 1959.

340. Kato, N.: Location of vitamin B$_{12}$ in human erythrocytes. J. Vitamin., 4:226, 1958.

340A. Katz, J. H., J. DiMase, and R. M. Donaldson, Jr.: Simultaneous administration of gastric juice–bound and free radioactive cyanocobalamin: Rapid procedure for differentiating between intrinsic factor deficiency and other causes of vitamin B$_{12}$ malabsorption. J. Lab. Clin. Med., 61:266, 1963.

341. Kidd, P., and D. L. Mollin: Megaloblastic anaemia and vitamin-B$_{12}$ deficiency after anticonvulsant therapy. Brit. Med. J., 2:974, 1957.

342. Killander, A.: B$_{12}$-vitaminhalt i serum vid akut och kronisk leukemi. Nord. Med., 52:1513, 1954.

343. ———: Megaloblastic anaemia associated with pregnancy or puerperium: report of three cases with normal serum vitamin B$_{12}$ levels and a subsequent response to treatment with vitamin B$_{12}$. Acta Haemat., 19:9, 1958.

344. ———: Mikrobiologisk bestämning av vitamin B$_{12}$ i serum och urin med Euglena gracilis var. bacillaris. Svensk Läkartidn., 50:2264, 1953.

345. ———: Studies on serum B$_{12}$ assay with special reference to its use in the diagnosis of vitamin B$_{12}$ deficiency. Acta Soc. Med. Upsal., 63:14, 1958.

346. ———: Subacute combined degeneration of the spinal cord. The diagnostic value of serum vitamin B$_{12}$ assay. Acta Med. Scand., 160:75, 1958.

347. ———: The use of the serum vitamin B$_{12}$ assay in the diagnosis of vitamin B$_{12}$ deficiency. Acta Med. Scand., 159:307, 1957.

348. Kinnory, D. S., E. Kaplan, Y. T. Oester, and A. A. Imperato: Determination of urinary excretion of radiocobalt-labeled vitamin B$_{12}$ by cobalt sulfide precipitation. J. Lab. Clin. Med., 50:913, 1957.

349. Klayman, M. I., and L. Brandborg: Clinical application of cobalt^{60}-labeled vitamin B$_{12}$ urine test. New Engl. J. Med., 253:808, 1955.

350. Kline, D. L., and E. E. Cliffton: Lifespan of leucocytes in man. J. Appl. Physiol., 5:79, 1952.

351. Knox, J. D. E., and I. W. Delamore: Subacute combined degeneration of the cord after partial gastrectomy. Brit. Med. J., 2:1494, 1960.

352. Kogan, E., A. Schapira, H. D. Janowitz, and D. Adlersberg: Malabsorption following extensive small intestinal resection including inadvertent gastro-ileostomy. J. Mt. Sinai Hosp. (New York), 24:399, 1957. Simultaneously published in D. Adlersberg: The Malabsorption Syndrome. Grune & Stratton, New York, 1957.

353. Krevans, J. R., C. L. Conley, and C. R. Barrows: Observations of the absorption and excretion of vitamin B_{12}. Bull. Johns Hopkins Hosp., 88:568, 1951.

354. Krevans, J. R., C. L. Conley, and M. V. Sachs: Radioactive tracer tests for the recognition and identification of vitamin B_{12} deficiency states. J. Chron. Dis., 3:234, 1956.

355. Kuhlbäck, B., and R. Gräsbeck: The urinary excretion of parenterally administered radiovitamin B_{12} in renal failure. Scand. J. Clin. Lab. Invest., 10:231, 1958.

356. Kuhlbäck, B., W. Nyberg, and R. Gräsbeck: The Schilling test in renal failure. Scand. J. Clin. Lab. Invest., 12:140, 1960.

357. Latner, A. L.: Absorption of bound radioactive vitamin B_{12}. Lancet, 2:961, 1958.

358. ————: Intrinsic factor and vitamin B_{12} absorption. Brit. Med. J., 2:278, 1958.

359. ————: Possible mode of action of intrinsic factor. Lancet, 1:1077, 1958.

360. ————, and R. J. Merrills: Further observations related to the isolation of intrinsic factor mucoprotein. Vitamin B_{12} und Intrinsic Factor, 1. Europäisches Symposion, Hamburg, 1956, Ferdinand Enke Verlag, Stuttgart, 456, 1957.

361. Latner, A. L., and L. Raine: The uptake of vitamin B_{12} by rat liver slices. Biochem. J., 66:53P, 1957.

362. ————: The vitamin B_{12}-binding systems of isolated intestine of the rat. Biochem. J., 68:592, 1958.

363. Lear, A. A., J. W. Harris, W. B. Castle, and E. M. Fleming: The serum vitamin B_{12} concentration in pernicious anemia. J. Lab. Clin. Med., 44:715, 1954.

364. Lees, F.: Radioactive vitamin B_{12} absorption in the megaloblastic anaemia caused by anticonvulsant drugs. Quart. J. Med., 30:231, 1961.

365. Leithold, S. L., D. David, and W. R. Best: Hypothyroidism with anemia demonstrating abnormal vitamin B_{12} absorption. Amer. J. Med., 24:535, 1958.

366. Ley, A. B., and L. E. Sharpe: The absorption of vitamin B_{12} after total gastrectomy. Clin. Res. Proc., 2:31, 1954.

366A. Li, J. G., S. R. Mettier, H. A. Harper, and A. McBride: Pernicious anemia due to the presence of intrinsic factor inhibitor diagnosed in childhood, with a 25-year follow-up. Clin. Res., 7:90, 1959.

367. Lichtman, H., V. Ginsberg, and J. Watson: Therapeutic effect of Aureomycin in pernicious anemia. Proc. Soc. Exp. Biol. Med., 74:884, 1950.

368. Little, W. D., L. G. Zerfas, and H. M. Trusler: Chronic obstruction of the small bowel. J.A.M.A., 93:1290, 1929.

370. London, I. M., D. Shemin, R. West, and D. Rittenberg: Heme synthesis and red blood cell dynamics in normal humans and in subjects with polycythemia vera, sickle-cell anemia, and pernicious anemia. J. Biol. Chem., 179:463, 1949.

371. Lous, P., and M. Schwartz: Radioaktivt maerket vitamin B_{12} anvendt i klinisk diagnostik. Ugeskr. Laeg., 119:477, 1957.

372. ————: The absorption of vitamin B_{12} following partial gastrectomy. Acta Med. Scand., 164:407, 1959.

372A. Lowenstein, F.: Absorption of cobalt^{60}-labeled vitamin B_{12} after subtotal gastrectomy. Blood, 13:339, 1958.

373. Lowenstein, L., L. Brunton, L. Shapiro, N. DeLeeuw, and M. Dufresne: Maintenance therapy of pernicious anaemia with oral administration of intrinsic factor and vitamin B_{12}. Canad. Med. Ass. J., 77:923, 1957.

374. Lowenstein, L., C. Pick, and N. Philpott: Megaloblastic anemia of pregnancy and the puerperium. Amer. J. Obstet. Gynec., 70:1309, 1955.

374A. Lushbaugh, C. C., and D. B. Hale: Clinical applications of whole body scintillometry. VI. Determination of cobalt^{60} vitamin B_{12} absorption and retention. Univ. Calif. Los Alamos Sci. Lab., 2627:280, 1961.

375. Lustberg, A., D. Goldman, and O. H. Dreskin: Megaloblastic anemia due to Dilantin therapy. Ann. Intern. Med., 54:153, 1961.

376. MacIntosh, P. C., and J. L. Hutchison: Megaloblastic anaemia due to anticonvulsant therapy: report of a case responding to vitamin B_{12}. Canad. Med. Ass. J., 82:365, 1960.

377. MacLean, L. D.: Incidence of megaloblastic anemia after subtotal gastrectomy. New Engl. J. Med., 257:262, 1957.

378. ———: Studies with vitamin B$_{12}$-Co^{60}. Surg. Forum, 5:470, 1954–55.

379. ———: The differentiation of achylia gastrica and achlorhydria by means of radioactive vitamin B$_{12}$. Gastroenterology, 29:653, 1955.

380. ———, and H. S. Bloch: Gastrointestinal absorption and urinary excretion of vitamin B$_{12}$-Co^{60}. Proc. Soc. Exp. Biol. Med., 87:171, 1954.

381. MacLean, L. D., and R. D. Sundberg: Incidence of megaloblastic anemia after total gastrectomy. New Engl. J. Med., 254:885, 1956.

382. Magnus, H. A.: A re-assessment of the gastric lesion in pernicious anaemia. J. Clin. Path., 11:289, 1958.

383. ———: Gastritis, in F. A. Jones (ed.): Modern Trends in Gastroenterology. Butterworth, London, 323, 1952.

384. ———, and C. C. Ungley: The gastric lesion in pernicious anaemia. Lancet, 1:420, 1938.

384A. Mainland, D.: Elementary Medical Statistics. W. B. Saunders Company, Philadelphia, 1952.

385. Maloney, M. A., and H. M. Patt: Neutrophil life cycle with tritiated thymidine. Proc. Soc. Exp. Biol. Med., 98:801, 1958.

386. Markson, J. L., and W. M. B. Davidson: Gastric biopsy in the megaloblastic anaemias. Scot. Med. J., 1:259, 1956.

386A. Markson, J. L., and J. M. Moore: Autoimmunity in pernicious anaemia and iron-deficiency anaemia. A complement-fixation test using human gastric mucosa. Lancet, 2:1240, 1962.

387. Marshall, R. A., and J. H. Jandl: Responses to "physiologic" doses of folic acid in the megaloblastic anemias. A.M.A. Arch. Intern. Med., 105:352, 1960.

388. Maslow, W. G., W. Donnelly, D. M. Koppel, and S. Schwartz: Observations on the use of cobalt^{60}-labeled vitamin B$_{12}$ in the urinary excretion test: clinical implications of the radioisotope technique. Acta Haemat., 18:137, 1957.

389. Massey, B. W., and C. E. Rubin: The stomach in pernicious anemia. Amer. J. Med. Sci., 227:481, 1954.

390. McIntyre, P. A., R. Hahn, C. L. Conley, and B. Glass: Genetic factors in predisposition to pernicious anemia. Bull. Johns Hopkins Hosp., 104:309, 1959.

391. McIntyre, P. A., R. Hahn, J. M. Masters, and J. R. Krevans: Treatment of pernicious anemia with orally administered cyanocobalamin (vitamin B$_{12}$). Arch. Intern. Med., 106:280, 1960.

392. McIntyre, P. A., M. V. Sachs, J. R. Krevans, and C. L. Conley: Pathogenesis and treatment of macrocytic anemia. Information obtained with radioactive vitamin B$_{12}$. Arch. Intern. Med., 98:541, 1956.

393. Meade, B. W., and P. F. J. Sewell: Anaemia after gastrectomy. Brit. Med. J., 2:367, 1959.

394. Mendelsohn, R. S., D. M. Watkin, A. P. Horbett, and J. L. Fahey: Identification of the vitamin B$_{12}$-binding protein in the serum of normals and of patients with chronic myelocytic leukemia. Blood, 13:740, 1958.

395. Metz, J., S. M. Lewis, K. J. Keeley, and D. Hart: The absorption of vitamin B$_{12}$ in megaloblastic anaemia associated with pregnancy. J. Clin. Path., 13:394, 1960.

396. Meulengracht, E.: Darmstriktur und perniziöse Anämie. Arch. f. Verdauungs., 28:216, 1921.

397. ———: Dünndarmstrikturen und perniziöse Anämie. Darmresection. Acta Med. Scand., 56:432, 1922.

398. ———: Histologic investigation into the pyloric gland organ in pernicious anemia. Amer. J. Med. Sci., 197:201, 1939.

399. ———: Pernicious anemia in intestinal stricture. Acta Med. Scand., 72:231, 1929.

400. ———: Perniciös anaemi refraktaer overfor Cycoplex Mco. Ugeskr. Laeg., 117:883, 1955.

401. Meyer, L. M.: Oral administration of Co^{60} vitamin B_{12} in pernicious anemia. Proc. Soc. Exp. Biol. Med., 82:490, 1953.
402. ———, S. N. Arkun, and M. Jiminez-Casado: Further observations on distribution of radioactivity following parenteral administration of Co^{60} vitamin B_{12}. Proc. Soc. Exp. Biol. Med., 92:515, 1956.
403. Meyer, L. M., N. I. Berlin, M. Jiminez-Casado, and S. N. Arkun: Vitamin B_{12} distribution determined, by surface body counting following parenteral administration of Co^{60} vitamin B_{12}. Proc. Soc. Exp. Biol. Med., 91:129, 1956.
404. Meyer, L. M., R. W. Bertcher, and E. P. Cronkite: Serum Co^{60} vitamin B_{12} binding capacity in some hematologic disorders. Proc. Soc. Exp. Biol. Med., 96:360, 1957.
405. ———, R. M. Suarez, I. F. Miller, C. W. Mulzac, and S. T. Olivarreta: Co^{60} vitamin B_{12} binding capacity of serum in persons with hematologic disorders, various medical diseases and neoplasms. Acta Med. Scand., 169:557, 1961.
406. Meyer, L. M., R. W. Bertcher, and C. Mulzac: Co^{60} vitamin B_{12} binding capacity of normal human cerebrospinal fluid. Proc. Soc. Exp. Biol. Med., 100:607, 1959.
407. Meyer, L. M., A. B. Garcia, A. Goldman, and P. A. Stern: Oral administration of Co^{60} vitamin B_{12} to normal persons, patients with pernicious anemia, and subjects with various medical disorders. J. Appl. Physiol., 6:263, 1953–54.
408. Meyer. L. M., A. Sawitsky, B. S. Cohen, M. Krim, and R. Fadem: Oral treatment of pernicious anemia with vitamin B_{12}. Amer. J. Med. Sci., 220:604, 1950.
408A. ———, and N. D. Ritz: Oral treatment of pernicious anemia with vitamin B_{12}. Bull. N.Y. Acad. Med., 26:263, 1952.
409. Meyer, L. M., A. Sawitsky, N. D. Ritz, and M. Krim: Oral treatment of pernicious anemia with subminimal doses of folic acid and vitamin B_{12}. Amer. J. Clin. Path., 20:454, 1950.
410. Meyer, L. M., R. M. Suarez, Jr., R. Buso, J. Sabater, and R. M. Suarez: Oral administration of Co^{60} vitamin B_{12} in tropical sprue and hepatic cirrhosis and diarrhea. Proc. Soc. Exp. Biol. Med., 83:681, 1953.
412. Meynell, M. J., W. T. Cooke, E. V. Cox, and R. Gaddie: Serum-cyanocobalamin level in chronic intestinal disorders. Lancet, 1:901, 1957.
413. Milhaud, G.: Intestinal absorption of vitamin B_{12} and of a vitamin B_{12}-peptide complex in normal subjects and in patients with partial gastrectomy. Nature, 189:33, 1961.
414. Miller, A.: The in vitro binding of cobalt^{60} labeled vitamin B_{12} by normal and leukemic sera. J. Clin. Invest., 37:556, 1958.
415. ———, H. F. Corbus, and J. F. Sullivan: A modified urinary excretion test for measuring oral cobalt^{60} labeled vitamin B_{12} absorption and its application in certain disease states. Blood, 12:347, 1957.
416. ———: The plasma disappearance, excretion, and tissue distribution of cobalt^{60} labelled vitamin B_{12} in normal subjects and patients with chronic myelogenous leukemia. J. Clin. Invest., 36:18, 1957.
417. Miller, A., and J. F. Sullivan: Excretion of a vitamin B_{12} binding substance in chronic myelogenous leukemic urine. Clin. Res. Proc., 7:209, 1959.
418. ———: Electrophoretic studies of the vitamin B_{12} binding protein of normal and chronic myelogenous leukemia serum. J. Clin. Invest., 38:2135, 1959.
419. ———: Some physicochemical properties of the vitamin B_{12} binding substances of normal and chronic myelogenous leukemic sera. J. Lab. Clin. Med., 53:607, 1959.
420. Miller, D., and R. K. Crane: The concept of a digestive surface in the small intestine: cellular nature of disaccharide and phosphate ester hydrolysis. J. Lab. Clin. Med., 56:928, 1960.
421. Miller, O. N.: Determination of bound vitamin B_{12}. Arch. Biochem., 68:255, 1957.
422. ———: Recent concept of Castle's intrinsic factor. Bull. Tulane Med. Fac., 16:115, 1957.

423. ———: Studies on an interaction among serum protein, materials containing intrinsic factor and vitamin B$_{12}$. Arch. Biochem., 72:8, 1957.

424. ———, and F. M. Hunter: Effect of intrinsic factor concentrates on vitamin B$_{12}$ receptor protein of tissues. Proc. Soc. Exp. Biol. Med., 97:863, 1958.

425. ———: Stimulation of vitamin B$_{12}$ uptake in tissue slices by intrinsic factor concentrate. Proc. Soc. Exp. Biol. Med., 96:39, 1957.

426. Miller, O. N., J. L. Raney, and F. M. Hunter: Effect of intrinsic factor on uptake of radioactive vitamin B$_{12}$ by slices of rat liver. Fed. Proc., 16:393, 1957.

427. Minard, F. N., and C. L. Wagner: In vitro assay of hog intrinsic factor with rat liver homogenates. Proc. Soc. Exp. Biol. Med., 98:684, 1958.

428. Minot, G. R., E. J. Cohn, W. P. Murphy, and H. A. Lawson: Treatment of pernicious anemia with liver extract: effect upon the production of immature and mature red blood cells. Amer. J. Med. Sci., 175:599, 1928.

429. Minot, G. R., and W. P. Murphy: Treatment of pernicious anemia by a special diet. J.A.M.A., 87:470, 1926.

430. ———: A diet rich in liver in the treatment of pernicious anemia. J.A.M.A., 89:759, 1927.

431. Moertel, C. G., H. H. Scudamore, C. A. Owen, Jr., and J. L. Bollman: Intestinal absorption of cobalt^{60}-labeled vitamin B$_{12}$ in the normal male albino rat. Amer. J. Physiol., 197:347, 1959.

432. ———: Site of absorption of Co^{60}-labeled vitamin B$_{12}$ in the male albino rat. Amer. J. Physiol., 199:289, 1960.

433. Mollin, D. L.: Radioactive vitamin B$_{12}$ in the study of blood diseases. Brit. Med. Bull., 15:8, 1959.

434. ———, and S. J. Baker: The absorption and excretion of vitamin B$_{12}$ in man, in Biochemical Society Symposia, No. 13, The Biochemistry of Vitamin B$_{12}$, R. T. Williams (ed.), University Press, Cambridge, 52, 1955.

435. ———, and I. Doniach: Addisonian pernicious anaemia without gastric atrophy in a young man. Brit. J. Haemat., 1:278, 1955.

436. Mollin, D. L., C. C. Booth, and S. J. Baker: The absorption of vitamin B$_{12}$ in control subjects, in Addisonian pernicious anaemia and in the malabsorption syndrome. Brit. J. Haemat., 3:412, 1957.

437. Mollin, D. L., W. R. Pitney, S. J. Baker, and J. E. Bradley: The plasma clearance and urinary excretion of parenterally administered ^{58}Co-B$_{12}$. Blood, 11:31, 1956.

441. Mollin, D. L., and G. I. M. Ross: The vitamin B$_{12}$ concentrations of serum and urine of normals and of patients with megaloblastic anaemias and other diseases. J. Clin. Path., 5:129, 1952.

442. ———: Vitamin B$_{12}$ concentrations of serum and urine in the first 72 hours after intramuscular injections of the vitamin. J. Clin. Path., 6:54, 1953.

442A. ———: Serum vitamin B$_{12}$ concentrations of patients with megaloblastic anaemia after treatment with vitamin B$_{12}$, folic acid, or folinic acid. Brit. Med. J., 2:640, 1953.

443. ———: Vitamin B$_{12}$ deficiency in the megaloblastic anaemias. Proc. Roy. Soc. Med., 47:428, 1954.

443A. ———: Serum vitamin B$_{12}$ concentrations in leukemia and in some other haematological conditions. Brit. J. Haemat., 1:155, 1955.

443B. ———: The pathophysiology of vitamin B$_{12}$ deficiency in the megaloblastic anaemias. Vitamin B$_{12}$ und Intrinsic Factor, 1. Europäisches Symposion, Hamburg, 1956, Ferdinand Enke Verlag, Stuttgart, 413, 1957.

444. Mollison, P. L.: Blood Transfusion in Clinical Medicine. Blackwell Scientific Publications, Oxford, 47, 1951.

445. Montuschi, E.: Jejunal diverticulosis with megaloblastic anaemia. Brit. Med. J., 2:301, 1959.

446. Mooney, F. S., and J. G. Heathcote: Oral treatment of pernicious anaemia with low doses of H.P.P./1. Lancet, 2:291, 1960.

447. ———: Oral treatment of pernicious anaemia. Lancet, 2:371, 1958.
448. ———: Oral treatment of pernicious anaemia. Lancet, 2:909, 1958.
449. ———: Oral treatment of pernicious anaemia. Lancet, 2:1016, 1958.
450. ———: Oral treatment of pernicious anaemia: further studies. Brit. Med. J., 1:232, 1961.
451. Moore, C. V., W. R. Arrowsmith, J. Welch, and V. Minnich: Studies in iron transportation and metabolism. IV. Observations on the absorption of iron from the gastro-intestinal tract. J. Clin. Invest., 18:553, 1939.
452. Moore, H. C., E. W. Lillie, and P. B. B. Gatenby: The response of megaloblastic anaemia of pregnancy to vitamin B_{12}. Irish J. Med. Sci., 6:106, 1955.
453. Morris, H.: Human Anatomy; A Complete Systematic Treatise, 11th ed. Blakiston Co., New York, 43, 1953.
454. Motteram, R.: A biopsy study of chronic gastritis and gastric atrophy. J. Path. Bact., 63:389, 1951.
455. Motulsky, A. G., M. H. Paul, and E. L. Durrum: Paper electrophoresis of abnormal hemoglobins and its clinical applications. A simple semiquantitative method for the study of the hereditary hemoglobinopathies. Blood, 9:897, 1954.
456. Mueller, J. F., and J. J. Will: Interrelationship of folic acid, vitamin B_{12} and ascorbic acid in patients with megaloblastic anemia. Amer. J. Clin. Nutr., 3:30, 1955.
456A. Nabet, P., and R. Wolff: L'ultrafiltration de la vitamine B_{12} libre et combinée. C. R. Soc. Biol. (Paris), 155:565, 1961.
457. Naish, J., and W. M. Capper: Intestinal cul-de-sac phenomena in man. Lancet, 2:597, 1953.
458. Narbeshuber, K.: Strikturanämie und Leberdiät. Med. Klin., 27:389, 1931.
458A. Nelp, W. B., H. N. Wagner, Jr., and R. C. Reba: Renal excretion of vitamin B_{12} and its use in measurement of glomerular filtration rate in man. J. Lab. Clin. Med., 63:480, 1964.
459. Nelson, R. S., and V. M. Doctor: The vitamin B_{12} content of human liver as determined by bio-assay of needle biopsy material. Ann. Intern. Med., 49:1361, 1958.
460. Nichol, C. A., and A. D. Welch: Synthesis of citrovorum factor from folic acid by liver slices; augmentation by ascorbic acid. Proc. Soc. Exp. Biol. Med., 74:52, 1950.
461. Nieweg, H. O.: Megaloblastic anaemia of pregnancy. Lancet, 2:491, 1952.
462. ———, J. Abels, W. Veeger, and N. Hellemans: The defective absorption of vitamin B_{12} in pancreatic insufficiency. Vitamin B_{12} und Intrinsic Factor, 2. Europäisches Symposion, Hamburg, 1961, Ferdinand Enke Verlag, Stuttgart, 610, 1962.
463. Nieweg, H. O., A. Arends, E. Mandema, and W. B. Castle: Enhanced absorption of vitamin B_{12} in gastrectomized rat by rat intrinsic factor. Proc. Soc. Exp. Biol. Med., 91:328, 1956.
464. Nieweg, H. O., J. G. Faber, J. A. De Vries, and W. F. S. Kroese: The relationship of vitamin B_{12} and folic acid in megaloblastic anemias. J. Lab. Clin. Med., 44:118, 1954.
465. Nieweg, H. O., S. C. Shen, and W. B. Castle: Mechanism of intrinsic factor action in the gastrectomized rat. Proc. Soc. Exp. Biol. Med., 94:223, 1957.
466. Nyberg, W.: B_{12}-vitaminbrist hos maskbärare. Finska Läkaresällskapets Handlingar, 104:150, 1960.
467. ———: Absorption and excretion of vitamin B_{12} in subjects infected with Diphyllobothrium latum and in noninfected subjects following oral administration of radioactive B_{12}. Acta Haemat., 19:90, 1958.
468. ———: The absorption of radioactive vitamin B_{12} in persons infested with the fish tapeworm, Diphyllobothrium latum. Vitamin B_{12} und Intrinsic Factor, 1. Europäisches Symposion, Hamburg, 1956, Ferdinand Enke Verlag, Stuttgart, 328, 1957.

469. ———: The influence of Diphyllobothrium latum on the vitamin B$_{12}$-intrinsic factor complex. I. In vivo studies with Schilling test technique. Acta Med. Scand., 167:185, 1960.

470. ———: The influence of Diphyllobothrium latum on the vitamin B$_{12}$-intrinsic factor complex. II. In vitro studies. Acta Med. Scand., 167:189, 1960.

471. ———, R. Gräsbeck, and V. Sippola: Urinary excretion of radio-vitamin B$_{12}$ in carriers of Diphyllobothrium latum. New Engl. J. Med., 259:216, 1958.

472. Nyberg, W., and P. Reizenstein: Intestinal absorption of radio-vitamin B$_{12}$ bound in pig liver. Lancet, 2:832, 1958.

472A. Nyberg, W., M. Saarni, and R. Gräsbeck: The releasing of vitamin B$_{12}$ from complex bound form by a principle contained in various human organs. Vitamin B$_{12}$ und Intrinsic Factor, 2. Europäisches Symposion, Hamburg, 1961, Ferdinand Enke Verlag, Stuttgart, 469, 1962.

473. Okuda, K.: Vitamin B$_{12}$ absorption in rats, studied by a "loop" technique. Amer. J. Physiol., 199:84, 1960.

474. ———, E. Duran, and B. F. Chow: Effects of physico-chemical state of vit. B$_{12}$ preparation in digestive tract on its absorption. Proc. Soc. Exp. Biol. Med., 103:588, 1960.

475. Okuda, K., R. Gräsbeck, and B. F. Chow: Bile and vitamin B$_{12}$ absorption. J. Lab. Clin. Med., 51:17, 1958.

476. Okuda, K., J. M. Hsu, and B. F. Chow: Effect of feeding D-sorbitol on the intestinal absorption of vitamin B$_6$ and vitamin B$_{12}$ in rats. J. Nutr., 72:99, 1960.

477. Okuda, K., J. A. Wider, and B. F. Chow: The effect of intrinsic factor on the hepatic uptake of vitamin B$_{12}$ following intravenous injection. J. Lab. Clin. Med., 54:535, 1959.

478. Østergaard Kristensen, H. P., and T. Friis: Effect of prednisone on B$_{12}$ absorption in pernicious anaemia. Acta Med. Scand., 166:249, 1960.

479. ———: The mechanism of the prednisone effect upon B$_{12}$ absorption in pernicious anaemia. Acta Med. Scand., 168:457, 1960.

480. ———: Mekanismen ved prednisons virkning på B$_{12}$-absorptionen ved perniciös anaemi. Ugeskr. Laeg., 122:1323, 1960.

481. Østergaard Kristensen, H. P., and H. Gormsen: Vitamin B$_{12}$ deficiency in uncharacteristic macrocytic anaemia. Acta Med. Scand., 162:415, 1958.

482. Østergaard Kristensen, H. P., L. Korsgaard Christensen, T. Friis, and A. Søeborg Ohlsen: The diagnosis of latent megaloblastic anaemia. A comparison between the estimation of plasma vitamin B$_{12}$ and the Schilling test. Danish Med. Bull., 5:32, 1958.

483. Østergaard Kristensen, H. P., J. Lund, A. Søeborg Ohlsen, and J. Pedersen: Maintenance therapy in pernicious anaemia controlled by determining vitamin-B$_{12}$ level in plasma. Lancet, 1:1266, 1957.

484. Ottesen, J.: On the age of human white cells in peripheral blood. Acta Physiol. Scand., 32:75, 1954.

485. Oxenhorn, S., S. Estren, L. R. Wasserman, and D. Adlersberg: Malabsorption syndrome: intestinal absorption of vitamin B$_{12}$. Ann. Intern. Med., 48:30, 1958.

487. Passey, R. M.: The gastric mucous membrane in Addison's anaemia. Guy's Hosp. Rep., 72:172, 1922.

488. Patel, J. C., and B. R. Kocher: Vitamin B$_{12}$ in macrocytic anaemia of pregnancy and the puerperium. Brit. Med. J., 1:924, 1950.

489. Paulley, J. W.: Observations on the aetiology of idiopathic steatorrhoea. Brit. Med. J., 2:1318, 1954.

490. Paulson, M., C. L. Conley, and E. S. Gladsden: Absence of intrinsic factor from intestinal juice of patients following total gastrectomy. Amer. J. Med. Sci., 220:310, 1950.

490A. Pawelkiewicz, J., M. Górna, W. Fenrych, and S. Magas: Conversion of cyanocobalamin in vivo and in vitro into its coenzyme form in humans and animals, in Vitamin B$_{12}$ Coenzymes. Ann. N.Y. Acad. Sci., 112:641, 1964.

491. Pearson, R. D.: Macrocytic anemia associated with intestinal strictures and anastomoses: report of two cases. Ann. Intern. Med., 40:600, 1954.

492. Pedersen, J., and I. Ebbesen: Radioactive vitamin B_{12} tests in pernicious anaemia after oral maintenance therapy. Acta Med. Scand., 161:413, 1958.

493. Pendl, I., W. Franz, and D. Hunkel-Trees: Vitamin B_{12} mit Vitamin B_{12}-bindendem Protein als antianämisch wirksames Prinzip. Hoppe Seyler Z. Physiol. Chem., 313:259, 1958.

494. Perman, G., R. Gullberg, P. G. Reizenstein, B. Snellman, and L.-G. Allgén: A study of absorption patterns in malabsorption syndromes. Acta Med. Scand., 168:117, 1960.

495. Perry, S., C. G. Craddock, Jr., and J. S. Lawrence: Rates of appearance and disappearance of white blood cells in normal and in various disease states. J. Lab. Clin. Med., 51:501, 1958.

496. Pitney, W. R., and M. F. Beard: Serum and urine concentrations of vitamin B_{12} following oral administration of the vitamin. Amer. J. Clin. Nutr., 2:89, 1954.

497. ————: Vitamin B_{12} deficiency following total gastrectomy. Arch. Intern. Med., 95:591, 1955.

498. ————, and E. J. Van Loon: Observations on the bound form of vitamin B_{12} in human serum. J. Biol. Chem., 207:143, 1954.

498A. Pitts, R. F.: Physiology of the Kidney and Body Fluids. Year Book Medical Publishers, Inc., Chicago, Illinois, 66, 1963.

499. Plum, P., and E. Warburg: Hematological changes, especially megalocytic anemia, in regional ileitis. Acta Med. Scand., 102:449, 1939.

500. Polachek, A. A., W. J. Pijanowski, and J. M. Miller: Diverticulosis of the jejunum with macrocytic anemia and steatorrhea. Ann. Intern. Med., 54:636, 1961.

501. Poliner, I. J., and H. M. Spiro: Confirmation of achylia by radioactive B_{12} uptake and blood pepsin measurement. Amer. J. Med., 23:894, 1957.

502. ————: The independent secretion of acid, pepsin, and "intrinsic factor" by the human stomach. Gastroenterology, 34:196, 1956.

503. Pollycove, M., and L. Apt: Absorption, elimination and excretion of orally administered vitamin B_{12} in normal subjects and in patients with pernicious anemia. New Engl. J. Med., 255:207, 1956.

504. ————, and M. J. Colbert: Pernicious anemia due to dietary deficiency of vitamin B_{12}. New Engl. J. Med., 255:164, 1956.

505. Prasad, A. S.: Studies on ultrafiltrable calcium. Ph.D. Thesis, University of Minnesota, Minneapolis, 1957.

506. ————, and E. B. Flink: Effect of carbon dioxide on concentration of calcium in an ultrafiltrate of serum obtained by centrifugation. J. Appl. Physiol., 10:103, 1957.

507. Pribilla, W., and H.-E. Posth: Untersuchungen mit radioaktivem Vitamin B_{12} bei partieller und totaler Gastrektomie unter besonderer Berücksichtigung der Intrinsic-factor-Produktion. Schweiz. Med. Wschr., 88:1, 1958.

507A. Quimby, E. H., S. Feitelberg, and S. Silver: Radioactive Isotopes in Clinical Practice. Lea & Febiger, Philadelphia, 1959.

508. Quinby, W. C., and J. J. McGovern: Surgical correction of defective absorption of vitamin B_{12} in a child. New Engl. J. Med., 259:755, 1958.

509. Rabiner, S. F., H. C. Lichtman, J. Messite, R. J. Watson, V. Ginsberg, L. Ellenbogen, and W. L. Williams: The urinary excretion test in the diagnosis of Addisonian pernicious anemia. Ann. Intern. Med., 44:437, 1956.

510. Raccuglia, G., and M. S. Sacks: Vitamin B_{12} binding capacity of normal and leukemic sera. J. Lab. Clin. Med., 50:69, 1957.

511. Rachmilewitz, M., and N. Grossowicz: Comparative microbiological investigations of vitamin B_{12} in human sera. Acta Med. Scand., Suppl. 312:540, 1956.

512. Rachmilewitz, M., G. Izak, A. Hochman, J. Aronovitch, and N. Grossowicz: Serum vitamin B_{12} in leukemias and malignant lymphomas. Blood, 12:804, 1957.

515. Raney, L. J., H. J. Hansen, and O. N. Miller: Studies on the possible absorption of intrinsic factor (IF). Fed. Proc., 18:542, 1959.
516. Rath, C. E., P. R. McCurdy, and B. J. Duffy: Effect of renal disease on the Schilling test. New Engl. J. Med., 256:111, 1957.
517. Rath, C. E., P. R. McCurdy, G. E. Schreiner, and B. J. Duffy: The effect of renal disease on the urinary excretion of cobalt[60] vitamin B_{12}. Proceedings of the Sixth International Congress of the International Society of Hematology. Grune & Stratton, New York, 329, 1958.
518. Reimers, C., and W. Tönnis: IV. Chemische und physikalisch-chemische Untersuchungen am Darm und im Blut bei intestinaler Autointoxikation. Z. Ges. Exp. Med., 84:765, 1932.
519. Reisner, E. H., Jr., J. P. Gilbert, C. Rosenblum, and M. C. Morgan: Applications of the urinary tracer test (of Schilling) as an index of vitamin B_{12} absorption. Amer. J. Clin. Nutr., 4:134, 1956.
521. Reizenstein, P. G.: Body distribution, turnover rate, and radiation dose after the parenteral administration of radiovitamin B_{12}. Acta Med. Scand., 165:467, 1959.
522. ———: Effect of digestive enzymes on bound vitamin B_{12}. Acta Med. Scand., 165:481, 1959.
523. ———: Excretion, enterohepatic circulation and retention of radiovitamin B_{12} in pernicious anemia and in controls. Proc. Soc. Exp. Biol. Med., 101:703, 1959.
524. ———: Excretion of non-labeled vitamin B_{12} in man. Acta Med. Scand., 165:313, 1959.
525. ———: Vitamin B_{12} metabolism, some studies on the absorption, excretion, enterohepatic circulation, turnover rate, body distribution and tissue-binding of B_{12}. Acta Med. Scand., Suppl. 347, 165:1, 1959.
525A. ———, E. P. Cronkite, and S. H. Cohn: Measurement of absorption of vitamin B_{12} by whole-body gamma spectrometry. Blood, 18:95, 1961.
526. Reizenstein, P. G., and W. Nyberg: Intestinal absorption of liver-bound radiovitamin B_{12} in patients with pernicious anaemia and in controls. Lancet, 5:248, 1959.
526A. Reubi, F. C.: Clearance Tests in Clinical Medicine. Charles C. Thomas, Springfield, Illinois, 13, 1963.
527. Reynell, P. C., G. H. Spray, and K. B. Taylor: The site of absorption of vitamin B_{12} in the rat. Clin. Sci., 16:663, 1957.
528. Rice, E. G., S. M. Greenberg, J. F. Herndon, and E. J. Van Loon: Effect of ethylenediamine tetra-acetate on vitamin B_{12} absorption in the rat. Nature, 184:1948, 1959.
529. Rice, E. G., J. F. Herndon, E. J. Van Loon, and S. M. Greenberg: Enhancement of vitamin B_{12}-absorption by D-sorbitol as measured by maternal and fetal tissue levels in pregnant rats. Amer. J. Physiol., 193:513, 1958.
530. Richardson, J. E.: Addisonian anaemia following entero-anastomosis. Brit. J. Surg., 33:71, 1946.
531. Richardson, W.: Pernicious anemia due to enteroenterostomy. New Engl. J. Med., 218:374, 1938.
532. Richmond, J., and S. Davidson: Subacute combined degeneration of the spinal cord in non-Addisonian megaloblastic anaemia. Quart. J. Med., 27:517, 1958.
533. Richter, O., A. C. Ivy, and M. S. Kim: Action of human "pernicious anemia liver extract." Proc. Soc. Exp. Biol. Med., 29:1093, 1932.
534. Rickes, E. L., N. G. Brink, F. R. Koniuszy, T. R. Wood, and K. Folkers: Comparative data on vitamin B_{12} from liver and from a new source, Streptomyces griseus. Science, 108:634, 1948.
535. ———: Crystalline vitamin B_{12}. Science, 107:396, 1948.
536. Ritz, N. D., and L. M. Meyer: Clearance of intravenously injected radioactive cobalt-labeled vitamin B_{12} in chronic myeloid leukemia and other conditions. Cancer, 13:1000, 1960.

537. Rodriguez-Rosado, A. L., and T. W. Sheehy: The role of calcium on the intestinal absorption of vitamin B_{12} in tropical sprue. Amer. J. Med. Sci., 242:548, 1961.

538. Rosenblum, C.: Radiation comparison of cobalt isotopes. Amer. J. Clin. Nutr., 8:276, 1960.

539. ———, R. L. Davis, and B. F. Chow: Comparative absorption of vitamin B_{12} analogues by normal humans. III. 5,6-Dichlorobenzimidazole, 5,6-Desdimethyl-benzimidazole and 5-Hydroxybenzimidazole analogues. Proc. Soc. Exp. Biol. Med., 95:30, 1957.

540. Rosenblum, C., D. T. Woodbury, J. P. Gilbert, K. Okuda, and B. F. Chow: Comparative absorption of vitamin B_{12} analogues by normal humans. I. Chlorocobalamin vs. cyanocobalamin. Proc. Soc. Exp. Biol. Med., 89:63, 1955.

541. Rosenblum, C., D. T. Woodbury, and E. H. Reisner, Jr.: The use of cobalt[60]-labelled vitamin B_{12} for the evaluation of intrinsic factor activity. Proc. 2nd Oxford Radioisotope Conf., July, 1954. Butterworth's, London, 1:287, 1954.

542. Rosenblum, C., R. S. Yamamato, R. Wood, D. T. Woodbury, K. Okuda, and B. F. Chow: Comparative absorption of vitamin B_{12} analogues by normal humans. II. Chloro-, sulfato-, nitro- and thiocyanato- vs. cyanocobalamin. Proc. Soc. Exp. Biol. Med., 91:364, 1956.

543. Rosenthal, H. L.: Absorption, excretion and tissue distribution of oral cyanocobalamin in rabbits. Amer. J. Physiol., 197:1048, 1959.

544. ———: Plasma disappearance rate and tissue distribution of radioactive cobalt labelled cyanocobalamin injected into various animals. Proc. Soc. Exp. Biol. Med., 105:6, 1960.

545. ———: The uptake and turnover of radioactive vitamin B_{12} in rabbit tissues. J. Nutr., 68:297, 1959.

546. ———, and J. K. Hampton, Jr.: The absorption of cyanocobalamin (vitamin B_{12}) from the gastrointestinal tract of dogs. J. Nutr., 56:67, 1955.

546A. Rosenthal, H. L., P. R. Myers, and G. O. O'Brien: The determination of serum vitamin B_{12} binding capacity. Vitamin B_{12} und Intrinsic Factor, 2. Europäisches Symposion, H. C. Heinrich, editor, Ferdinand Enke Verlag, Stuttgart, 410, 1962.

547. Ross, G. I. M.: Vitamin B_{12} assay in body fluids. Nature, 166:270, 1950.

548. ———: Vitamin B_{12} assay in body fluids using Euglena gracilis. J. Clin. Path., 5:250, 1952.

550. ———, and D. L. Mollin: Vitamin B_{12} in tissues in pernicious anemia and other conditions. Vitamin B_{12} und Intrinsic Factor, 1. Europäisches Symposion, Hamburg, 1956, Ferdinand Enke Verlag, Stuttgart, 437, 1957.

551. ———, E. V. Cox, and C. C. Ungley: Hematologic responses and concentration of vitamin B_{12} in serum and urine following oral administration of vitamin B_{12} without intrinsic factor. Blood, 9:473, 1954.

551A. Ross, J. F., H. Belding, and B. L. Paegel: The development and progression of subacute combined degeneration of the spinal cord in patients with pernicious anemia treated with synthetic pteroylglutamic (folic) acid. Blood, 3:68, 1948.

552. Rubin, C. E.: Observations on the pathogenesis of juvenile pernicious anemia. J. Clin. Invest., 36:925, 1957.

553. Rüdel, C., and W. Tönnis: III. Histologische Befunde an Leber und Nieren bei experimenteller intestinaler Autointoxikation. Z. Ges. Exp. Med., 84:752, 1932.

554. Schauman, O.: Zur Kenntniss der sogenannten Bothriocephalus-Anämie. Weilin & Goos, Helsingfors, 1894.

555. Scheid, H. E., and B. S. Schweigert: Vitamin B_{12} content of organ meats. J. Nutr., 53:419, 1954.

556. Scherer, E.: Hyperchrome Anämie und Dünndarmstriktur. Klin. Wschr., 9:790, 1930.

557. Schilling, R. F.: Intrinsic factor studies. II. The effect of gastric juice on the urinary excretion of radioactivity after the oral administration of radioactive vitamin B_{12}. J. Lab. Clin. Med., 42:860, 1953.

558. ———: Recent studies of intrinsic factor and the utilization of radioactive vitamin B$_{12}$. Fed. Proc., 13:769, 1954.

559. ———: The absorption and utilization of vitamin B$_{12}$. Amer. J. Clin. Nutr., 3:45, 1955.

560. ———, D. V. Clatanoff, and D. R. Korst: Intrinsic factor studies. III. Further observations utilizing the urinary radioactivity test in subjects with achlorhydria, pernicious anemia, or a total gastrectomy. J. Lab. Clin. Med., 45:926, 1955.

561. Schilling, R. F., and L. L. Schloesser: Intrinsic factor studies. V. Some aspects of the quantitative relationship between vitamin B$_{12}$, intrinsic factor, binding, and the absorption of vitamin B$_{12}$. Vitamin B$_{12}$ und Intrinsic Factor, 1. Europäisches Symposion, Hamburg, 1956, Ferdinand Enke Verlag, Stuttgart, 194, 1957.

562. Schlesinger, A.: Nachweis des antiperniciosa-Prinzips im Magensaft einer Patientin mit perniziös-anämischem Blutbild bei Dünndarmstenose. Klin. Wschr., 12:298, 1933.

563. Schloesser, L. L., P. Deshpande, and R. F. Schilling: Biologic turnover rate of cyanocobalamin (vitamin B$_{12}$) in human liver. Arch. Intern. Med., 101:306, 1958.

564. Schwartz, M.: Inhibition of intrinsic factor by pernicious anaemia sera. Lancet, 2:239, 1959.

565. ———: Intrinsic-factor-inhibiting substance in serum of orally treated patients with pernicious anaemia. Lancet, 2:61, 1958.

566. ———, P. Lous, and E. Meulengracht: Absorption of vitamin B$_{12}$ in pernicious anaemia. Defective absorption induced by prolonged oral treatment. Lancet, 2:1200, 1958.

567. ———: Reduced effect of heterologous intrinsic factor after prolonged oral treatment in pernicious anaemia. Lancet, 1:751, 1957.

568. Scudamore, H. H., A. B. Hagedorn, E. E. Wollaeger, and C. A. Owen, Jr.: Diverticulosis of the small intestine, and macrocytic anemia with report of two cases and studies on absorption of radioactive vitamin B$_{12}$. Gastroenterology, 34:66, 1958.

569. Scudamore, H. H., J. H. Thompson, Jr., and C. A. Owen, Jr.: Absorption of Co^{60}-labeled vitamin B$_{12}$ in man and uptake by parasites, including Diphyllobothrium latum. J. Lab. Clin. Med., 57:240, 1961.

570. Seyderhelm, R.: Verhandlungen ärzlicher Gesellschaften. Klin. Wschr., 2:1816, 1923.

571. ———: Die Pathogenese der perniziösen Anämie. Ergebn. Inn. Med. Kinderheilk., 21:361, 1922.

572. ———, W. Lehmann, and P. Wichels: Experimentelle intestinale perniziöse Anämie beim Hund. Klin. Wschr., 32:1439, 1924.

573. ———: Intestinale, perniziöse Anämie beim Hund durch experimentelle Dünndarmstriktur. Krankheitsforschung, 4:263, 1927.

574. Sheehy, T. W., E. Perez-Santiago, and M. E. Rubini: Tropical sprue and vitamin B$_{12}$. New Engl. J. Med., 265:1232, 1961.

576. Shemin, D., and D. Rittenberg: The life span of the human red blood cell. J. Biol. Chem., 166:627, 1946.

578. Shenoy, K. G., and G. B. Ramasarma: Extraction procedure and determination of the vitamin B$_{12}$ content of some animal livers. Arch. Biochem., 51:371, 1954.

579. Shiner, M., and I. Doniach: Study of X-ray negative dyspepsia with reference to histologic changes in the gastric mucosa. Gastroenterology, 32:313, 1957.

580. Shinton, N. K.: Oral treatment of pernicious anaemia with vitamin B$_{12}$-peptide. Brit. Med. J., 1:1579, 1961.

581. Siegel, S., B. F. Chow, K. Okuda, S. Chen, and E. J. Hanus: Effect of food on the absorption of vitamin B$_{12}$. Amer. J. Clin. Nutr., 9:705, 1961.

582. Siurala, M.: Gastric lesion in some megaloblastic anemias. Acta Med. Scand., 154:337, 1956.

583. ———: Gastric lesion in some megaloblastic anemias: with special reference to

the mucosal lesion in pernicious tapeworm anemia. Acta Med. Scand., Suppl. 299:1, 1954.

584. ———, E. Erämaa, and W. Nyberg: Pernicious anemia and atrophic gastritis. Acta Med. Scand., 166:213, 1960.

585. Siurala, M., and W. J. Kaipainen: Intestinal megaloblastic anaemia, treated with Aureomycin and Terramycin. Acta Med. Scand., 147:197, 1953.

586. Siurala, M., and W. Nyberg: Vitamin B₁₂ absorption in atrophic gastritis. Acta Med. Scand., 157:435, 1957.

586A. Siurala, M., and K. Sepälä: Atrophic gastritis as a possible precursor of gastric carcinoma and pernicious anemia. Acta Med. Scand., 166:455, 1960.

587. Skouby, A. P., and H. P. Østergaard Kristensen: Five years' treatment of Addison's anaemia with purified intrinsic factor and vitamin B₁₂. Acta Med. Scand., 164:233, 1959.

588. Smith, E. L.: Isolation and chemistry and vitamin B₁₂ in Biochemistry of Vitamin B₁₂. Biochem. Soc. Symposia, No. 13:3, 1955.

589. ———: Crystalline anti-pernicious-anaemia factor. Brit. Med. J., 2:1367, 1949.

590. ———: Radioactive penicillin and vitamin B₁₂. Brit. Med. Bull., 8:203, 1952.

591. ———: Purification of anti-pernicious anaemia factors from liver. Nature, 161:638, 1948.

592. ———, D. J. D. Hockenhull, and A. R. J. Quilter: Tracer studies with the B₁₂ vitamins. 2. Biosynthesis of vitamin B₁₂ labelled with ⁶⁰Co and ³²P. Biochem. J., 52:387, 1952.

593. Sobotka, H., H. Baker, and H. Ziffer: Distribution of vitamin B₁₂ between plasma and cells. Amer. J. Clin. Nutr., 8:283, 1960.

594. Söderlund, S.: Meckel's diverticulum. A clinical and histologic study. Acta Chir. Scand., Suppl. 248, 1959.

595. Sokoloff, M. F., E. H. Sanneman, Jr., and M. F. Beard: Urinary excretion of vitamin B₁₂. Blood, 7:243, 1952.

596. Spang, A.: Ungewöhnlich ausgedehnte Diverticulosis des Dünndarms mit megaloblastischer Anämie. Fortschr. Röntgenstr., 81:55, 1954.

597. Spies, T. D., R. E. Stone, G. G. Lopez, F. Milanes, R. L. Toca, and T. Aramburu: Vitamin B₁₂ by mouth in pernicious and nutritional macrocytic anaemia and sprue. Lancet, 2:454, 1949.

598. Spray, G. H.: An improved method for the rapid estimation of vitamin B₁₂ in serum. Clin. Sci., 14:661, 1955.

599. ———, and L. J. Witts: Results of three years' experience with microbiological assay of vitamin B₁₂ in serum. Brit. Med. J., 1:295, 1958.

600. Stevenson, T. D., and M. F. Beard: Serum vitamin B₁₂ content in liver disease. New Engl. J. Med., 260:206, 1959.

601. Stevenson, T. D., J. A. Little, and L. Langley: Pernicious anemia in childhood. New Engl. J. Med., 255:1219, 1956.

602. Stokes," J. B., and W. R. Pitney: Pernicious anaemia treated orally with "Bifacton." Refractoriness to potent animal intrinsic factor. Brit. Med. J., 1:322, 1958.

603. Stone, H. H., and B. F. Chow: Absorption and excretion of radioactive vitamin B₁₂ in diabetes. A study in patients with and without retinopathy. Diabetes, 6:418, 1957.

604. Strauss, M. B., and W. B. Castle: Studies of anemia in pregnancy. III. The etiologic relationship of gastric secretory defects and dietary deficiency to the hypochromic and macrocytic (pernicious) anemias of pregnancy and the treatment of these conditions. Amer. J. Med. Sci., 185:539, 1933.

605. Strauss, E. W., and T. H. Wilson: Effect of intrinsic factor on vitamin B₁₂ uptake by rat intestine in vitro. Proc. Soc. Exp. Biol. Med., 99:224, 1958.

606. Strength, D. R., W. F. Alexander, and J. P. Wack: Intracellular distribution of vitamin B₁₂-Co⁶⁰ in liver and kidney of B₁₂ deficient and normal rats. Proc. Soc. Exp. Biol. Med., 102:15, 1959.

607. Sturgis, C. C., and S. M. Goldhamer: Macrocytic anemia, other than pernicious

anemia associated with lesions of the gastrointestinal tract. Ann. Intern. Med., 12:1245, 1939.

608. Suhrland, L. G., D. Rubin, A. S. Weisberger, and G. C. Meacham: Failure of oral therapy in the maintenance of pernicious anemia. A.M.A. Arch. Intern. Med., 104:411, 1959.

609. Swedberg, B.: Perniciosa-neuropati utan anemi: betydelsen av säker diagnos före insättande av B$_{12}$-behandling vid neurologiska symtom. Svensk. Läkartidn., 57: 1277, 1960.

610. Swendseid, M. E., M. Gasster, and J. A. Halsted: Limits of absorption of orally administered vitamin B$_{12}$: Effect of intrinsic factor sources. Proc. Soc. Exp. Biol. Med., 86:834, 1954.

611. Swendseid, M. E., J. A. Halsted, and R. L. Libby: Excretion of cobalt^{60}-labeled vitamin B$_{12}$ after total gastrectomy. Proc. Soc. Exp. Biol. Med., 83:226, 1953.

612. Swendseid, M. E., E. Hvollboll, G. Schick, and J. A. Halsted: The vitamin B$_{12}$ content of human liver tissue and its nutritional significance; a comparison study of various age groups. Blood, 12:24, 1957.

613. Taylor, K. B.: Chronic atrophic gastritis and pernicious anemia. Gastroenterology, 41:147, 1961.

614. ———: Pernicious anaemia. Postgrad. Med. J., 37:468, 1961.

615. ———: Inhibition of intrinsic factor by pernicious anaemia sera. Lancet, 2:106, 1959.

616. ———, B. J. Mallett, and G. H. Spray: Observations on the inhibitory effects of intrinsic factor preparations on vitamin B$_{12}$ absorption. Clin. Sci., 17:647, 1958.

617. Taylor, K. B., B. J. Mallett, L. J. Witts, and W. H. Taylor: Observations on vitamin B$_{12}$ absorption in the rat. Brit. J. Haemat., 4:63, 1958.

618. Taylor, K. B., and J. A. Morton: An antibody to Castle's intrinsic factor. Lancet, 1:29, 1958.

618A. Taylor, K. B., I. M. Roitt, D. Doniach, K. G. Couchman, and C. Shapland: Autoimmune phenomena in pernicious anaemia: Gastric antibodies. Brit. Med. J., 2:1347, 1962.

619. Ternberg, J. L., and R. Eakin: Erythein and apoerythein and their relation to the antipernicious anemia principle. J. Amer. Chem. Soc., 71:3858, 1949.

620. Thompson, R. B., and C. C. Ungley: Megaloblastic anemia associated with anatomic lesions in the small intestine. Blood, 10:771, 1955.

621. ———: Megaloblastic anaemia of pregnancy and the puerperium. Quart. J. Med., 20:187, 1951.

622. Tönnis, W.: I. Experimentelle Erzeugung einer intestinalen Autointoxikation und ihre klinische Wirkung. Z. Ges. Exp. Med., 84:728, 1932.

623. ———, and A. Brusis: Veränderungen des morphologischen Blutbildes bei akuter und chronischer Darminhaltsstauung. (Ein Beitrag zur intestinalen Autointoxikation.) Deutsch. Z. Chir., 233:133, 1931.

624. Tönnis, W., H. Horster, C. Reimers, and C. Rüdel: VI. Zusammenfassende Darstellung der Versuchsergebnisse. Z. Ges. Exp. Med., 84:782, 1932.

625. Toon, R. W., and O. H. Wangensteen: Anemia associated with blind intestinal segments and its prevention with Aureomycin. Proc. Soc. Exp. Biol. Med., 75:762, 1950.

626. Toporek, M.: The relation of binding power to intrinsic factor activity. Effect of pseudovitamin B$_{12}$ on absorption of vitamin B$_{12}$. Amer. J. Clin. Nutr., 8:297, 1960.

627. ———, R. C. Bishop, N. A. Nelson, and F. H. Bethell: Urinary excretion of Co^{60}-vitamin B$_{12}$ as a test for effectiveness of intrinsic factor preparations. J. Lab. Clin. Med., 46:665, 1955.

628. Townsend, S. R., and D. G. Cameron: Megaloblastic anemia associated with diverticula of the small bowel. Amer. J. Med., 23:668, 1957.

629. Turnbull, A.: Experience with labelled vitamin B$_{12}$. Proc. Roy. Soc. Med., 47:424, 1954.

630. Unglaub, W. G., O. N. Miller, and G. A. Goldsmith: Saturation studies with vitamin B_{12} in human subjects. Fed. Proc., 15:374, 1956.

631. ————: "Saturation" studies with vitamin B_{12} in human subjects. Amer. J. Clin. Nutr., 6:535, 1958.

632. Unglaub, W. G., H. L. Rosenthal, and G. A. Goldsmith: Studies of vitamin B_{12} in serum and urine following oral and parenteral administration. J. Lab. Clin. Med., 43:143, 1954.

633. Ungley, C. C.: The chemotherapeutic action of vitamin B_{12}. Vitamins Hormones, 13:137, 1955.

634. ————, and R. B. Thompson: Vitamin B_{12} and folic acid in megaloblastic anaemias of pregnancy and the puerperium. Brit. Med. J., 1:919, 1950.

635. U.S. Department of Commerce, National Bureau of Standards: Maximum permissible amounts of radioisotopes in the human body and maximum permissible concentrations in air and water. National Bureau of Standards Handbook, 52, March 20, 1953.

636. Van Buchem, F. S. P.: L'anemia megaloblastica in corso di gravidanza e puerperio. Minerva Med., 45:1513, 1954.

637. ————, and H. O. Nieweg: Anaemia in pregnancy. Lancet, 1:153, 1959.

638. Verloop, M. C., and E. Florijn: Megaloblastaire anaemie bij darnstricturen en -anastomoses. Ned. T. Geneesk, 95:454, 1951.

639. Victor, M., and A. A. Lear: Subacute combined degeneration of the spinal cord. Current concepts of the disease process. Value of serum vitamin B_{12} determinations in clarifying some of the common clinical problems. Amer. J. Med., 20:896, 1956.

640. Vilter, C. F., R. W. Vilter, and T. D. Spies: The treatment of pernicious and related anemias with synthetic folic acid. I. Observations on the maintenance of a normal hematologic status and on the occurrence of combined system disease at the end of one year. J. Lab. Clin. Med., 32:262, 1947.

641. Wallerstein, R. O., J. W. Harris, R. F. Schilling, and W. B. Castle: Observations on the etiologic relationship of achylia gastrica to pernicious anemia. XV. Hematopoietic effects of simultaneous intravenous and of simultaneous or serial oral administration of intrinsic factor and vitamin B_{12}. J. Lab. Clin. Med., 41:363, 1953.

642. Wallgren, I.: Ueber die Veränderungen des Verdauungskanals bei der perniziösen Anämie. Arb. Path. Inst. Univ. Helsingfors, 3:275, 1923–25, as cited by Magnus and Ungley (384).

642A. Watkin, D. M., C. H. Barrows, Jr., B. F. Chow, and N. W. Schock: Renal clearance of intravenously administered vitamin B_{12}. Proc. Soc. Exp. Biol. Med., 107:219, 1961.

643. Watkinson, G., D. B. Feather, F. G. W. Marson, and J. A. Dossett: Massive jejunal diverticulosis with steatorrhoea and megaloblastic anaemia improved by excision of diverticula. Brit. Med. J., 2:58, 1959.

644. Watson, G. M., and H. W. Florey: The absorption of vitamin B_{12} in gastrectomized rats. Brit. J. Exp. Path., 36:479, 1955.

645. Watson, G. M., and L. J. Witts: Intestinal macrocytic anaemia. Brit. Med. J., 1:13, 1952.

646. Weinstein, I. B., and D. M. Watkin: $Co^{58}B_{12}$ absorption, plasma transport and excretion in patients with myeloproliferative disorders, solid tumors and nonneoplastic diseases. J. Clin. Invest., 39:1667, 1960.

647. Weinstein, I. B., S. M. Weissman, and D. M. Watkin: The plasma vitamin B_{12} binding substance: I. Its detection in the seromucoid fraction of plasma from normal subjects and patients with chronic myelocytic leukemia. J. Clin. Invest., 38:1904, 1959.

648. Weisberger, A. S., and B. Levine: Incorporation of radioactive L-cystine by normal and leukemic leukocytes in vivo. Blood, 9:1082, 1954.

649. Weygand, F., H. Klebe, and A. Trebst: Einbau von 5,6-Dimethyl-benzimidazol-(2-^{14}C) in Vitamin B$_{12}$ durch Streptomyces olivaceus. J. Naturf., 9B: 449, 1954.

650. Whipple, G. H., F. S. Robscheit-Robbins, and W. F. Bale: Red cell stroma protein rich in vitamin B$_{12}$ during active regeneration. J. Exp. Med., 102: 725, 1955.

651. Wijmenga, H. G.: Intrinsic factor and vitamin B$_{12}$-binding substances. Purification, properties and possible relationship. Vitamin B$_{12}$ und Intrinsic Factor, 1. Europäisches Symposion, Hamburg, 1956, Ferdinand Enke Verlag, Stuttgart, 156, 1957.

652. Wilkinson, R. W., and M. B. Leeds: Subacute combined degeneration of the spinal cord. Lancet, 1: 74, 1955.

653. Will, J. J., J. F. Mueller, C. Brodine, C. E. Kiely, B. Friedman, V. R. Hawkins, J. Dutra, and R. W. Vilter: Folic acid and vitamin B$_{12}$ in pernicious anemia. J. Lab. Clin. Med., 53: 22, 1959.

654. Williams, A. W., N. F. Coghill, and F. Edwards: The gastric mucosa in pernicious anaemia: biopsy studies. Brit. J. Haemat., 4: 457, 1958.

655. Williams, W. L., B. F. Chow, L. Ellenbogen, and K. Okuda: Intrinsic factor preparations which augment and inhibit absorption of vitamin B$_{12}$ in healthy individuals. Vitamin B$_{12}$ und Intrinsic Factor, 1. Europäisches Symposion, Hamburg, 1956, Ferdinand Enke Verlag, Stuttgart, 250, 1957.

656. Williams, W. L., L. Ellenbogen, and R. G. Esposito: Preparation of highly purified intrinsic factor. Proc. Soc. Exp. Biol. Med., 87: 400, 1954.

657. Williams, W. L., L. Ellenbogen, S. F. Rabiner, and H. C. Lichtman: An improved urinary excretion test as an assay for intrinsic factor. III. Comparison of results of this method with the classical clinical method. J. Lab. Clin. Med., 48: 511, 1956.

658. Wilson, T. H., and E. W. Strauss: Some species differences in the intrinsic factor stimulation of B$_{12}$ uptake by small intestine in vitro. Amer. J. Physiol., 197: 926, 1959.

659. Wintrobe, M. M.: Clinical Hematology. Lea & Febiger, Philadelphia, 1961.

660. Wokes, F.: Anaemia and vitamin B$_{12}$ dietary deficiency. Proc. Nutr. Soc., 15: 134, 1956.

661. ———, J. Badenoch, and H. M. Sinclair: Human dietary deficiency of vitamin B$_{12}$. Amer. J. Clin. Nutr., 3: 375, 1955.

663. Wolff, R., P. L. Drouet, and R. Karlin-Weissman: L'emploi de la ponction-biopsie pour l'étude de la vitamine B$_{12}$ hépatique chez l'Homme. R. Comp. Rend. Acad., 232: 568, 1951.

663A. Wolff, R. L.: The uptake of radioactive vitamin B$_{12}$ by perfused rat intestine in situ. Amer. J. Clin. Nutr., 8: 295, 1960.

664. ———, and J. Vuillemin-Weis: The mode of action of intrinsic factor in vitamin B$_{12}$ absorption by rat intestine. Amer. J. Clin. Nutr., 8: 293, 1960.

665. Wood, I. J.: Value of gastric biopsy in the study of chronic gastritis and pernicious anaemia. Brit. Med. J., 2: 823, 1951.

666. Zalusky, R., V. Herbert, and W. B. Castle: Cyanocobalamin therapy effect in folic acid deficiency. Arch. Intern. Med., 109: 545, 1962.

INDEX

Abels, J., 22, 135, 209

Absorption indices: normal subjects, 126; chronic lymphatic leukemia, 126, 127; chronic myeloid leukemia, 126, 127; acute/subacute myeloid leukemia, 126, 130; nonleukemic leukocytosis, 126, 130

Absorption of B_{12}: results in total gastrectomy, 6, 21, 22, 27, 40, 61, 62, 120–122; results in partial gastrectomy, 6, 21, 30, 31, 40, 63–67, 120–122; results in selective malabsorption, 7; results in sprue, 7, 19, 29, 40, 81, 82, 83; results in secondary steatorrhea, 7, 19, 29, 82, 83; results in pernicious anemia, 17, 26, 39, 42, 43, 51, 99, 108, 114, 116; results in histamine-fast achlorhydria, 19, 21, 27, 67–69; results with varying doses in control subjects, 19, 22, 27, 34, 41, 45–51; results with varying doses in pernicious anemia, 19, 23, 27, 34, 35, 50–58; results in regional ileitis, 19, 29, 40, 81, 82; effect of carbamylcholine chloride in, 19, 32, 111, 112, 113; results in epileptics with megaloblastic anemia, 22; inhibition by stomach or gastric juice, 22, 23, 35; relation between oral dose and absorption, 22–24, 34, 35, 41; effect of food intake on, 22, 31, 132–135; limit of, 22, 34, 35, 41; results in megaloblastic anemia of pregnancy, 22, 83, 84; results in pernicious anemia with constant amount of intrinsic factor, 23; inefficiency of absorption at high dosage levels, 23, 24, 34, 35, 41; results in pernicious anemia with varying amounts of intrinsic factor, 23, 24, 38, 42, 61; stoichiometric relation between B_{12} and intrinsic factor, 23, 24, 42; absorption gradient in pernicious anemia, 23, 24, 146; inhibition by intrinsic factor concentrate

or gastric juice, 24, 25, 30, 42, 175, 201; effect of "flooding" doses of "cold" B_{12}, 24, 86, 87, 88; inhibition by massive doses of parenteral B_{12}, 24, 86, 87, 88; B_{12}-polypeptide complexes, 25; liver-bound radio-B_{12}, 25; effect of age on, 26, 40, 51; results in familial B_{12} malabsorption with proteinuria, 29; results in juvenile pernicious anemia, 29; results in harborers of fish tapeworm, 29, 33, 34; effect of intrinsic factor in normal subjects, 30, 40; effect of steroids in pernicious anemia, 33; effect of calcium on, 35–36; inhibition by EDTA, 35–36; site of absorption of, 35, 172, 175, 176; binding of B_{12} and intrinsic factor action, 37–38; free vs. intrinsic-factor-bound B_{12}, 37, 38; analogues, 39; intestinal mucosal block, 41; results in cirrhosis of the liver, 41, 84, 85; "intestinal B_{12} acceptor," 42; results in posterolateral column disease of the spinal cord, 69–71; results in Faber's pernicious anemia, 71–81; effect of pancreatin on, 83; effect of sodium bicarbonate, 83; results in nutritional B_{12} deficiency, 84, 85; results in nutritional folic acid deficiency, 84, 85; results in neuritis, 84, 85, 86; results in leukemia, 84, 85, 122–132; discharge of "free" vs. "bound" B_{12} into the blood stream, 166–169. See also Fecal excretion test, Glass test, Plasma absorption test, Total body counting, Urinary excretion test

Achlorhydria: 19, 21, 27, 67–69; histamine-fast, 19, 21, 26, 27, 28, 39, 40, 56, 67–69, 77, 78, 113, 224

Achromycin, 7, 77, 78

Achylia gastrica, 4, 5, 32, 33

Adams, J. F., 29

Made in the USA
Monee, IL
07 July 2026

56552256R00155